Shelter Behavior Medicine of the Dog and Cat

Shelter Behavior Medicine of the Dog and Cat

Wailani Sung, MS, PhD, DVM, DACVB, FFCP
Joybound People and Pets, Walnut Creek, CA

Jeannine Berger, DVM, DACVB, DACAW
Monticello Veterinary Practice, Winters, CA

WILEY

Published by John Wiley & Sons, Inc., Hoboken, New Jersey.

For general information on our other products and services or for technical support, please contact our Customer Care Department within the United States at (800) 762-2974, outside the United States at (317) 572-3993 or fax (317) 572-4002.

Wiley also publishes its books in a variety of electronic formats. Some content that appears in print may not be available in electronic formats. For more information about Wiley products, visit our web site at www.wiley.com.

Library of Congress Cataloging-in-Publication Data applied for:

Paperback ISBN: 9781394291212

Cover Design: Wiley
Cover Images: Joy Bound, Ieva Gigele/Getty Images

Set in 9.5/12.5pt STIXTwoText by Straive, Pondicherry, India

SKY10170423_100126

"Never say 'I can't do it.' Say 'I haven't done it yet.'"

– attributed to Carol S. Dweck, Growth Mindset

Contents

Foreword

By Dr. Bonnie Beaver

For years, the staff of animal shelters around the world have worked hard to do what is right for the animals in their care. The flow of unwanted dogs and cats into these shelters continues, leaving staff to struggle with placing them into forever homes. This book answers the need for help with these efforts. It provides guidance in promoting positive welfare for animals while in a shelter and insights into realistic ways to reduce behavior problems that might undermine successful adoption.

Within the past few decades, animal welfare has gradually changed from the "I know it when I see it" philosophy to one based on science and focused on understanding the animal's perspective. Of course, we do not have all the answers yet, but science continues to make discoveries that change perspectives. Sentience has become a subject of much research – can animals feel pain and pleasure; do they have emotions? Based on recent research findings, even species with a nervous system very different from that of vertebrates, like octopuses and various types of fish, are now considered to be sentient.

Having sentience means an animal can experience the world in ways that are unique to its species. As an example, domestic animals have dichromatic rather than trichromatic vision. Their visual world is different than ours. The olfactory capability of the dog is almost unconceivable to us. These differences result in unique interpretations of the environment, requiring consideration of the animal's perspective when considering their behavior and welfare.

It is difficult to consider all of this and then add in the constraints associated with a shelter environment. At the heart of sheltering is a true love for the animal and a strong desire to do what is best. There are limitations, however, such as budgets, space, and differences of opinion. Setting up a program that is realistic, while providing the best animal welfare and behavioral assessments, is difficult, but this book provides suggestions across the breadth of subjects important for sheltered animals and the dedicated people who care for them.

Shelter Behavior Medicine of the Dog and Cat was written by two experts in animal behavior, with both Drs. Sung and Berger being board certified by the American College of Veterinary Behaviorists. To complement this behavioral expertise, both have an intense interest in animal welfare, with Dr. Berger also being board certified by the American College of Animal Welfare. But their expertise extends far beyond behavior and welfare; together, they bring more than two and a half decades of combined experience working across multiple levels of animal shelter operations. They have "been there, done that."

January 2026
College Station

Bonnie V. Beaver, BS, DVM, MS, DSc (hon)
Fellow, National Academies of Practice
Diplomate, American College of Veterinary Behaviorists
Diplomate, American College of Animal Welfare
Professor, Texas A&M University College of Veterinary Medicine and Biomedical Science

About the Authors

Wailani Sung, MS, PhD, DVM, DACVB
Joybound People and Pets
Senior Director of Animal Admissions and Well-being

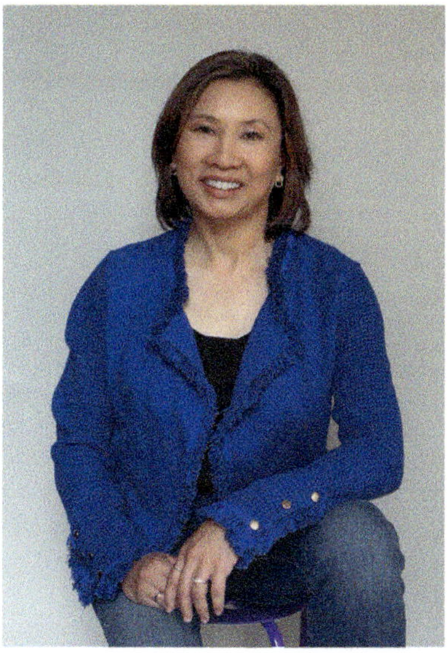

Dr. Wailani Sung, DVM, MS, PhD, DACVB is a board-certified veterinary behaviorist dedicated to improving the well being of animals and strengthening the human–animal bond. She earned both a Master's degree and a Ph.D. in psychology, with a focus on animal behavior, before completing her doctorate in veterinary medicine at The University of Georgia College of Veterinary Medicine. Following her residency, she achieved Board Certification in Veterinary Behavioral Medicine.

Dr. Sung currently serves as Senior Director of Animal Admissions and Wellbeing at Joybound People and Pets in Walnut Creek, California. In this role, she oversees three key areas: the transfer of pets from municipal shelters, the assessment and management of the shelter's behavior population, and the training classes and consultations provided to privately owned pets. She also advises animal shelters nationwide on individual case evaluations and the development of effective behavior programs.

An accomplished author and speaker, Dr. Sung is a co-author of *From Fearful to Fear Free* (with Dr. Marty Becker, Dr. Lisa Radosta, and Mikkel Becker) and a contributing author to *Decoding Your Cat*. She has also written extensively for veterinary textbooks, including *Feline Behavior and Welfare, Handbook of Feline Behavior, Behavior of Exotic Pets, Blackwell's Five-Minute Veterinary Consult: Canine and Feline Behavior*, and *Animal Behavior for Shelter Veterinarians and Staff*. Her insights have appeared on PetMD, PetCoach, Reader's Digest, and more.

A frequent lecturer at major conferences – including the American Veterinary Medical Association Conference, Western Veterinary Conference, Midwest Veterinary Conference, Humane World Expo, Aggression in Dogs Conference, and Fear Free Pet Behavior Symposium – Dr. Sung is recognized internationally for her expertise. She has also been featured in the PBS NOVA documentary *Cat Tales* and the Netflix documentary *Inside the Mind of a Cat*.

Driven by a passion for animal welfare, Dr. Sung continues to inspire veterinarians, trainers, shelters, and pet guardians with her science-based, compassionate approach to animal behavior.

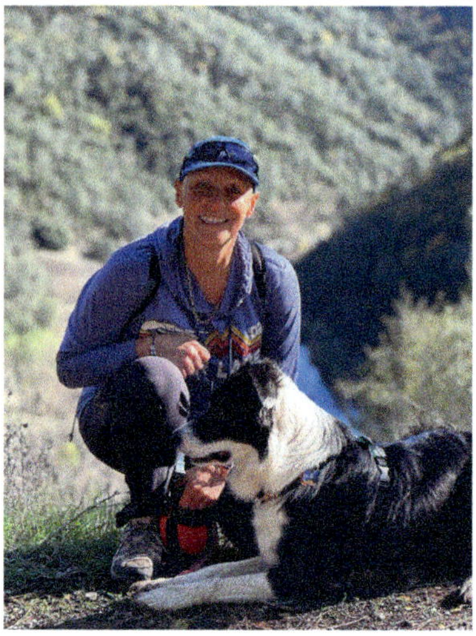

Dr. Jeannine Berger, DVM, DACVB, DACAW, is a strategic leader in veterinary medicine and animal welfare with more than 30 years of experience advancing both animal well-being and operational excellence. She earned her veterinary degree and completed her doctoral thesis at the University of Zurich before relocating to California in 1998.

After moving to the United States, Dr. Berger held multiple roles in medicine and epidemiology at the University of California, Davis Veterinary Medical Teaching Hospital, followed by private small-animal practice. She then served for more than 12 years at the San Francisco SPCA, holding multiple leadership roles – from Director of Behavior Services to Senior Vice President of Rescue and Welfare – where she oversaw all aspects of shelter animal care.

Dr. Berger is among the small number of veterinarians dual-boarded by the American College of Veterinary Behaviorists and the American College for Animal Welfare, underscoring her unique expertise in behavior, welfare, and systems-level leadership. Her contributions span clinical practice, research, education, and organizational leadership, unified by a commitment to improving animal well-being and strengthening the institutions that serve them.

She is currently the CEO and practicing veterinarian at Mayfair Vet Care, Dixon's only urgent care clinic and at Monticello Veterinary Practice, a community-focused small-animal practice in Winters, California – both created to expand access to veterinary care. Dr. Berger also operates a veterinary behavior consulting service, offering behavior consultations, professional education, and expert-witness support.

In recognition of her global impact, Dr. Berger received the Bronze Medal for Global Animal Welfare from the World Veterinary Association in 2019.

Preface-The Shoreline

Working in animal welfare often feels like standing on an endless shoreline. The need is vast, the resources finite, and the outcomes uncertain. Every day brings more animals than any system can fully serve, and every decision is made under the weight of knowing that effort alone will never be enough.

The *starfish* parable – adapted from *The Star Thrower* – is frequently invoked in animal welfare ethics (Eiseley 1969). In the story, thousands of starfish lie stranded on a beach, the scale of the problem seemingly insurmountable. A young person bends down, picks up a single starfish, and throws it back into the sea. When an older bystander remarks the act cannot possibly make a difference, the response is simple: *it mattered to that one.*

This narrative powerfully reflects the emotional motivation behind individual rescue efforts, while also underscoring the ethical tension between individual lives and population-level responsibility. In shelters and rescues, this exchange often plays out between generations. Newer professionals arrive driven by urgency and optimism, eager to try new approaches and unwilling to accept suffering as inevitable. Seasoned leaders – shaped by years of constraint, hard choices, and repeated exposure to loss – may sound like the voice of the man on the beach, questioning whether individual efforts can truly move the needle. Both perspectives come from experience. Both are rooted in caring. Effective shelter leadership lives in the space between them.

The work is not about denying the scale of the problem, nor about clinging to idealism without structure. It is about recognizing that while we may not save them all, the choices made for each pet still carry full moral weight. For the pet whose stress is reduced, whose behavior improves, or whose outcome shifts because someone took the time to act differently, the impact is absolute.

Progress in shelters rarely comes from sweeping reform alone. It comes from thousands of small, intentional decisions made daily by leaders who validate innovation without dismissing experience and teams who understand that compassion and realism are not opposing forces. This book is about that balance: how leadership, grounded in evidence and empathy, can turn individual actions into sustainable change.

Effective leaders do not stand on the shoreline debating whether the problem is too large to address. They acknowledge the scale, remove barriers to thoughtful action, and empower their teams to keep picking up starfishes – one informed, humane decision at a time.

Reference

Eiseley, L. (1969). *The Star Thrower*. New York: Times Books.

Declaration of Generative AI Use

Scite (December 2025 version) and Notebook LM (December 2025 and January 2026 versions) were used to summarize related research materials. The artificial intelligence (AI) helped identify recurring themes, author needs, and common concerns regarding AI use in writing. All AI-generated analyses were validated against original research data.

The AI-assisted reviews complemented human expert review across editorial, legal, and AI expert teams. All AI feedback was evaluated and selectively incorporated based on human judgment.

Sincerely,
Wailani Sung

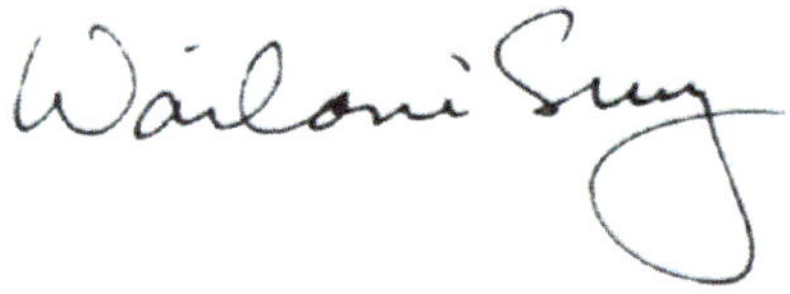

Generative AI tools were used in a limited and supportive capacity during the preparation of this manuscript. Specifically, ChatGPT was utilized to assist with language editing, structural refinement, and summarization of selected sections. Wordtune was additionally used for synonym suggestions and phrasing optimization.

AI-assisted outputs contributed to the identification of recurring themes, clarification of complex concepts, and refinement of written expression. All AI-generated content was critically reviewed and cross-checked against the original source material, clinical experience, and supporting literature to ensure accuracy, consistency, and alignment with the author's intent.

The use of AI served to complement, not replace, human expertise. All interpretations, conclusions, and final content decisions were made by the author. AI-assisted suggestions were selectively incorporated based on professional judgment and were subject to review within the broader editorial process, including input from subject-matter experts and peer reviewers where applicable.

The author assumes full responsibility for the integrity, accuracy, and originality of the content presented in this manuscript.

Sincerely,
Jeannine Berger

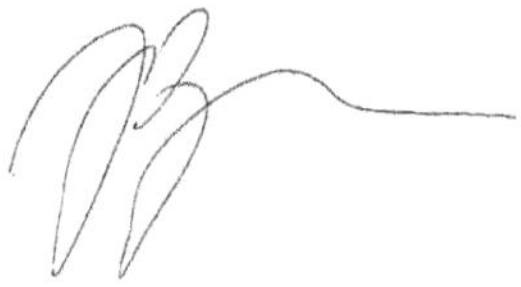

Acknowledgments

To my husband, **Jeff Shamrock** – thank you for 20 years of unwavering support through endless hours of studying, quiet (and not so quiet) determination, and every twist of my professional path. You kept me grounded through the setbacks and celebrated every success. And thank you for embracing the countless foster dogs and cats who came through our home – many of whom never left. You welcomed them into our house and into your heart. I would not want to navigate my personal or professional journey without you on my side.

To **my family**, who supported my dreams long before they made sense to anyone else – thank you for giving me the freedom to dream big and follow my passion. If I had listened to my dad, who suggested I should "become a real doctor" because surely no one could make a living doing their hobby, I would have missed the greatest joy of my life. They say that if you do what you love, you'll never work a day in your life – and even after more than 40 years in this wonderful, endlessly diverse profession, that is exactly how I feel. Sometimes, it's more than okay not to listen and carve your own path.

To my coauthor, colleague, and – above all – friend, **Dr. Wailani Sung**. Thank you for pushing me to do better, for helping me see things in new ways, and for relentlessly, lovingly talking me into writing this book with you.

To all the **shelter pets** who have taught me everything I know – and everything I still need to learn. My hope for each of you is simple: that you find the forever home you deserve.

My sincerest thanks to the **senior leadership at the San Francisco SPCA** from 2010 to 2022 – you know who you are. You taught me what matters, what doesn't, when to push, and when to let things be. You helped me learn how to keep my eye on the prize and never waver from my values. Your influences shaped the professional I am today.

To **every team member,** I have and had the privilege of working with and learning from along the way – thank you. Each of you has taught me valuable lessons, and I promise to carry your feedback with me as I continue to grow.

A profound thank you to **Dr. Bonnie Beaver**, not only for carving the path in veterinary behavior and welfare – especially for women in this field – but also for being a true mentor and role model. I have never attended a lecture of yours without learning something new, even on topics I thought I knew well. It is the mark of a master to continually inspire new ways of thinking and to elevate the well-being of animals and people alike. Thank you for writing the foreword to our book.

To my business partners, **Dr. Sara Ogren** and **Jodie Moeding**, thank you for giving me the opportunity and time to write this book – often while you carried more than your share at three very busy clinics. I know how many times you stepped up so I could do this.

And last, but never least, to **Dr. Verena Affolter** and **Dr. Bridgid Twomey**, thank you for the countless hours of review, edits, and thoughtful feedback. Your guidance made this book immeasurably better.

Jeannine Berger

First and foremost, my deepest gratitude goes to my husband, Jeff Paulson, who has been my unwavering supporter and steadfast champion. His encouragement has carried me through the inevitable challenges of this work, and his belief in me – especially, when I set my sights on ambitious goals – has made every achievement possible. I am profoundly thankful for his partnership, patience, and constant reminder to reach for the "big brass ring."

There are not enough words to express my respect and gratitude for my first mentor, Dr. Katherine Houpt, one of the true pioneers of veterinary behavioral medicine. She ignited my passion for animal behavior and demonstrated, through both scholarship and example, the depth and scientific validity of this specialty. Her influence shaped not only my career path but also my intellectual curiosity and clinical approach.

I was exceptionally fortunate early in my career to learn from two extraordinary veterinary behaviorists, Dr. Sharon Crowell-Davis and Dr. Lynne Seibert. As trailblazers in the field, they set a high standard for clinical excellence, scientific rigor, and professional integrity. Their mentorship made it possible for me to envision my own path forward in a specialty that was still defining itself.

To my parents, thank you for supporting me – even when my aspirations seemed unconventional or difficult to understand. Your willingness to stand behind my choices gave me the confidence to pursue a life devoted to animals and the people who care for them.

Finally, this book would not exist without my dear friend and mentor, Dr. Jeannine Berger. In many ways, it is a reflection of her vision. She gave me the opportunity to work in an animal non-profit organization and encouraged me to immerse myself in shelter behavior medicine. Her guidance, insight, and belief in the importance of this work profoundly shaped my professional trajectory. I would not be where I am today without her mentorship and friendship.

Striving to improve the lives of pets and the people connected to them has always been my purpose in life. To the many friends and colleagues who have supported, challenged, and inspired me along the way – thank you. Your collective dedication to advancing veterinary behavioral medicine continues to elevate this field and the lives it touches.

Wailani Sung

About the Companion Website

This book is accompanied by a companion website.

www.wiley.com/go/sbmedofdogcat1e

To access the website materials, click on the link under Related Resources on the book's page on wiley.com. You can also find this by searching www.wiley.com for the ISBN 9781394291212.

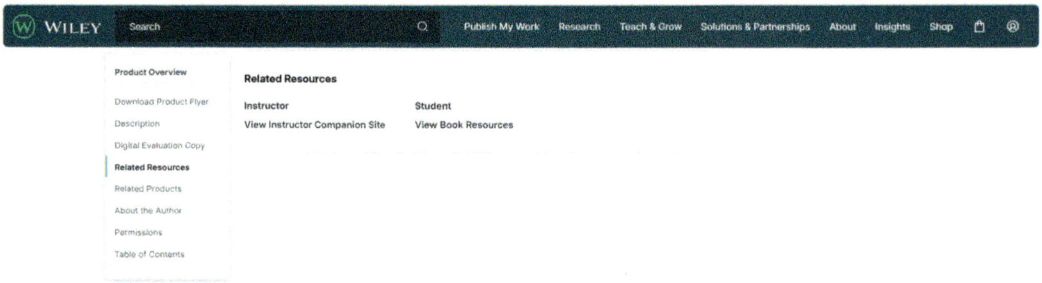

This website includes:

- Appendix

1

Introduction

It was later in my career – after becoming board certified in veterinary behavior – that I discovered my passion for shelter medicine. My first love had not been shelter work at all, but large-animal reproduction and population management. So, what makes a large-animal veterinarian from Switzerland study, practice, and ultimately write a book on shelter behavior medicine for dogs and cats in the United States?

The answer lies in an unconventional, yet deeply fulfilling career path. My journey has carried me across continents and disciplines – from Switzerland to America, from small-animal technician to large-animal veterinarian, and through academia and nonprofit work to becoming the owner of a small-animal general practice and urgent care clinic.

Along the way, I developed a strong interest in medicine and epidemiology, which eventually guided me toward the specialized fields of behavior and welfare – where I earned my two specialty certifications.

Each step in this journey has provided me with unique perspectives and tools to ultimately understand animals not only as patients but also as individuals living within broader systems, including families, shelters, and communities. My experiences have shaped the way I approach both clinical cases and population-level challenges. I am especially passionate about using data-driven decision-making to improve how animals are cared for and how we, as professionals, can continually evolve our understanding of animal welfare, in the past, present, and future.

This career has brought me and continues to bring me tremendous joy. The journey I began in the mid-1980s has led me to where I am today: coauthoring this book with my highly respected colleague and dear friend, Dr. Wailani Sung. Together, we share a vision of creating a much-needed, practical resource for shelters of all sizes and budgets.

We believe that every shelter, regardless of its resources, can design an intentional and compassionate journey from admission to adoption success. That journey begins with comprehensive behavioral and medical assessments and continues through thoughtful population management, strategic flow management planning, and making informed decisions that serve the best interests of each animal, the organization, and the community it supports.

My dedication to leadership has deepened over the years. I've learned that true leadership requires setting the tone, modeling empathy and accountability, and remaining open to innovation, even when it means taking risks. It is crucial that organizations are supported with the proper funding, structure, and a clear vision to achieve lasting and sustainable success in their mission to help animals. As senior vice president of Rescue and Welfare at the San Francisco Society for Prevention of Cruelty to Animals (SFSPCA), I had the opportunity to put these principles into practice on a large scale. There, I learned firsthand how strategic planning, collaboration, and data-driven decision-making could unite teams and transform shelter animal care destinations. That experience strengthened my belief that leadership in animal welfare must be both compassionate and evidence-based, balancing heart and science to create meaningful change.

When I was first asked to evaluate a well-established and successful shelter behavior program, I imagined my work would center on reviewing training protocols, providing postadoption behavioral support, and helping teams navigate difficult euthanasia decisions for severely aggressive dogs. But during my initial interview, I was asked a pivotal question: "Do you believe all pets can be behaviorally rehabilitated?" My answer was simple but honest: "It depends."

Because the truth is, shelter pets and owned pets are fundamentally different. Pets living in homes receive individualized care by very dedicated owners and therefore have different emotional and environmental contexts when compared to animals living in shelters. What works for one pet in a dedicated home may not work for others. That distinction between treatment and management, rehabilitation, welfare, and wellbeing has become central to my philosophy and to the pages of this book.

This book outlines how a problem-oriented approach can equip shelter practitioners, leadership, and teams with the knowledge and confidence to address behavioral and medical challenges in shelter pets effectively. Fostering collaboration among all levels of the organization – from executive leadership to frontline caregivers – is crucial to support a guided and unified framework for decision-making, ensuring sustainability, consistency, and clarity in care.

As a shelter professional, you will learn how to approach behavior and medical concerns in shelter pets using a problem-oriented approach. Data-driven approaches will assist in assessing the scope of sustainability (SoS) and designing medical and behavioral care trajectory strategies (CTS) and treatment plans. Using a practical resource like this book can protect an organization's resources and increase positive case resolution and overall productivity.

Our book will also be of great value to veterinarians in general practice. There are countless ways a veterinarian can influence the fate of a shelter pet, and for that reason, we have dedicated an entire subchapter (see Section 13.4) to this topic. With nearly half of the 5–6 million pets entering U.S. shelters each year eventually being adopted, the role of veterinarians extends far beyond the shelter walls (Shelter Animals Count 2025). Whether working in general practice, urgent care, or emergency medicine, veterinarians are often the first professionals to identify behavioral or medical challenges that may later determine a pet's likelihood of being surrendered or successfully staying in a home. By recognizing and addressing these issues early, veterinarians can play a pivotal role in preventing shelter admission, improving adoptability, and supporting long-term success for pets and their families.

Ultimately, this book serves as a practical guide for the entire shelter team – helping to improve adoption matches, increase positive case resolution, protect organizational resources, and strengthen the shelter's overall impact within the community. Through unified practices and compassionate leadership, shelters can save more lives while ensuring health, wellbeing, and humane care for every pet.

1.1 Background and Importance of Behavioral Medicine in Animal Shelters

The journey from animal admission to outcome begins with behavioral and medical assessments and continues through an intentional CTS informed by population-level welfare, public safety, and available resources. This process ensures that every pet receives the care needed and the best possible chance for a successful resolution. To best serve the pets, the organization, and the community, a proactive and transparent approach is essential. Decisions are guided by herd-health principles while remaining attentive to the needs and risks presented by each pet. At times, this process involves complex decisions regarding treatment, behavior management, and, in some cases, humane end points, all made with the goal of reducing suffering and supporting ethical, defensible outcomes at scale. While shelter models vary, ethical decision-making requires aligning animal welfare, human safety, and organizational capacity within each operational context. Achieving this requires collaboration and commitment across all levels of any organization – including leadership, the executive team, and the board of directors – to ensure that decisions are ethically grounded, evidence-based, and aligned with the organization's mission, vision, and SoS.

Medical and behavioral assessments of pets entering a shelter are crucial to balance individual care and population health. Adoption success depends on a number of factors, many of which are out of the control of the shelter organization. To prevent unnecessary euthanasia while also ensuring public safety and protecting other animals, shelters must strive to make informed, evidence-based evaluations about each pet's prospective wellbeing and behavior. This requires carefully assessing both the physical and psychological health of each pet before making life-and-death decisions. Beyond the needs of any single pet, shelters must consider the broader impact on the entire population and the organization's sustainability. Decisions should balance individual welfare with available resources and community responsibility, ensuring humane care while preserving the shelter's ability to fulfill its mission.

Through data-driven strategies, organizations can better assess the SoS and implement well-structured case trajectory strategies. Integrated trajectory strategies and individualized treatment planning ensure that each pet receives care tailored to its unique medical, behavioral, and emotional needs, thereby increasing their chance of successful adoption. By aligning leadership goals with daily shelter operations, this framework promotes a shared understanding of priorities, efficient resource allocation, and improved communication across departments. The result is a compassionate, sustainable, and scientifically grounded approach that enhances operational efficiency, animal wellbeing, and team morale.

Behavioral rehabilitation differs significantly from treating a physical condition, such as a broken leg, where financial resources are often the primary limiting factor. In contrast, the success of behavioral treatment depends heavily on management and environmental control. Addressing emotional or behavioral concerns requires preventing exposure to situations that trigger fear, anxiety, or aggression.

For example, a dog that is fearful of crowds should not be taken to busy public places, such as farmers markets. Similarly, a dog that becomes destructive when left alone should not be left unsupervised until the underlying anxiety is addressed, potentially with the support of antianxiety medication and behavior modification. A dog that exhibits aggression toward unfamiliar dogs should not be taken to dog parks or other high-risk environments.

By proactively managing the environment, caretakers can prevent the rehearsal of unwanted behaviors and create conditions that support learning, safety, and emotional recovery. Environmental management is therefore a cornerstone of successful behavioral rehabilitation and should accompany any behavior modification or pharmacologic plan.

Many pets arrive at shelters already experiencing some type of behavior challenges, may it be fear, anxiety, or even aggression. Once in the shelter, these pets are placed in an environment that is inherently stressful. These stressors can intensify preexisting behavioral and emotional challenges, making assessment and rehabilitation particularly difficult. In certain cases, the shelter environment may prevent effective behavioral intervention altogether. High levels of arousal, sensory overstimulation, or lack of consistent one-on-one interaction can interfere with learning and adaptation. For these reasons, the prognosis for rehabilitation in a shelter setting can range from good to guarded or poor, depending on the pet's condition, history, and available resources.

It is also important to recognize that, despite the best intentions, prolonged shelter stays can inadvertently worsen behavioral and emotional health, leading to a decline in overall wellbeing. To prevent further suffering, the humane and ethical approach may be to consider alternative placement resolution, such as foster care or sanctuary settings or, when appropriate, compassionate euthanasia.

Ultimately, each case must be evaluated individually, with decisions guided by welfare science, behavior assessment, and realistic expectations with a focus on the organization's SoS.

1.2 Overview of Animal Welfare

1.2.1 Why Are Animal Welfare Concerns Becoming Increasingly Important?

Animal welfare discussions are fundamental because they reflect a society's values and compassion toward living beings. Ensuring the wellbeing of the animals in our care by promoting ethical treatments and prevention of cruelty, first and foremost, ensures that they are not subjected to unnecessary suffering. Moreover, humane care for animals is also important from a public health perspective. Not only can animal diseases be passed on to humans, but also the animals we focus on in this book provide us with companionship and emotional support. Our treatment of animals has a direct impact on the quality of the environment we live in.

1.2.2 What Is Animal Welfare?

Let's start by defining it. To define animal welfare, we must recognize the following.

An animal's welfare must be considered from the animal's point of view rather than from an anthropomorphic perspective. An anthropomorphic perspective attributes human emotions and characteristics to animals, which can lead to mischaracterization of their true needs and experiences. The welfare of an animal can be defined as the *state* of the animal at any given moment. It refers to how the animal copes in any given situation and at any particular moment. Hence, evaluating an animal's state requires an understanding of its species-specific characteristics. By focusing on the animal's perspective, we can ensure that their actual needs are met and promote their wellbeing more effectively.

We all have to recognize and admit to our personal biases and preconceived notions. Once we are aware that we have them, they should consciously be put aside and not be used to determine what *we* think is most appropriate for the animal. Instead, we should focus on understanding their *species-specific needs* and behaviors in order to make the best decisions on their behalf.

1.2.3 How Should Animal Welfare Be Measured in Terms of the Animal's State?

A difficult aspect of assessing welfare is that animals do not have "*good*" or "*bad*" welfare – such as whether they *have* food (present or not) or *have* an elevated core temperature (as measured with a thermometer and considered normal or abnormal by medically defined standards). Assessing animal welfare is far more complex. Focusing on animal welfare must be intentional and requires knowledge and a set of skills. Generally speaking, veterinarians are uniquely positioned to assess

Box 1.1 ACAW Definition of Animal Welfare
Animal welfare refers to the state of the animal. Assessment of welfare includes consideration of the animal's health, behavior, and biological function. **ACAW Definition of Animal Welfare (Adopted March 05, 2010).**

and address animal welfare concerns. Nevertheless, as animal welfare science and ethics have become increasingly complex in today's environment, the American Veterinary Medical Association (AVMA) has recognized that veterinarians should be educated to advanced levels so they can provide evidence-based information and expertise to the public, veterinary professionals, and other stakeholders. As a result, the American College of Animal Welfare (ACAW) was founded to address the deeper understanding of animal welfare's impact on favorable medical and lifestyle outcomes (see Box 1.1; ACAW 2010).

The goal of this book is to provide practical tools and guidance for animal care professionals who are committed to improving the wellbeing of animals in their care. It starts with making animal welfare a priority and putting the tools available to all of us to work. As Ruth Harrison illustrated with her 1964 book *Animal Machines*, dedication and commitment can lead to a brighter future for all animals (Harrison 1964). This book led us to one of the various frameworks available in today's practice to assess animal welfare. These models are interconnected and can help us make daily welfare-centric animal care decisions.

1.2.4 Animal Welfare Assessment Framework

There are multiple valid approaches to assessing animal welfare. Health, disease, productivity, and reproductive success were historically used to measure farm animal welfare. As interest in and science of animal welfare has gained traction in the past century, the concept has expanded to include other aspects, such as behavior and stress, in the framework. Physiologically, the homeostatic view examines whether an animal can maintain a balance under stressful conditions. Bernard Rollin's concept of *telos* emphasizes the inherent nature of an animal – the species-specific set of biological and psychological interests that define how an animal is meant to live, such as the "dogness" of a dog or the "pigness" of a pig (Rollin 1981, 2007). Welfare, in this framework, is compromised when an animal is prevented from expressing behaviors and living conditions consistent with its nature.

In contrast, David Mellor's work focuses on the animal's *affective states* – the subjective emotional experiences that arise from both internal and external conditions. Mellor argues that welfare assessment must extend beyond the absence of pain or distress to include the presence of positive experiences and the mitigation of negative emotions such as fear, frustration, anxiety, and helplessness (Mellor 2016; Mellor and Beausoleil 2015).

Together, these frameworks offer a complementary approach to shelter animal welfare: Rollin's *telos* helps define what an animal needs to be and do, while Mellor's affective states help assess how the animal is actually feeling in its current environment. Integrating both perspectives allows shelters to evaluate welfare not only by physical health and behavior but also by emotional experience – an essential consideration for animals living in our care.

Temple Grandin proposes yet another aspect of animal welfare. She argues in her book *Animals Make Us Human: Creating the Best Life for Animals* that animals should be given a choice about whether or not to participate in an activity (Grandin and Johnson 2009). They should be given a choice about their environment, such as access to natural sunlight and fresh air.

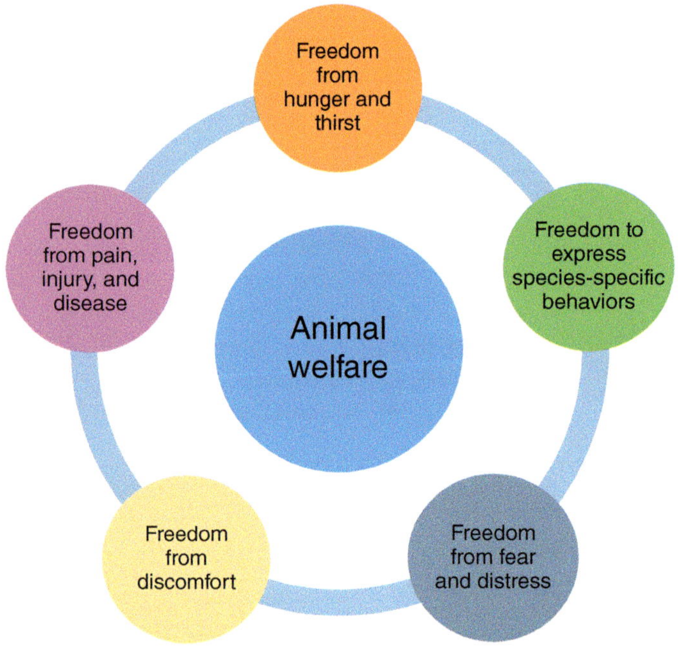

Figure 1.1 The Five Freedoms – Centered Around Minimal Welfare Standards

In 1965, the British Government appointed a committee led by Professor Roger Brambell to evaluate the welfare of farm animals in the United Kingdom. The committee's findings were published in what is now known as the *Brambell Report*, which emphasized that animals should have access to specific necessities and the freedom to express normal behaviors (Brambell 1965). This work laid the foundation for modern animal welfare science and ultimately led to the development of the *Five Freedoms* framework (see Figure 1.1). This work outlines the minimum requirements to ensure animal welfare.

It emphasizes the importance of providing animals with the ability to express natural behaviors and ensuring their physical and mental wellbeing. These principles have since become the framework for *minimal animal welfare standards* not only for farm animals but also for laboratory animals and pets globally. The SFSPCA, the American Society for Prevention of Cruelty to Animals (ASPCA), The Humane World for Animals (formerly The Humane Society of the United States [HSUS]), and many other animal welfare organizations have adopted this framework. It is helpful to improve public awareness of the needs of animals we care for. It is a very practical approach to assessing animal welfare and has become the foundation for animal welfare laws and regulations around the world.

Similarly, the *Five Domains Model*, developed by Mellor and Reid (1994), was initially created to evaluate the welfare impacts of experimental and husbandry procedures on animals. This framework assesses welfare across four physical or functional domains – nutrition, environment, health, and behavior – and a fifth domain representing the animal's mental or affective state, which reflects its overall subjective experience (see Figure 1.2).

The model has since been expanded and refined. An international panel of experts – including the author (JB) – adapted the Five Domains framework to evaluate the negative welfare consequences associated with common interventions in equine care and training (McGreevy et al. 2018).

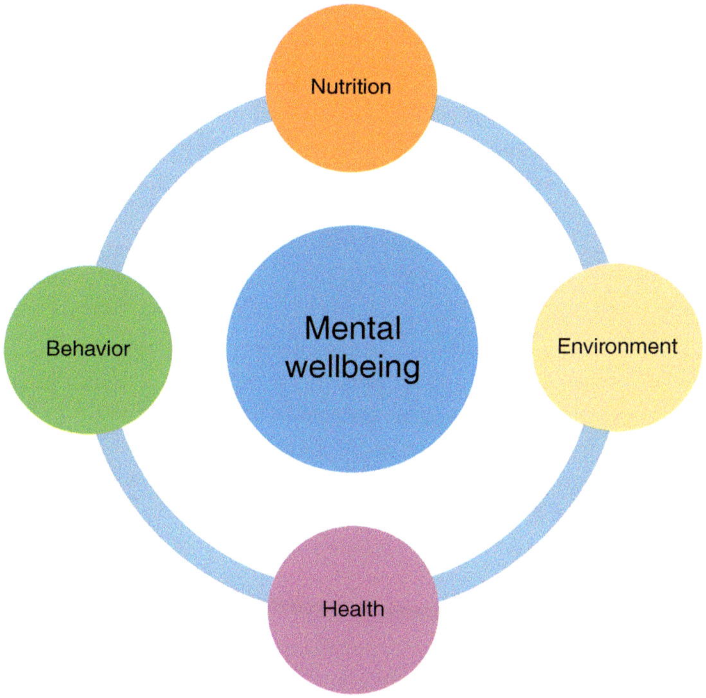

Figure 1.2 The Five Domains – Centered Around Mental WellBeing

By applying this structured, science-based approach, caretakers and professionals can more consistently assess, monitor, and improve the overall wellbeing of animals across a wide range of management contexts.

While the Five Freedoms have served as the foundation of animal welfare for decades, they represent a baseline – a *minimum standard of care* designed to prevent suffering. The framework is fundamentally rooted in ensuring animals are free from negative states such as hunger, discomfort, injury, fear, and the inability to express normal behavior. As such, it focuses primarily on the absence of harm, rather than the presence of positive experiences or emotional wellbeing.

Importantly, the Five Freedoms remain a tried-and-true, practical, and widely accepted model, particularly in field services and animal control, where they are frequently used to assess neglect and determine whether conditions meet the legal threshold for cruelty. Their clarity and simplicity make them highly effective for enforcement, education, and establishing minimum welfare expectations. However, when applied as the sole framework for evaluating overall quality of life, they may fall short of capturing the full spectrum of an animal's lived experience, particularly mental and emotional wellbeing.

For example, the freedom from hunger and thirst essentially asks:

Is food available and is the animal maintaining a body condition score around 5/9?

It does *not* ask deeper qualitative questions such as:

- *How does the animal feel about the food?*
- *Is it palatable and enjoyable?*
- *Is it the correct diet for this individual's health needs?*

- *Does the animal get to experience treats or variety?*
- *If the animal is obese, how does this impact comfort, mobility, or mood?*

In other words, the Five Freedoms safeguard basic physical needs, but they do not fully address the emotional, sensory, and cognitive dimensions that contribute to an animal's overall *wellbeing*.

The Five Domains Model is considered a more modern, nuanced, and comprehensive approach. Instead of asking only whether basic needs are being met, the domains integrate both physical and emotional components of welfare. The four functional domains – nutrition, environment, health, and behavior – directly influence the fifth domain: the animal's mental or affective state, which captures the full range of positive and negative emotional experiences.

This shift is important. The domains framework recognizes that welfare is not simply the avoidance of suffering, but the promotion of positive states such as pleasure, comfort, curiosity, contentment, and social satisfaction. It accounts for how animals *feel*, not just how they function.

For organizations with the capacity to elevate their welfare practices, adopting the Five Domains as an operational framework allows them to move beyond meeting basic needs and begin actively supporting high-quality wellbeing. The model encourages caretakers to consider sensory enrichment, choice, agency, emotional fulfillment, and individualized care – elements that are not captured in the traditional Five Freedoms.

In this way, the focus shifts from ensuring "acceptable welfare" to promoting optimal wellbeing, representing a more compassionate, evidence-based, and forward-thinking approach to animal care.

Overall, there are no perfect assessment tools to objectively quantify this complex topic. Regardless of the circumstances or species, the key to using any tool is to understand that they provide a framework for discussions around animal welfare impacts. These tools should not be used as a substitute for informed decision-making and should be applied to identify potential negative impacts on animal welfare and prioritize areas of concern. For establishing consistent standards of welfare for animals over time, the authors recommend adopting one tool that fits the organization best.

While the Five Freedoms are simple, intuitive, and easy for a wide audience to understand – including team members, volunteers, adopters, and pet owners – they remain an effective tool for communicating the fundamentals of animal welfare. Their straightforward structure reinforces the core essentials of humane care. By keeping attention on these foundational needs, organizations can reliably prioritize what matters most for animals, ensuring that basic requirements are consistently met and resources are allocated responsibly.

In contrast – and in complement – the Five Domains Model offers a more advanced, comprehensive welfare framework that elevates both the depth and sustainability of care. The Five Domains encourage teams to evaluate not only the absence of suffering but also the presence of positive experiences, emotional states, and factors that influence long-term wellbeing. This approach provides a richer, more accurate picture of each pet's shelter experience and current and future needs.

Using the Five Domains can significantly enhance the case trajectory strategy and decision-making, because it:

- Reflects the animal's *true overall state*, not just observable behavior.
- Helps identify subtle wellbeing deficits that influence behavior.
- Supports individualized treatment and management plans.
- Highlights areas where improvements will meaningfully impact quality of life.
- Guides more sustainable resource allocation by clarifying what will or won't improve outcomes.
- Promotes professional, transparent welfare assessments across teams.

Table 1.1 Comparison Five Freedoms vs. Five Domains

Category	Five Freedoms	Five Domains
Origin	Developed in the 1960s–1990s as a foundational welfare guideline	Developed by Mellor and Reid (1994); updated as a modern, science-based framework
Primary Purpose	Prevent suffering and ensure basic needs are met	Evaluate both negative and positive welfare experiences to promote optimal wellbeing
Focus	Absence of harm	Presence of positive experiences + reduction of negatives
Approach	Binary checklist (Freedom from X)	Multidimensional assessment linking physical states to emotional experiences
Structure	Five statements of basic care and protection	Four physical domains (nutrition, environment, health, behavior) + one mental/affective domain
Behavioral Considerations	Considers "Freedom to express normal behavior," but limited assessment depth	Evaluates quality, diversity, and motivation behind behaviors, including agency and choice
Emotional/Mental State	Mostly implied, minimally addressed	Central to the model – affective experiences are the ultimate welfare indicator
Examples of Questions Asked	"Is the animal free from hunger?" "Is it free from pain?"	"Does the animal enjoy its food?" "Does it experience comfort, pleasure, curiosity, and engagement?"
Level of Welfare Targeted	Minimum acceptable standard (baseline)	High-level wellbeing; aims for enrichment, positive emotions, and improved quality of life
Usefulness in Shelters	Ensures fundamental care but limited in guiding enrichment or emotional support	Helps identify welfare deficits and opportunities to enhance physical and emotional wellbeing
Modern Relevance	Considers basic essentials	Considers modern wellbeing standards
Examples	Meeting Body Condition Score requirements, providing shelter, preventing distress	Evaluating sensory environment, promoting choice, reducing fear, fostering positive social interactions

Together, the Five Domains help organizations pursue not only humane care but also *optimal* care, benefiting both animals and the professionals responsible for them. The comparison table provides a visual overview of how the Five Freedoms and Five Domains complement each other and how each framework supports different levels of welfare assessment (see Table 1.1).

1.3 Discussion of the Alignment of the Shelter and Their Goals

1.3.1 The Organizations' Mission, Vision, and Strategic Plan

Every successful organization or business is guided by a clearly defined mission, and this is especially critical for animal welfare organizations. A mission statement provides the foundation for all decision-making and activities by clearly defining an organization's purpose and values. It should actively guide daily operations, strategic planning, and ethical choices, rather than exist as a static statement. Regular review and thoughtful revision of the mission help ensure it remains relevant as societal expectations, animal welfare science, and organizational capacity evolve.

For a mission to be effective, it must be clearly communicated and consistently shared with all stakeholders – both internal and external – so that teams, leadership, partners, and the community understand and align with the organization's goals. The mission explains the existence of the organization and projects its long-term goals.

While the mission defines the organization's reason for existing, the vision describes what the organization seeks to become or achieve in the future. Together, they create a cohesive framework for decision-making and long-term planning.

A clear vision provides direction and serves as a guiding force for an organization's strategic plan. It acts as a motivational tool that inspires stakeholders and aligns their efforts toward shared goals. A well-defined vision also helps organizations prioritize initiatives and allocate resources effectively, supporting the efficient and intentional execution of strategic plans.

Animal welfare organizations – particularly animal shelters and rescue groups – benefit greatly from having a clear and compelling vision. It energizes teams, volunteers, and donors; fosters consistency in decision-making; and provides a roadmap for navigating complex ethical and operational challenges.

Effective strategic planning is the strongest when it is grounded in both a clear mission and a clear vision. The mission defines *why* the organization exists, while the vision articulates *where* it is going. Together, they inform goals, guide priorities, and ensure that programs, policies, and resource allocation are aligned with organizational values. A well-defined mission leads to a coherent vision, which in turn supports a strategic plan that promotes sustainability, accountability, and meaningful progress toward achieving the organization's objectives. This alignment ensures that goals, programs, and resources are used sustainably and effectively, allowing the organization to achieve its objectives while staying true to its core purpose.

1.3.2 The Importance of the Scope of Sustainability (SoS) and Care Trajectory Strategies (CTS)

An organization's, individual's, family's, or community's capacity refers to their ability to provide physical, emotional, and social services to those under their care. Beyond evaluating the needs of a single pet, shelters must also consider the broader impact of each decision on the entire animal population under their care – referred to here as the organization's *scope of sustainability* (SoS).

Traditionally, shelters have used *capacity for care* (C4C) to describe an organization's ability to meet animals' basic physical and medical needs within available space, staffing, and operational resources. While C4C remains a critical framework for ensuring minimum standards of care, SoS is intentionally broader.

The SoS encompasses not only immediate care capacity but also the cumulative effects of decisions on team wellbeing, public safety, animal flow, length of stay (LOS), resource allocation, community trust, and the organization's long-term ability to fulfill its mission. This approach recognizes that decisions made for one animal can meaningfully affect outcomes for many others.

By integrating individual animal welfare with population-level impacts and organizational sustainability, shelters can make ethical, defensible decisions that support both the wellbeing of individual animals and the shelter's capacity to continue serving the community effectively.

The SoS refers to the resources, skills, and support systems available to effectively fulfill and sustain the mission of the organizations. It ensures that the needs of the pets as well as the individuals caring for them within an organization are consistently met. It is essential for welfare agencies to define and adhere closely to their SoS in order to achieve their objectives within their means.

It involves continuously evaluating the ability to provide comprehensive care that addresses various aspects of the wellbeing of pets and humans alike. This requires adequate infrastructure, trained personnel, and emotional support to be in place to deliver optimal care. A primary cause of professional burnout and compassion fatigue in animal sheltering is that organizations often exceed their SoS. This is due to the tremendous, seemingly never-ending need to help animals and people who go above and beyond to care for them.

Assessing the SoS can be challenging due to the subjective nature of care needs and the diverse factors influencing them. Sustainability is significantly influenced by personal biases and cultural factors since they influence beliefs about caregiving responsibilities and acceptable forms of support. Different cultures or communities may have varying expectations about who should provide care and how it should be delivered, affecting both the availability and the type of care offered. Understanding these nuances is crucial for developing an effective and inclusive scope for CTS that respect the values of the individuals and the communities involved in caring for shelter pets. Each situation requires a personalized approach, considering cultural, social, and economic contexts. Additionally, resources are almost always limited, making it often challenging to accurately address all aspects of care needs. It is therefore important to prioritize the most essential welfare needs and create realistic, achievable goals that align with the organization's available resources. Doing so supports sustainable operations, prevents overextension of teams and budget, and ensures that animals receive consistent, high-quality care. Clear prioritization also helps teams make thoughtful, ethical decisions – especially for animals with complex behavioral or medical needs – by aligning care plans with what can truly be delivered safely, effectively, and in sustainable ways.

Additionally, it is important to involve all stakeholders in the process taking into consideration everyone's perspectives. When organizations have limited resources, they are pressed to make difficult decisions about how to allocate funds, personnel, and the community support initiatives they can reasonably support. This can lead to care gaps when certain programs are missing. For example, when resources are not allocated to public facing spay/neuter programs, this may have a significant negative impact on communities and animal welfare organizations. Additionally, the absence of low-cost positive reinforcement–based training and behavior programs in a community can have an adverse impact by potentially increasing the number of unhoused animals, driving higher shelter admissions, and ultimately contributing to increased euthanasia. Consequently, animal rescue organizations may face ethical dilemmas as they strive to meet the needs of both animals and the community. This can create a ripple effect, leading to increased stress for care teams, decrease in animal welfare, and consequently a decrease in quality of life for animals and the overall quality of life in the community.

It is crucial for organizations to identify and map out the steps they will need to take to reach their goals through strategic case trajectory planning. It involves assessing the current situation, setting goals, and developing strategies to achieve those goals. Medical and behavioral treatment trajectory planning is essential to secure the right care for shelter pets in a timely manner. A clinical movement plan is the process of creating a roadmap to help the various programs in an animal shelter reach their objectives. An admission to a resolution flow plan helps to identify the right resources, support, and services needed to care for the organization as a whole, the animals in their care, and each individual team member.

Only then can care capacity be allocated sustainably, ensuring SoS through the availability of appropriate resources, staffing, and support systems that meet animals' needs while safeguarding the health and wellbeing of the caregivers responsible for their daily care.

1.4 Access to Veterinary Care and the Impact on Animal Welfare

Limited access to veterinary medical and behavioral care in a community negatively affects both animal welfare and public wellbeing. When owned animals do not receive timely, appropriate care, they are more likely to experience preventable suffering, untreated disease, and escalating behavior issues. These conditions can contribute to the spread of infectious disease, increase safety risks through aggression or accidents, and pose broader public health concerns.

The lack of accessible veterinary and behavior services strains community resources – particularly in rural or remote areas – and is not limited to feral or stray animal populations. The author (JB) observed this firsthand while providing free vaccine clinics in rural communities, where some owned animals presented with severe matting because owners could not obtain the required rabies vaccinations. Consequently, owners were unable to access grooming services. Providing vaccination services (free or low-cost) not only supported disease prevention and reduced public health risk but also enabled caregivers to better meet basic welfare needs for their animals by removing barriers to essential follow-up care. Barriers to basic care can increase neglect or cruelty and result in higher numbers of pets surrendered with significant medical or behavioral needs. In some communities, few or no shelters or rescue resources are available to accept these animals. As a result, existing shelters and rescues may become overwhelmed, further compromising animal welfare and increasing the likelihood of euthanasia.

Affordable animal health services are crucial to guarantee that animals receive the necessary medical care to maintain their health and wellbeing. By making veterinary care more accessible and cost-effective, pet owners are more likely to seek preventative treatments, spay and neuter, and address health issues before they escalate. It affects the broader community as lack of animal health services can positively impact animals, humans, and ecosystems.

Similarly, early intervention in animal health leads to lower care costs due to less severe clinical signs when illnesses occur, ultimately resulting in quicker recovery times. It also allows for the rapid detection of potential health issues, which can be treated before they become more serious and costly problems.

By addressing behavioral concerns early, owners can prevent the development of permanent or serious behavioral concerns and help their pets thrive. Early intervention is key to helping pets adjust and cope with their environment. Animals are more likely to respond quickly to positive reinforcement and training, so it's important to address behavioral issues as soon as possible. Veterinarians play a crucial role in early intervention by providing expert guidance and care to address health and behavioral issues in animals. Veterinarians are trained to offer advice or resources on training and behavior management, helping pet owners create a positive and supportive environment for their animals.

Education plays a pivotal role in veterinary care by equipping pet owners with the knowledge they need to care for their pets. By understanding the importance of regular check-ups, vaccinations, and preventative measures, owners can better manage their pets' health and wellbeing. Additionally, educational programs can raise awareness about common behavioral issues and effective and humane training techniques. This leads to more harmonious interactions between animals and humans, tightening the human–animal bond and decreasing owner surrender (Kwan and Bain 2013).

One of the ways to improve accessibility to veterinary services is offering mobile clinics that travel to underserved areas, providing on-site care at a reduced cost. Subsidizing veterinary services through government funding or partnerships with animal welfare organizations can also make treatments more affordable for low-income families. Additionally, implementing telemedicine options for routine consultations can help pet owners access veterinary advice without the need for in-person visits.

Telemedicine in veterinary care offers numerous benefits, such as increased accessibility for pet owners who live in remote areas or have limited mobility. This is also true for pets with behavior challenges. It allows veterinarians to provide timely advice and follow-up consultations, reducing the need for travel and minimizing stress for both pets and their owners. Furthermore, telemedicine can facilitate early detection of health issues, triage medical and behavior cases, and enable prompt intervention and potentially prevent more serious conditions from developing. However, implementing telemedicine in veterinary care does come with its own challenges. One major obstacle is ensuring that both veterinarians and pet owners have access to reliable technology and internet connectivity. Additionally, there can be limitations in accurately diagnosing certain conditions without a physical examination, which may require a follow-up in-person visit. Legal and regulatory considerations for telemedicine in veterinary care require compliance with state and national veterinary practice acts. Veterinarians must be licensed in the state where the pet resides, and telemedicine consultations must adhere to established standards of care. Additionally, maintaining the confidentiality of pet owners' and patients' information is crucial, necessitating secure communication platforms and data protection measures. Veterinarians should ensure that they understand any state-specific regulations that may apply to telemedicine in their state.

In summary, access to veterinary care is essential because it ensures pets receive timely medical attention, preventing minor issues from escalating into serious health and/or behavior problems. It also supports animals' wellbeing by providing essential support, particularly for those in underserved or remote areas. Ultimately, improved access to regular veterinary care results in healthier pets that remain in their homes. It reduces the burden on pet owners and local shelters, promoting community health and wellbeing and strengthening the human–animal bond.

References

American College of Animal Welfare (ACAW) (2010). Definition of animal welfare. Adopted 5 March 2010. Available at: https://www.acaw.org/main/welfare-topics (accessed 28 December 2025).

Brambell, F.W.R. (1965). *Report of the Technical Committee to Enquire into the Welfare of Animals Kept Under Intensive Livestock Husbandry Systems*. London: Her Majesty's Stationery Office.

Grandin, T. and Johnson, C. (2009). *Animals Make Us Human: Creating the Best Life for Animals*. Boston, MA: Houghton Mifflin Harcourt.

Harrison, R. (1964). *Animal Machines: The New Factory Farming Industry*. London: Vincent Stuart.

Kwan, J.Y. and Bain, M.J. (2013). Owner attachment and problem behaviors related to relinquishment and training techniques of dogs. *Journal of Applied Animal Welfare Science* 16 (2): 168–183. https://doi.org/10.1080/10888705.2013.768923.

McGreevy, P.D., Berger, J.M., de Brauwere, N. et al. (2018). Using the Five Domains Model to assess the welfare impact of equestrian sports on horses. *Animals* 8 (10): 176. https://doi.org/10.3390/ani8100176.

Mellor, D.J. (2016). Updating animal welfare thinking: moving beyond the "Five Freedoms" towards "A Life Worth Living". *Animals* 6 (3): 21. https://doi.org/10.3390/ani6030021.

Mellor, D.J. and Beausoleil, N.J. (2015). Extending the "Five Domains" model for animal welfare assessment to incorporate positive welfare states. *Animal Welfare* 24: 241–253. https://doi.org/10.7120/09627286.24.3.241.

Mellor, D. J., & Reid, C. S. W. (1994). Concepts of animal well-being and predicting the impact of procedures on experimental animals. Improving the well-being of animals in the research environment, 3–18. https://www.wellbeingintlstudiesrepository.org/exprawel/7/

Rollin, B.E. (1981). *Animal Rights and Human Morality*. Buffalo, NY: Prometheus Books.

Rollin, B.E. (2007). Cultural variation, animal welfare and telos. *Animal Welfare* 16: 129–136.

Shelter Animals Count (2025). *2025 mid-year analysis: national shelter data report*. New York: Shelter Animals Count/ASPCA. Available at: https://www.shelteranimalscount.org/ (accessed 19 January 2026).

2

Communication and Education for Success

2.1 Building a Collaborative Team

The world of animal sheltering is emotionally, financially, and physically demanding. Teams, volunteers, and animals depend on consistent leadership and compassionate care 365 days a year. People drawn to this work come from diverse backgrounds and bring with them varying levels of experience, education, personal motivation, and live perspectives. This diversity enriches an organization by fostering innovative problem-solving, creative collaboration, and a culture of inclusion, all qualities essential to long-term success. However, these same differences can also create misunderstandings or conflicts when roles and responsibilities are not clearly defined and consistently reinforced.

Establishing and communicating clear expectations allows each team member to focus on their specific responsibilities, supporting efficiency, collaboration, and workplace harmony. Effective leaders help the team understand the "bigger picture" – that the shared mission outweighs individual roles and that every person contributes uniquely to the organization's success. As John C. Maxwell emphasizes in *The 17 Indisputable Laws of Teamwork*, strong leadership unites individuals under a common vision where collaboration drives collective achievement (Maxwell 2001).

When goals are unclear or communication is inconsistent, conflict becomes inevitable. In an environment already burdened by emotional intensity and difficult decision-making, these challenges can accelerate professional burnout and compassion fatigue. Financial strain, high caseloads, and frequent exposure to suffering compound these pressures, making strong leadership and clear organizational structure even more critical.

To ensure the success of any animal shelter or animal welfare organization, leaders must build and nurture teams that are aligned, collaborative, and committed to a shared defined mission. Collaboration requires a clearly articulated vision, consistent communication, and an inclusive environment, where team members, volunteers, board members, and donors all feel safe expressing ideas and are confident that their contributions matter. Leaders must not only cast the vision, they must also align teams, coordinate cross-departmental efforts, and ensure accountability.

When team members recognize that their work directly advances the organization's mission and when they feel valued, they become more invested and collaborative. The key to organizational success is collaboration, not competition. A shared sense of purpose improves overall outcomes for animals, enhances the wellbeing of teams and volunteers, and strengthens the organization's reputation and sustainability.

An effective leader clarifies roles, responsibilities, and lines of communication; this sets the seal for everyone's understanding and accountability. This transparency builds trust and encourages a positive, respectful work culture. In turn, donors and external partners gain confidence that their investments are being used wisely and that the organization remains mission-driven.

A well-designed mission statement is essential for any animal welfare organization. It serves as the guiding star for core values, priorities, and long-term objectives. When the mission is clearly understood, teams can make better decisions, allocate resources more effectively, and maintain alignment even during challenging times. A strong mission unifies the team, supports collaboration, reduces conflict, and attracts both dedicated team members and supportive donors. By grounding daily work in a shared purpose, leaders create stability, clarity, and a path toward sustainable success.

In summary, to build successful teams you need clear expectations, consistent communication, a shared mission, and leadership that cultivates trust, accountability, and collaboration.

2.2 Overcoming Common Implementation Challenges

One thing is certain: Implementing any plan will bring challenges. Effective leaders understand how to transform these challenges into opportunities for growth. Identifying and addressing potential obstacles as early as possible is the first step. To achieve this, organizations must have skilled leaders who prioritize cohesive teams, transparent communication, and a culture of openness. Earlier in this chapter, we discussed what it takes to build collaborative teams; now, we explore how to overcome obstacles and ensure long-term success.

When rolling out a plan or launching a new project, transparency and communication are essential. Early identification of problems allows teams to correct course quickly and maintain momentum. Open communication encourages team members to share concerns, ask questions, and provide honest feedback. This assures troubleshooting issues before they become major barriers.

Challenges frequently arise when teams are not aligned around a shared vision. Teams must feel inspired by the vision and guided toward the end goal, with clear expectations and consistent leadership. Influencing others is an essential leadership skill; it means earning trust through consistency, honesty, and transparency, not manipulating outcomes. As John C. Maxwell states, "Leadership is influence," and influence can be exercised from any level of the organization (Maxwell 2022). Many of the most impactful leaders lead without a formal title, using their reliability and subject matter knowledge to build credibility. When team members learn that you "*say what you do, and do what you say*," respect naturally follows.

Taking on challenges and working through roadblocks strengthens your legitimacy as a leader. Effective leaders set a positive example and foster an environment where people feel valued, supported, and empowered to work together. Over time, as trust deepens and expertise grows, the leader's network strengthens and collaboration becomes more natural. Leaders are expected to generate creative ideas, pursue new opportunities, and make informed decisions. They also recognize both the contributions and the gaps within their teams, understanding that success requires collective effort and shared accountability.

Honest, timely and direct feedback should occur at all levels of the organization. Creating a culture where feedback is welcomed – and where team members are regularly acknowledged for their insights and contributions – strengthens morale, trust, and collaboration.

In our experience, the keys to navigating challenges include setting clear expectations, using visual and measurable goals, demonstrating credibility, knowing your audience, and showing respect. These foundational elements enable leaders and teams to overcome obstacles effectively and remain aligned with the organization's mission.

Equally important is the use of consistent communication structures. Regular standing meetings should be established for team members who need shared information to make decisions or contribute critical insights. Rounds, daily or weekly huddles, and periodic town halls provide reliable forums for information exchange, alignment, and transparency. When communication is predictable and inclusive, teams are better equipped to act decisively, collaborate effectively, and adapt to change.

Challenges are an inevitable part of leadership. The following concepts outline practical steps leaders can use to address obstacles and sustain progress.

2.2.1 Lead Yourself

Once a challenge has been identified, it is crucial to recognize that you are the first – and often the most difficult – person you must learn to lead. Effective leadership begins with a deep understanding of your own values, leadership style, strengths, and areas for growth. Self-awareness forms the foundation for every decision you make and every interaction you have with your team.

Leaders who understand their emotional triggers, communication tendencies, and natural decision-making patterns are better equipped to respond thoughtfully rather than react impulsively. This grounded approach promotes stability, which is especially vital in the high-stress environment of animal sheltering.

Developing this level of self-awareness is an ongoing process, not a one-time exercise. There are many leadership tools and frameworks available to support this growth, including personality assessments, emotional intelligence evaluations, leadership coaching, and reflective practices, such as journaling or after-action reviews. These tools help leaders gain clarity on how they influence others, how they respond under pressure, and how they can continue to develop into more effective, empathetic, and strategic decision-makers.

Strong leaders also invest in their own resilience. This includes setting healthy boundaries, seeking mentorship, and being willing to ask for feedback and help when needed. Leaders who model vulnerability and self-improvement create a culture where team members feel safe to do the same. This, in turn, fosters psychological safety – a shared belief within the team that individuals can speak up, ask questions, admit mistakes, raise concerns, and offer new ideas without fear of punishment, ridicule, or retaliation. In psychologically safe environments, team members are more likely to communicate openly, challenge assumptions, report errors early, and engage in constructive problem-solving. This trust-based climate supports creativity, collaboration, learning, and honest feedback, all of which are essential for effective teamwork and sustainable performance.

One moment that stands out for me (JB) occurred during a team meeting when I asked for honest feedback. A newer team member shared that team members and volunteers were often hesitant to approach me because, as I moved through the organization, I walked quickly, and appeared too busy to be interrupted. I was genuinely taken aback. From my perspective, I believed I was approachable.

This feedback revealed a significant blind spot. With this insight, I made a conscious change: I began walking more slowly, intentionally pausing, making eye contact, and stopping to engage in conversation. That small behavioral adjustment had a meaningful impact on approachability, trust, and communication.

This experience reinforced an essential leadership lesson for me – how we are perceived matters just as much as our intent and even subtle behaviors can either open or close the door to connection.

Ultimately, self-leadership is not optional; it is the cornerstone of organizational success. A leader who cannot manage their own reactions, workload or communication style, will struggle to guide others effectively. By committing to continuous self-reflection and growth, leaders build the credibility, consistency, and trust required to inspire their teams, navigate conflict, and successfully implement even the most challenging organizational initiatives.

Fortunately, many leadership tools and frameworks are available to help strengthen this awareness, build confidence, and continually refine our ability to lead with clarity and integrity.

2.2.2 Mission, Vision, and Value Alignment

Before moving forward with any initiative, it is essential to ask whether the project truly aligns with the organization's mission, values, and vision. This requires a clear understanding of what your organization stands for and the purpose it exists to fulfill. When leaders and team members have a shared understanding of these foundational elements, they are better equipped to make decisions that support long-term sustainability and meaningful impact.

Take time to review and articulate your organization's mission, values, and vision – and ensure the entire team understands them (see Chapter 1). Communicate these guiding principles clearly and consistently throughout the project. Doing so allows you to recognize any deviations from the intended direction early in the process, ensuring that misalignment can be addressed before valuable time, effort, and resources are spent or wasted on work which does not support the organization's goals.

2.2.3 Naming the Problem

The first step in driving any meaningful change is to clearly define the problem. Not everyone in the organization will immediately agree that a particular project or change is necessary, which is why clarity is essential. In his book, *Managing at the Speed of Change*, Daryl Conner introduced the term "burning platform," inspired by the 1988 Piper Alpha oil rig disaster in the North Sea (Conner 1993). He used the metaphor to illustrate that people are far more willing to embrace change when they perceive a compelling, urgent reason, such as staying the same is more dangerous than moving forward. While the "burning platform" represents a point of undeniable urgency, effective leaders strive to identify needs long before they reach this critical stage. This requires gathering data, talking with stakeholders, observing workflows, and deeply understanding the organization's environment so that potential issues are recognized and addressed early.

The concept of the burning platform underscores two key leadership responsibilities: *urgency and timing*. Leaders must know *when* to act, but they must also ensure that team members can clearly envision what will exist *after* the goal is achieved. One of the most common questions people have during any change is, *"What's in it for me?"* True buy-in requires understanding the individual you are speaking to. How an issue is framed, discussed, and motivated must reflect the perspectives, priorities, and experiences of the audience. The best leaders adapt their messaging to resonate with different audiences while staying grounded in shared values and objectives.

To strengthen alignment and motivate action, it is helpful to provide what Chip and Dan Heath call a "*destination postcard*" (Heath and Heath 2010). This is a vivid, compelling description of the future state one aims to create, something concrete enough for people to see, to feel, and to understand the benefits of reaching it. A clear and inspiring picture of future success can significantly improve engagement and reduce resistance. When team members understand where the organization is headed, why the change matters, and how they fit into the bigger picture, they are far more likely to stay committed and contribute meaningfully.

Helping people visualize the positive outcomes and not just the urgency creates shared motivation and reduces challenges along the way. In some cases, it will also reveal when a team member is not aligned with the mission or the change effort, allowing leaders to make informed decisions about adjusting roles or removing individuals from the project if necessary to preserve momentum.

Ultimately, by clearly articulating the problem, identifying needs early, and painting a compelling vision of the future, leaders create the clarity and alignment necessary for successful and sustainable change.

2.2.4 SMART

Specific, Measurable, Achievable, Relevant, and Time-bound goals (SMART goals) offer a widely recognized framework originally introduced by George T. Doran in 1981 as a practical tool for improving management effectiveness (Doran 1981). It has since become an essential practice for driving success in any project or organizational initiative. The structure and clarity established by SMART goals ensure that everyone understands what needs to be accomplished, how progress will be tracked, and when results are expected. By clearly defining expectations and timelines, SMART goals also strengthen accountability, ensuring that team members know their responsibilities and can evaluate their own progress objectively.

Equally important is the practice of recognizing and celebrating incremental success. Highlighting small wins not only boosts morale but also reinforces momentum and confidence within the team. These milestones serve as evidence that progress is being made, even if the end goal is still ahead.

By monitoring progress consistently, leaders can identify when the team is slightly off track and take corrective action early. It is far easier and far less costly to address small deviations early, than to wait until minor issues escalate into major setbacks. Early course corrections help preserve resources and reduce frustration. Moreover, they maintain alignment with the project's goals and the organization's mission.

Regular check-ins, transparent communication, and visual progress indicators can help teams stay focused on the objectives, while also allowing room to adjust strategies when necessary. This flexibility is a hallmark of effective leadership: understanding when to stay the course and when to refine the approach.

Ultimately, the combination of SMART goals, continuous evaluation, and celebration of milestones creates an environment where challenges become manageable, progress is visible, and team members remain engaged and motivated. This disciplined yet adaptive framework strengthens trust, enhances collaboration, and increases the likelihood of long-term project success.

2.2.5 Understanding Resistance

To overcome challenges effectively, it is essential to identify individuals who may resist the project or proposed change. In any organization, there will always be some who are not fully on board. These individuals – often referred to as "*resisters*" – can slow down progress or even derail a project if their concerns are not understood and addressed. The first step is to learn who they are, listen to their perspectives, and understand the reasoning behind their hesitation.

Not all stakeholders possess the same level of knowledge as the project leader, and some may not fully understand the scope, purpose, or urgency of the initiative. This knowledge gap can significantly hinder progress, which is why educating all stakeholders is critical. A project starts on solid ground only when leaders understand the viewpoints of individuals and teams. It is equally important that leaders know how those individuals perceive their own contributions and roles in the process.

This is where the concept of management by walking around (MBWA) becomes especially valuable. Originating at Hewlett-Packard in the 1970s under leaders such as Bill Hewlett and Dave Packard, and later popularized in *In Search of Excellence*, MBWA emphasizes spontaneous, informal interactions with team members across roles and departments (Peters and Waterman 1982). These interactions allow leaders to identify issues early, build trust, and encourage teams to surface challenges and propose solutions. Visibility, approachability, and genuine curiosity from leadership create conditions where communication flows freely and problems can be addressed before they escalate.

In the modern, post-COVID era, however, MBWA faces new challenges. Many animal welfare organizations – particularly those without brick-and-mortar facilities – now have leadership teams working remotely or largely off-site from day-to-day operations. While remote work may be appropriate or unavoidable in some foster-based or geographically dispersed models, its practice even in facility-based organizations can create significant disconnects. When leaders are not physically present where animals are cared for and teams have to perform emotionally demanding work, opportunities for informal communication, real-time observation, and relational trust-building can easily be reduced.

In remote or hybrid settings, leadership must aim to shift from *passive presence* to *intentional visibility*. This may include structured on-site time, routine walk-throughs during operational hours, scheduled but informal check-ins with frontline teams, and consistent engagement with volunteers – not just managers. In virtual spaces, it requires more than meetings and metrics; leaders must create forums where staff can speak candidly, raise concerns safely, and feel heard without bureaucratic barriers.

Ultimately, MBWA is not about physical walking alone – it is about accessibility, attentiveness, and relational leadership. In animal welfare organizations with physical operations, leaders who remain too far removed from daily realities risk missing early warning signs of burnout, workflow breakdowns, safety concerns, and animal welfare compromises. Effective leadership in this era requires adapting MBWA principles to ensure that proximity – whether physical or relational – is not lost and that trust, accountability, and shared purpose remain strong across all levels of the organization.

Another effective leadership practice for upper management that I (JB) learned from a former supervisor is the value of meeting not only with direct reports on a weekly basis but also scheduling regular check-ins – such as monthly meetings – with team members two levels down. These conversations offer invaluable insight into daily operational challenges, emerging needs, and team morale that may not surface through traditional reporting lines, strengthening both communication and organizational alignment.

Maintaining strong communication with middle management is especially critical. Middle managers are often responsible for translating upper management's ideas, policies, and procedures into daily practice. Keeping them informed, aligned, and supported improves consistency, strengthens execution, and reduces friction between strategic vision and frontline realities.

These practices also support effective succession planning. When middle managers are engaged, informed, and excited about the organization's vision and the changes needed to achieve it, they are more likely to develop leadership confidence, invest in long-term goals, and emerge as strong future leaders within the organization.

2.3 Achieving Win-Win-Win Solutions in Animal Welfare

Successfully advancing animal welfare goals depends on strong communication and negotiation skills – both of which can be learned, practiced, and strengthened over time. Although professionals in this field share a deep commitment to animals, differences in experience, perspective, and priorities can lead to conflict. When these challenges arise, the guiding question should always be: How do we achieve a win-win-win outcome? In our experience, one simple message helps keep everyone aligned: "*It's about the animals.*" When the animals win, the organization succeeds – and the people do too.

In summary, achieving win-win-win solutions in animal welfare depends on aligned teams, open communication, and a shared strategic vision. Turning principles into action requires intentional, consistent effort. By clearly defining the organization's mission, vision, and animal welfare philosophy – and by using objective, measurable indicators – leaders, teams, and volunteers can work toward common goals and consistent outcomes. Adopting a recognized, science-based framework such as the Five Domains Model provides a structured approach for evaluating welfare, guiding ethical decision-making, and allocating resources responsibly. Together, these elements support sustainable care while keeping organizations firmly grounded in their mission and values.

Throughout this chapter, we have emphasized that effective leadership in animal welfare is built through practice, reflection, and a willingness to grow through discomfort. Along the way, we have each relied on a set of books, frameworks, and tools that helped us navigate uncertainty, difficult decisions, and the everyday realities of leading mission-driven organizations.

To support readers on their own leadership journeys, we have created a Leadership Resource List, available in the appendix of this book. The materials listed proved useful in developing emotional intelligence, ethical decision-making, collaboration, negotiation, and sustainable leadership practices. These resources are not presented as abstract theory, but as practical guides that have informed our thinking, strengthened our communication, and provided clarity during challenging periods. Many were revisited repeatedly as circumstances changed, teams evolved, and new responsibilities emerged. We encourage readers to explore these resources with curiosity, adapt what resonates, and remain open to continuous learning. True leadership is not about having all the answers, but about asking thoughtful questions, listening with intention, and staying open to growth – especially when growth challenges us.

See Appendix A for Leadership Resources.

References

Conner, D.R. (1993). *Managing at the Speed of Change: How Resilient Managers Succeed and Prosper Where Others Fail*. New York: Villard Books.

Doran, G.T. (1981). There's a S.M.A.R.T. way to write management's goals and objectives. *Management Review* 70 (11): 35–36.

Heath, C. and Heath, D. (2010). *Switch: How to Change Things When Change Is Hard*. New York: Broadway Books.

Maxwell, J.C. (2001). *The 17 Indisputable Laws of Teamwork: Embrace Them and Empower Your Team*. Nashville, TN: Thomas Nelson.

Maxwell, J.C. (2022). *The 21 Irrefutable Laws of Leadership: Follow Them and People Will Follow You*. Nashville, TN: Thomas Nelson.

Peters, T.J. and Waterman, R.H. (1982). *In Search of Excellence: Lessons from America's Best-Run Companies*. New York: Harper & Row.

3A

Understanding Canine Behavior and Communication

3A.1 Basics of Canine Behavior

Understanding canine communication requires more than recognizing individual signals. It requires seeing behavior as an interconnected system shaped by evolution, context, and emotion. Dogs communicate using a rich tapestry of visual, auditory, olfactory, tactile, and gustatory cues, each influenced by the environment, the situation, and the intended recipient.

3A.1.1 Key Aspects of Visual Communication in Dogs

Dogs rely heavily on *visual* communication – arguably more than vocal or olfactory cues – because body language provides rapid, nuanced information that helps avoid conflict and maintain social harmony. Unlike static "signals," canine visual communication is *dynamic*: postures shift second-to-second, multiple body regions blend into a single emotional message, and subtle changes indicate internal physiological shifts. Understanding dog communication means observing these elements as a fluid system, rather than interpreting each feature in isolation.

Body language reflects not only a dog's outward expression but also their internal emotional and neurological state. For example, when a dog yawns in a tense situation, this isn't merely a "calming signal"; it's the outward expression of an autonomic nervous system shift. The body is attempting to self-regulate by increasing oxygen intake, lowering arousal, and dampening sympathetic activation. Similarly, a dog that freezes for one second before retreating is expressing a surge of internal conflict between fear and social inhibition.

When we teach visual communication, we emphasize patterns, context, and moment-to-moment transitions. A relaxed dog does not instantly become aggressive; arousal increases through a measurable continuum that can be seen in the tightening of facial muscles, the stiffening of the torso, the elevation of the tail, and the narrowing of the eyes. The observer should therefore look for *trends* in movement and posture rather than single "signs" (see Box 3A.1).

3A.1.1.1 Visual Communication

3A.1.1.1.1 Whole-Body Posture

How a dog arranges the entire body is one of the clearest indicators of emotional state (Simpson 1997; Siniscalchi et al. 2018).

Box 3A.1 Interpretation of Body Language Considerations

Interpretation of Body Language Must Consider

- Context: Environment, trigger, and social situation
- The dog's learning history and temperament
- The direction of the vocalization (what or whom it is aimed at)
- The dog's body language (posture, ear and tail position, and facial tension)

- Relaxed: Soft muscles, neutral head height, and even weight distribution (see Figure 3A.1).
- Uncertain: Slightly lowered head, shifting weight, and subtle tension along the spine (see Figure 3A.2).
- Fearful: Crouched posture, lowered body, and weight shifted backward (see Figure 3A.3).
- Threatened/aggressive: Forward-leaning, stiff legs, and enlarged silhouette.
- Submissive: Lowered posture or full-body crouch, curved spine, and reduced height (see Figure 3A.4).

Why it matters: Posture reflects sympathetic vs. parasympathetic activation, confidence, and social intent.

3A.1.1.1.2 Tail Position and Movement

The tail acts as a directional signal of emotional activation (Simpson 1997; Siniscalchi et al. 2018).

- Neutral: Low–mid height and relaxed sway (see Figure 3A.5).
- Excited/alert: Higher carriage and fast movement (see Figure 3A.6).
- Fearful/anxious: Tucked or held low (see Figure 3A.7).
- Agonistic: High, stiff, and rapid vibration at the tip ("flagging") (see Figure 3A.8).

Neurological tie-in: Tail height correlates with muscle tension driven by arousal pathways in the sympathetic nervous system.

Figure 3A.1 Neutral Dog

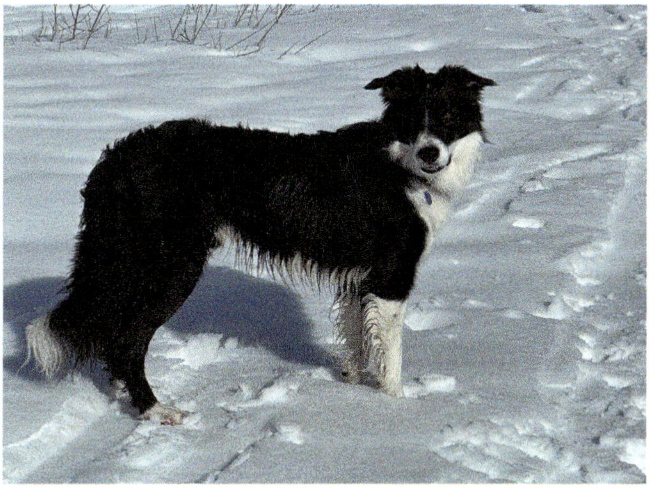

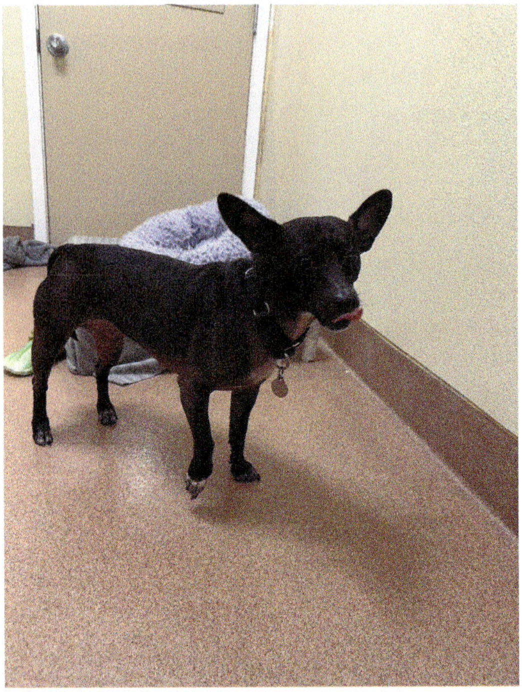

Figure 3A.2 Uncertain Body Posture with Paw Lift

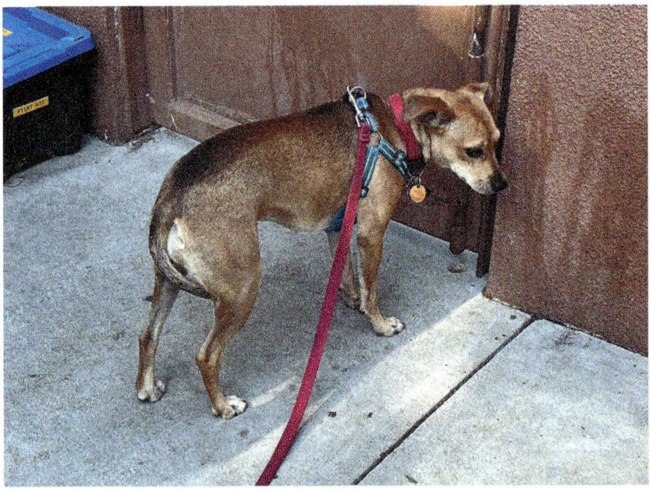

Figure 3A.3 Uncertain Body Posture with Tail Tucked

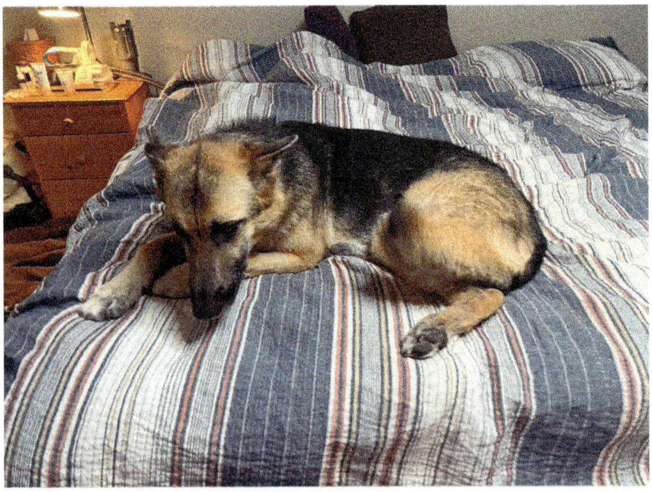

Figure 3A.4 Submissive/deferential Posture

Figure 3A.5 Neutral Tail with Mutual Sniff

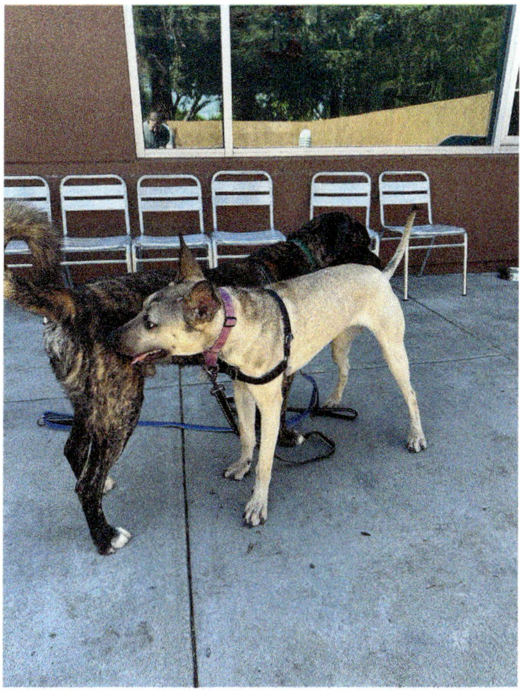

Figure 3A.6 Tail Up in Play

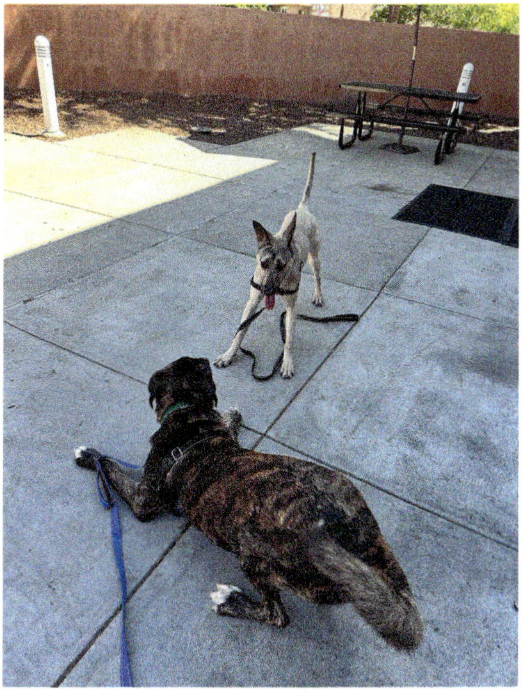

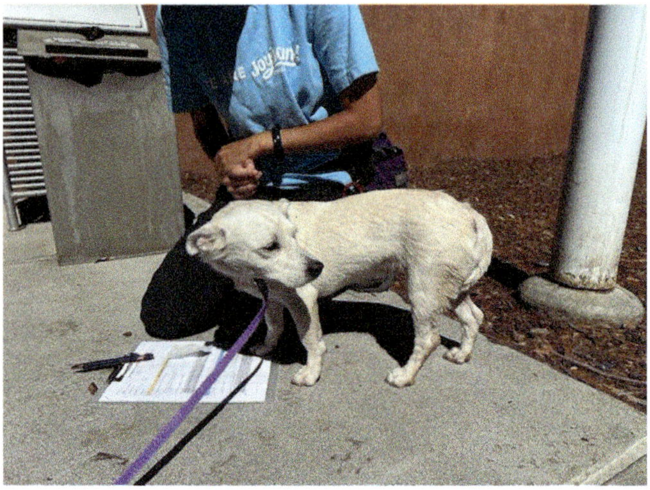

Figure 3A.7 Tail Tucked

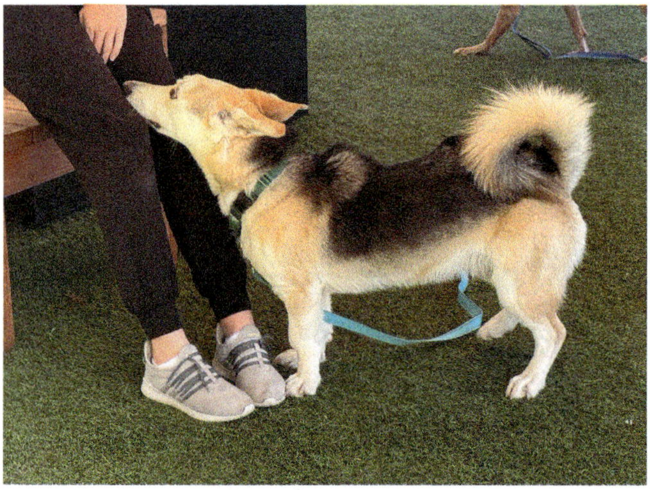

Figure 3A.8 Tail Stiff and Elevated, with Piloerection

3A.1.1.1.3 Ear Position

Ears adjust to collect auditory information *and* signal emotional tone (Simpson 1997; Siniscalchi et al. 2018).

- Neutral: Slight forward-side orientation (see Figure 3A.9).
- Forward/stiff: Focused, alert, and assessing (see Figure 3A.10).
- Flattened: Fear, appeasement, or defensive readiness (see Figure 3A.11).
- Rapidly changing and flicking: Heightened vigilance.

Physiology: Ear muscles respond instantly to threat appraisal and mediate both hearing acuity and communication.

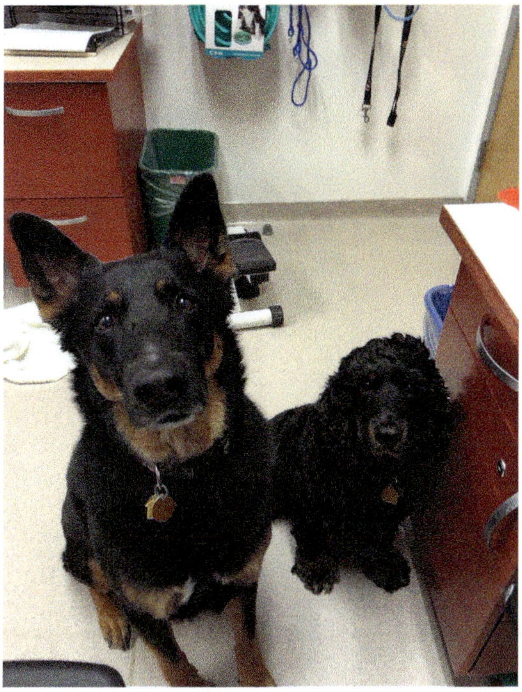

Figure 3A.9a Ears Forward, Erect and Floppy

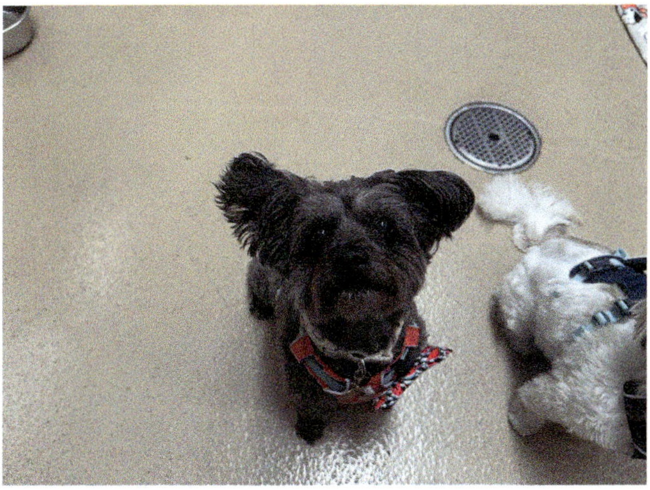

Figure 3A.9b Neutral small dog with ears forward

3A.1.1.1.4 Eyes and Facial Muscles

The face often gives the earliest indication of rising stress (Simpson 1997; Siniscalchi et al. 2018).

- Soft eyes: Relaxed orbicular muscles and slow blinking (see Figure 3A.12).
- Hard stare: Reduced blinking, focused pupils, and fixed gaze (see Figure 3A.13).
- Whale eye: Increased sclera visibility due to head–eye mismatch (see Figure 3A.14).
- Tension lines: Furrowing of brows and tightening around the muzzle.

What it represents: Shifts between parasympathetic regulation and sympathetic arousal; increased stare is a precursor to escalation.

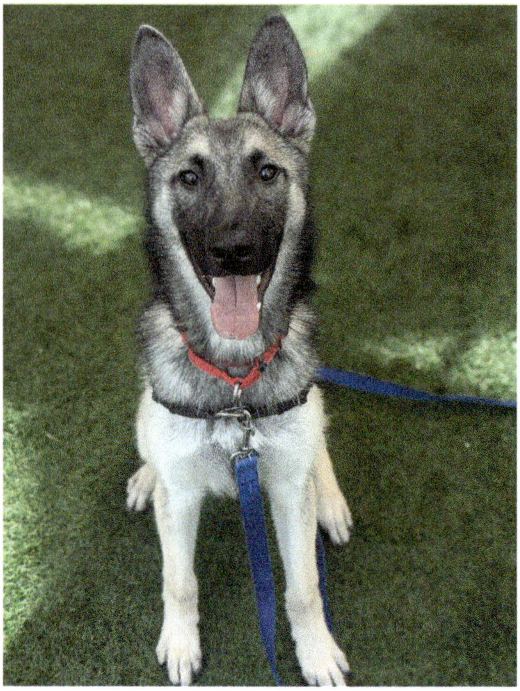

Figure 3A.10 Ears Forward and Alert

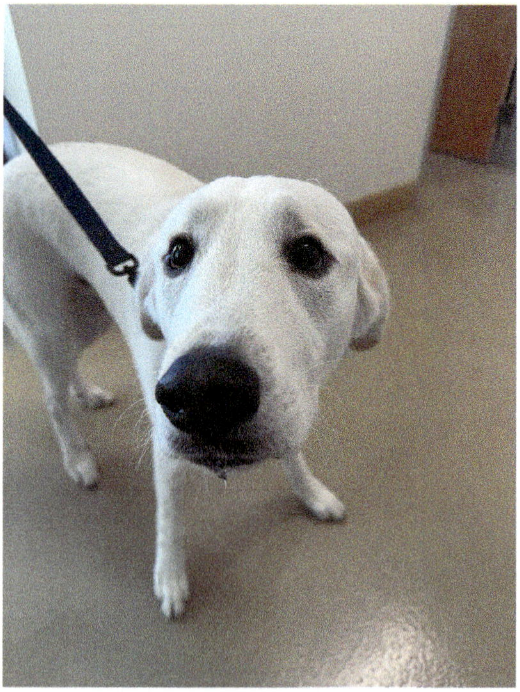

Figure 3A.11 Ears Flattened

Figure 3A.12 Soft Eyes

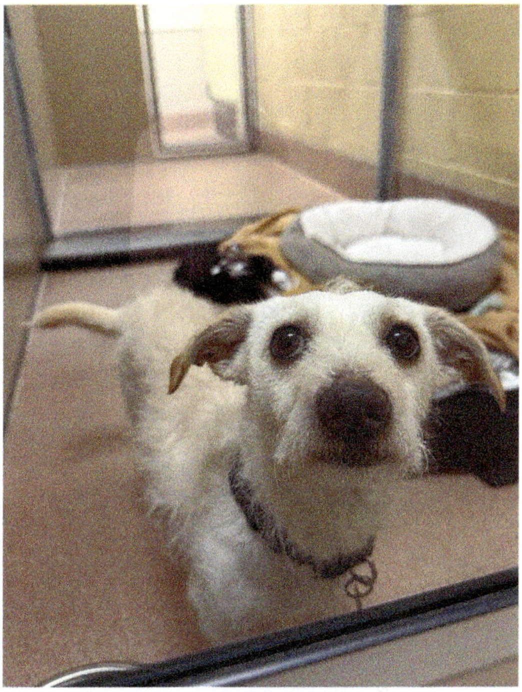

Figure 3A.13 Stare

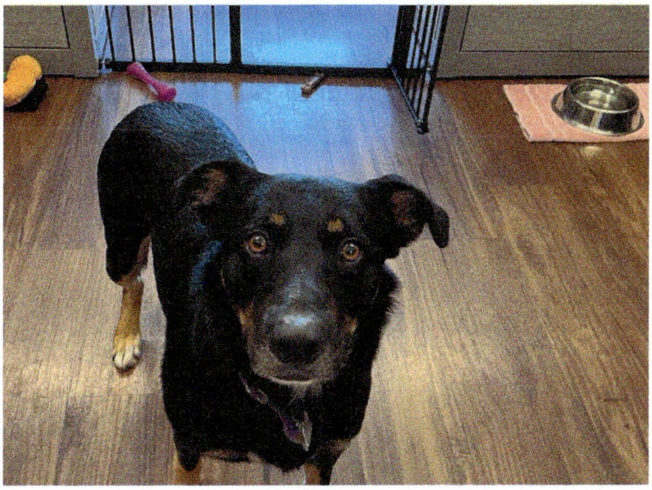

Figure 3A.14 Whale Eye

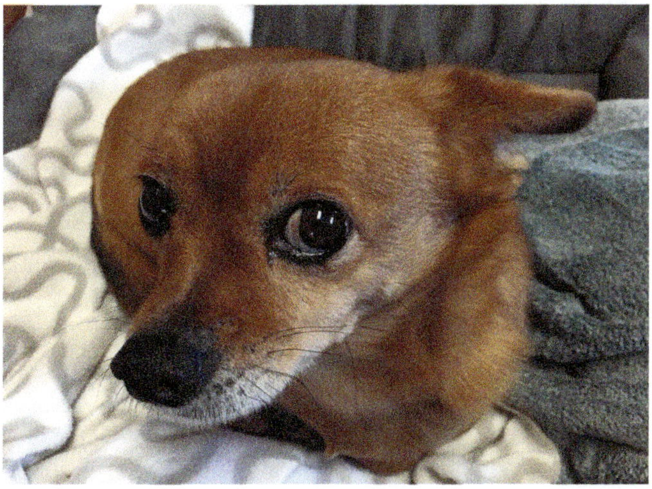

3A.1.1.1.5 Mouth and Oral Expressions

The mouth conveys relaxation vs. tension (Simpson 1997; Siniscalchi et al. 2018).

- Relaxed: Slightly open mouth and loose lips (see Figure 3A.15).
- Closed and still: Heightened focus or early stress (see Figure 3A.16).
- Panting: Stress response and thermoregulatory activation (see Figure 3A.17).
- Lip licking, yawning: Displacement behaviors linked to autonomic shifts (see Figure 3A.18)
- Showing teeth: May indicate fear, uncertainty, or agonistic intent; context is essential.

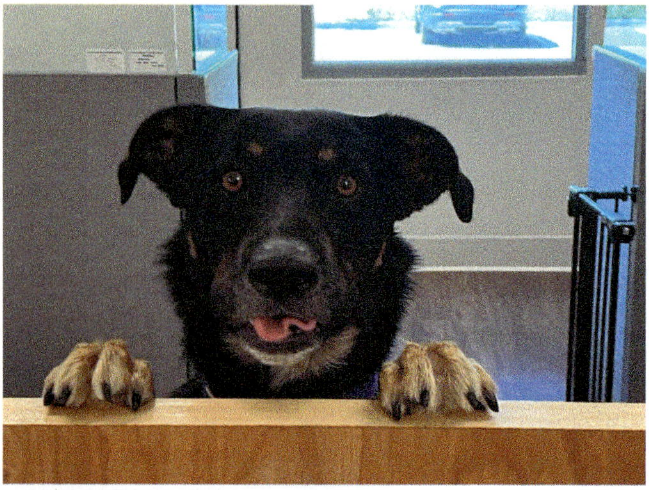

Figure 3A.15 Open Mouth

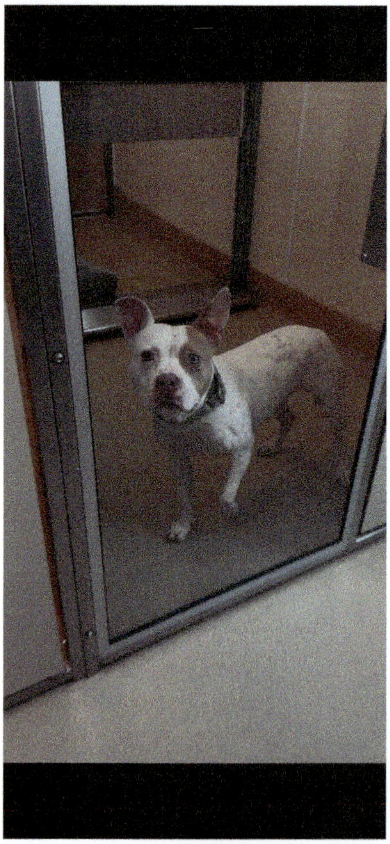

Figure 3A.16 Closed Mouth, Leg Lift and Stare

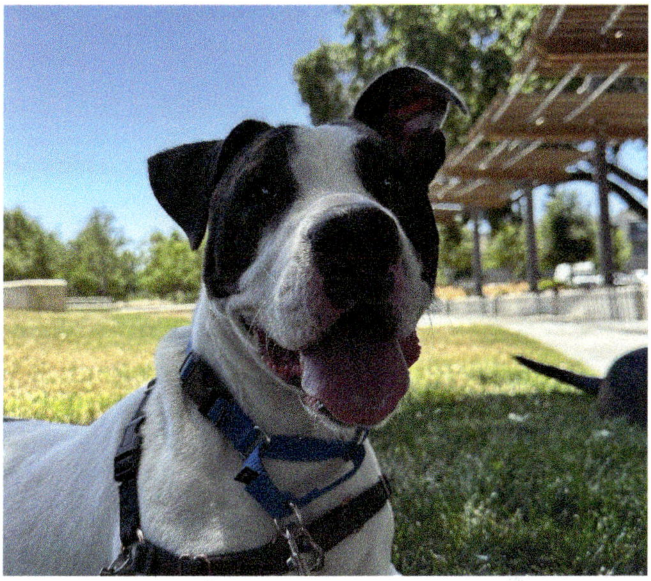

Figure 3A.17 Panting

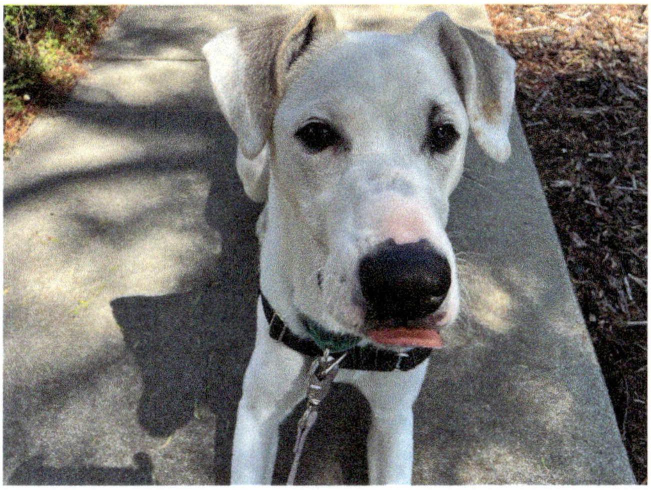

Figure 3A.18 Lip Lick

3A.1.1.1.6 Movement Patterns (Gait and Tempo)

The way a dog moves communicates readiness, avoidance, or conflict.

- Loose, bouncy movement: Play or affiliative intent.
- Slow approach and curved body: Non-threatening greeting.
- Stalking, stiff gait: Elevated arousal or predatory motor patterns.
- Retreating with short, quick steps: Fear or appeasement.

Movement reveals motivation: pursuit vs. withdrawal and confidence vs. conflict.

3A.1.1.1.7 Interaction of Signals (the "Communication Matrix")

Dogs rarely send one signal at a time. Instead, their communication must be understood as:

- Clusters (e.g. whale eye + still tail = tension)
- Transitions (relaxed → tense → freeze)
- Contradictions (wagging tail + stiff body = conflicted state)
- Escalation sequences (subtle → obvious → overt)

3A.1.1.1.8 Context and Environment

Body language must always be interpreted in context:

- Presence of another dog or person
- Resource-rich situations
- Social familiarity vs. novelty
- Pain or medical conditions
- Confined spaces or escape routes
- Noises, movement, and other signals in the environment
- Physical restraint or confinement

Context determines whether a behavior is affiliative, agonistic, playful, or fearful.

3A.1.1.1.9 Species-Specific Communication Skills

Dogs vary in their ability to communicate visually depending on:

- Breed morphology (brachycephalic faces, curled tails, and cropped ears) (see Figure 3A.19).
- Coat types (long fur obscuring signals)

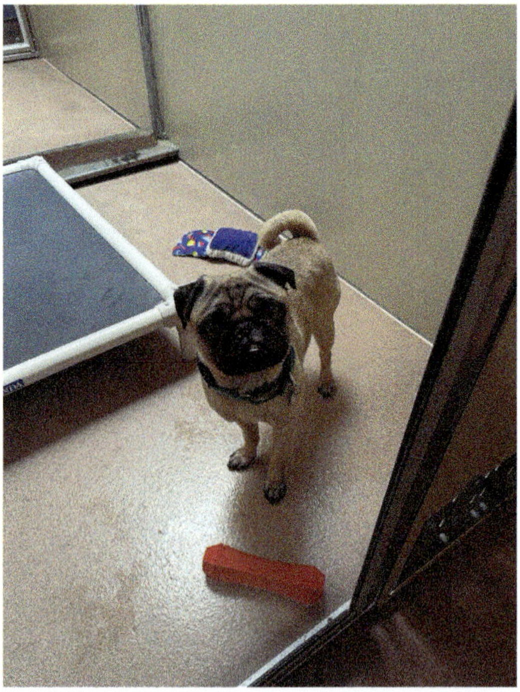

Figure 3A.19 Brachycephalic Face

- Individual experiences and socialization
- Learning history and reinforcement patterns

3A.1.1.1.10 The Internal State: Physiology Behind the Behaviors

Visual communication mirrors the dog's internal state:

- Sympathetic activation: Dilated pupils, forward posture, and faster movement.
- Parasympathetic shift: Relaxed posture, soft eyes, and open mouth.
- Stress hormones (cortisol and adrenaline): Create micro-tension and displacement behaviors.
- Pain states: Altered gait and facial expression and can be mistaken for fear or aggression.

3A.1.2 Auditory Communication in Dogs

While dogs communicate primarily through visual signals, auditory communication remains a powerful secondary system – especially over long distances or when visual cues are limited. Unlike human language, canine vocalizations do not form "words." Instead, dogs use variations in pitch, duration, repetition, volume, and context to convey internal emotional states and influence the behavior of others. Each vocalization reflects a combination of emotional arousal, motivation (approach, avoidance, defense, or social contact), and neurological activation (Yeon 2007). Importantly, auditory signals should never be interpreted in isolation; they must always be evaluated in conjunction with body language, environmental context, and the ongoing interaction. Vocalizations add information, but posture, movement, facial expression, and behavioral sequencing provide the critical framework for accurate interpretation.

Auditory communication is fluid, not fixed. A bark can shift from excitement to alarm within seconds; a growl may soften into a play rumble or escalate toward aggression depending on how interactions unfold. For example, a dog greeting a familiar person may bark with a high pitch, loose body posture, and wagging tail – signals consistent with excitement. The same dog, if startled by a sudden approach in a confined space, may produce a lower-pitched, repetitive bark accompanied by a stiffened body and weight shift forward, indicating heightened arousal or defensive concern. Similarly, a growl during play is often paired with exaggerated, bouncy movements and self-handicapping behaviors, whereas a growl accompanied by freezing, hard eye contact, and closed mouth signals a very different emotional state and requires immediate space.

3A.1.2.1 Expanded Key Vocalizations (Simpson 1997; Yin and McCowan 2004; Beaver 2009)

3A.1.2.1.1 Bark

The bark is the most flexible and context-dependent vocalization in dogs. It is unique in canids: domestic dogs bark more frequently and in more contexts than wolves, reflecting adaptation to living alongside humans.

Functions

- Alert/alarm: Signals the detection of something novel approaching the territory.
- Defensive threat: Used to deter another dog or person; paired with a forward posture.
- Excitement or anticipation: Rapid, high-pitched barks during play or before outings.
- Solicitation: Used to request attention, food, or play from caregivers.
- Contact call: Helps locate family members or seek reassurance ("*Where are you?*").

Biological significance: Barking is linked to emotional arousal, with pitch rising as sympathetic activation increases. The bark's variability makes context essential: the same dog may bark differently at a stranger vs. a favorite person (Yin and McCowan 2004).

3A.1.2.1.2 Whine

A high-pitched, narrow-band vocalization associated with emotional vulnerability.

Functions

- Solicitation: Puppies whine for maternal care; adults often whine for attention or comfort.
- Pain or illness: A dog may whine when physically uncomfortable.
- Stress, anxiety, or fear: Whining increases during separation, confinement, or social tension.
- Submissive gesture: Occurs during appeasement interactions with other dogs.

Physiology: Whining reflects parasympathetic and sympathetic co-activation – an internal "*conflict state,*" where the dog wants something but may feel insecure or uncomfortable.

3A.1.2.1.3 Yelp

A sudden, high-frequency vocalization typically produced in moments of acute distress.

Functions

- Pain response: Reaction to unexpected sudden pain (stepped on tail and rough play).
- Startle/fear shock: When a dog is frightened or overwhelmed.
- Overexcitement: Occurs in hyper-aroused states when self-regulation fails.

Social purpose: A yelp can inhibit the other party's behavior ("*Stop what you're doing!*"), especially in play, teaching others to moderate force. It is a key part of social development.

3A.1.2.1.4 Howl

A long-distance vocalization connected to social cohesion and environmental triggers.

Functions

- Group cohesion: Helps coordinate members across distances.
- Contact call: Dogs howl when left alone, attempting to locate social partners.
- Distress response: Some dogs howl when experiencing separation anxiety.
- Auditory trigger response: Sirens, music, or another dog's howl can initiate mimicry.

Biological background: Howling is rooted in wolf ancestry, though domestic dogs use it less often. It is associated with arousal and communication over large distances, especially when visual cues are unavailable.

3A.1.2.1.5 Growl

A low-pitched, broad-frequency vocalization that communicates distance-increasing intent (see Box 3A.2).

Functions

- Warning/threat: "*Back off*" signal when a dog feels threatened or needs space.
- Defensive aggression: Signals that the dog may escalate if pressure continues.

Box 3A.2 Important Note

Growling is *communication*, not disobedience. Punishing growls removes an important safety signal and can cause sudden, unsignaled bites.

- Resource guarding: Protecting food, valued objects, or resting spaces.
- Play growl: Occurs during rough-and-tumble play; looser body language distinguishes it from threat growls.

Additional auditory signals that are often overlooked.

3A.1.2.1.6 Baying

A deep, extended bark common in hounds.

Use: Trailing scents, alerting handlers, expressing excitement, or coordination during hunts.

3A.1.2.1.7 Grumbling/Grunting

Low-level rumbling noises often indicate mild displeasure, fatigue, or contentment depending on body language.

3A.1.2.1.8 Sighing

A long exhalation signaling relaxation, frustration, or disengagement. Paired with body posture, it can signify "I'm done interacting."

3A.1.2.1.9 Huffing/Snorting

Short forceful breaths used in:

- Mild irritation
- Uncertainty
- Attempts to gather better scent information
- Arousal during play

3A.1.2.1.10 "Talking" or "Muttering"

Breed-dependent vocal quirks (e.g. huskies) that reflect high social engagement and learned behavior reinforced by humans (see Table 3A.1; Simpson 1997; Yin and McCowan 2004; Beaver 2009).

Table 3A.1 Key Aspects of Auditory Communication in Dogs (Adapted from Simpson 1997; Yin and McCowan 2004; Beaver 2009)

Aspect	Description/Purpose	Context/Notes
Pitch	High pitch → fear, anxiety, pain, or excitement Low pitch → threat, confidence, defensive/offensive intent	Pitch alone is not sufficient; must be interpreted with context and body language
Duration	Short bursts → alerting or startle responses Long sustained tones → distress, contact calls, or prolonged arousal	Indicates intensity and type of emotional state
Frequency/Repetition	Rapid repetition → heightened arousal or urgency Single vocalization → momentary message	Repetition can amplify urgency or indicate persistent need

(*Continued*)

Table 3A.1 (Continued)

Aspect	Description/Purpose	Context/Notes
Volume	Loud → high arousal (alarm, fear, or threat) Soft → appeasement, uncertainty, or solicitation	Volume reflects emotional intensity and social intent
Context	Auditory cues require situational awareness, presence of triggers, and social relationships	Same sound can mean different things in different situations
Accompanying Body Language	Posture, tail height, facial expression, and movement patterns shape meaning	Combined signals provide the true "message" behind vocalizations
Purpose and Motivation	Vocalizations aim to increase/decrease distance, draw attention, stop behavior, express discomfort, or coordinate social interactions	Motivation must be interpreted alongside context and body language
Learning History	Dogs learn which vocalizations work with which humans; whining and barking may be reinforced	Past reinforcement influences how vocalizations are used and repeated

3A.1.3 Olfactory Communication in Dogs

Dogs live in a sensory world that is fundamentally different from our own. While humans rely heavily on vision, dogs experience their environment through *smell*. Their olfactory world is so rich, complex, and layered that it is almost unimaginable to the human brain. In daily interactions, humans often miss the primary conversations happening right under their noses, conversations entirely driven by scent.

Why humans are poorly equipped to understand canine scent communication: Compared to dogs, humans are sensory beginners. Anatomically, our olfactory system is not designed for nuance:

- Humans have 5–10 million olfactory receptors.
- Dogs have 200–300 million olfactory receptors (Buzek et al. 2022; Lee et al. 2023).
- The portion of the brain devoted to analyzing scent is, proportionally, 40 times larger in dogs.

Dogs also possess a specialized sensory structure that humans entirely lack: the vomeronasal organ (VNO), which analyzes pheromones and other chemical signalers. This gives dogs access to a layer of social information invisible to humans, including identity, emotional state, sex, reproductive status, diet, stress hormones, and even health conditions (Mills et al. 2013; McGlone et al. 2022). To humans, a fire hydrant is just a fire hydrant. To a dog, it is a *multimedia message board*: Who was here, what sex they are, how healthy they are, how confident they were, what they've eaten, how stressed they felt, and how long ago they passed by.

Olfactory communication is not merely "*smelling*," it is a full sensory dialogue, one that shapes how dogs navigate social relationships, territory, reproduction, and safety.

3A.1.3.1 Forms of Olfactory Communication

3A.1.3.1.1 Urine Marking

Urine is one of the most important mediums of canine scent communication. Unlike a simple excretion, urine deposits serve as chemical messages that persist long after the dog is gone. These marks help dogs exchange information without direct interaction, which is safer and more efficient than constant face-to-face encounters.

Research across canids shows that urine can encode:

- Identity (individual scent signature)
- Sex
- Age
- Social status/confidence
- Reproductive status (estrus and hormonal changes)
- Health condition
- Timing of the deposit – dogs can estimate how long ago the scent was left

When a dog encounters a urine mark, it typically pauses to analyze the scent before choosing whether to urinate over the existing urine. This "overmarking" behavior functions similarly to replying to a message or updating a status.

Sex Differences in Marking

- Male dogs are more likely to mark frequently and with a lifted leg. Neutering reduces frequency but does not eliminate the behavior.
- Female dogs also mark, typically by squatting, though some lift a hind leg slightly. Marking by females often increases around estrus or social tension.

Volume Matters

- Marking usually involves small amounts of urine. This is distinct from full bladder emptying, which is physiologically different and not primarily communicative.

Flehmen Response Occasionally, dogs will lick the urine – not as a taste test but to gather additional chemical information. This activates the VNO (also known as Jacobson's organ), a specialized chemosensory structure that allows animals to detect pheromones and other chemical signals important for social and reproductive behavior (Beaver 2009).

3A.1.3.1.2 Feces

Although dogs do not use feces for territorial marking in the same way that some other species do, fecal scent still carries meaningful information and dogs frequently examine the feces of other dogs. The interest suggests that feces may provide insights into:

- Dietary content
- Parasite load or illness
- Health and gastrointestinal function
- Emotional stress (stress hormones affect scent)
- Possibly identity cues, though research is limited

Even though the communicative role of feces may be less elaborate than that of urine, it still offers dogs a chemical snapshot of another individual's condition, information humans would never detect visually or olfactorily.

3A.1.3.1.3 Body Odor and Glandular Secretions

Both dogs and humans produce scent from multiple areas of the body, with each source conveying distinct biological and social information. In dogs, these olfactory signals play a critical role in communication, social recognition, and emotional assessment (Siniscalchi et al. 2018).

Key canine scent sources include:

- Sebaceous glands – produce skin oils that carry individual scent markers.
- Anal gland secretions – highly individualized chemical signatures used for identification.
- Interdigital glands – release scent deposited during scratching or ground-marking.
- Ear and skin microbiome odors – bacteria metabolize secretions, creating unique olfactory "*fingerprints*."
- Pheromonal changes – influenced by stress, reproductive hormones, health status, and emotional state.

For dogs, these scent cues provide information about identity, emotional intent, reproductive status, and social context. While humans are largely unaware of these chemical signals, dogs detect and interpret them rapidly and automatically, using scent as a primary channel for social communication and environmental assessment.

3A.1.3.1.4 Breath and Hormonal Chemosignals

Dogs gather information from breath odor, as well. Stress, fear, sickness, and metabolic changes all alter volatile organic compounds exhaled through respiration. To a dog, emotional experiences have scent signatures. This is why some specially trained dogs can detect (Table 3A.2):

- Cancer
- Seizure onset
- Hypoglycemia
- Stress and anxiety states

Table 3A.2 Key Aspects of Canine Olfactory Communication (Adapted from Beaver 2009; Siniscalchi et al. 2018; Buzek et al. 2022; McGlone et al. 2022; Lee et al. 2023)

Aspect	Description/Purpose	Context/Notes
High Sensory Resolution	Dogs can detect concentrations as low as one part per trillion	Equivalent to sensing a single drop of liquid in 20 Olympic-sized pools
Time Perception through Scent	Dogs can detect how long a scent has been present based on breakdown of volatile compounds	Biological ability humans do not possess
Individual Scent Fingerprints	Dogs recognize other dogs (and humans) by unique scent signatures	Similar to humans recognizing faces or voices
Long-Distance and Long-Duration Communication	Scent allows communication across space and time; messages persist even when the sender is gone	Enables asynchronous social interaction
Low-Risk Social Interaction	Olfactory exchange allows information gathering without direct confrontation	Reduces risk of aggression
Vomeronasal Organ Specialization	Processes pheromones and chemical markers related to reproduction, emotion, and identity	Signals humans cannot perceive
Context Dependency	Scent signals must be interpreted considering location, time since deposition, emotional state, and social environment	Meaning depends on situational context
Integration with Other Systems	Olfaction works in combination with visual cues, auditory cues, past experience, and environment	Dogs rarely rely on scent alone

3A.1.4 Tactile Communication in Dogs

Touch is one of the earliest and most fundamental forms of communication across mammalian species. For dogs, tactile interaction serves as a bridge between internal emotional states and external social relationships. Unlike humans – who primarily communicate through hand-based touch – dogs use their entire body as a tactile instrument. Every point of contact carries meaning, shaped by context, relationship, learning history, and physiology.

Where humans may touch deliberately with fingers and palms, dogs "*speak*" through:

- All four paws (pressure, weight shifts, or stepping onto another individual)
- Their muzzle and nose (nudging, prodding, or sniff-touch)
- Flank or shoulder contact (leaning, rubbing, or proximity signals)
- The head and neck (resting, nuzzling, or pushing forward)
- Tail contact (brushing against others)
- Full-body touch (play wrestling, cuddling, mounting, or social sleeping)

Touch is not simply physical. It is neurological, emotional, and relational. And for dogs – who evolved as social mammals living in cooperative packs – tactile communication is essential for survival, bonding, and social clarity (Siniscalchi et al. 2018).

Touch feels different to dogs than to humans. Humans rely on manual dexterity and fine touch via the hands, which are densely packed with mechanoreceptors. Dogs, however, distribute tactile sensation across their entire body. Their sensitivity varies by region, adapted to communication, coordination, and social behavior (Table 3A.3).

Just as humans use tone of voice, gesture, or facial expression, dogs use pressures, contacts, and tactile rhythms to express needs and intentions.

3A.1.4.1 Forms and Functions of Tactile Communication in Dogs

3A.1.4.1.1 Pawing and Physical Solicitation

Dogs use their paws as a social tool:

- Light pawing → solicitation of attention or closeness.
- Heavier pawing → urgency or solicitation of attention escalating ("*do something*" or "*look at me*").
- Resting a paw → affiliative bonding or reassurance (not dominance).
- Pawing during play → initiation or escalation.

Table 3A.3 Key Differences Touch Feels Different to Dogs than to Humans

Humans	Dogs
Touch is concentrated in hands and fingertips	Touch is whole-body, with heightened sensitivity in muzzle, paws, face, and tail base
Use touch intentionally to explore or communicate	Touch arises through movement, posture, play, leaning, grooming, and close contact
Cultural norms strongly shape touch	Touch varies by breed tendencies, early socialization, learning history, and individual preference
Touch is often linguistic ("tactile punctuation")	Touch is often emotional ("state signaling")

Paws are highly expressive because they combine pressure, movement, and direction, much like human gestures.

3A.1.4.1.2 Leaning, Pressing, and Full-Body Contact (Siniscalchi et al. 2018)

Leaning is one of the most overlooked forms of communication. It can mean:

- Seeking comfort or social closeness.
- Checking in with a trusted person.
- Requesting touch.
- Redirecting pressure to ground themselves emotionally.
- Anxious clinging or "contact seeking" in stress.

Body leaning activates neural networks associated with safety, oxytocin release, and emotional regulation, similar to how humans experience a comforting hug.

3A.1.4.1.3 Nose Touches, Nudges, and Muzzle Behavior

Dogs explore the world using their noses, but they also *communicate* with them:

- Soft nudges → greeting ritual or affection.
- Persistent muzzle punching → soliciting attention or action.
- Nose-to-face touches → social reassurance.
- Nose-to-dog or nose-to-human → conflict-reducing greeting.

The dog's muzzle contains a high concentration of mechanoreceptors and thermoreceptors that make nose-based touch both exploratory and emotional.

3A.1.4.1.4 Social Grooming and Mutual Touch

While dogs do not groom each other as regularly as cats, for example, they still engage in:

- Licking the face or ears of familiar dogs.
- Pressing or rubbing their heads into humans or other dogs.
- Nibble grooming (or called flea-biting) refers to a rapid series of gentle bites made with the incisors. This behavior uses quick, repeated, lightly applied bites – often directed toward their own skin, a social partner, bedding, or even a handler's clothing or skin. The movement is typically fast and rhythmic, resembling the way a dog might nibble at fleas and is usually associated with grooming, affiliative contact, or arousal.

These behaviors are associated with affiliation, bonding, and conflict reduction.

3A.1.4.1.5 Play Contact

Play incorporates an entire vocabulary of tactile signals:

- Biting (Bite Severity Classification, BSC Level 1–3) (see Chapter 5 for BSC)
- Wrestling
- Hip checks
- Shoulder bumps
- Pinning and releasing
- Chasing followed by body tagging

Healthy play is rhythmic and reciprocal. It teaches dogs tolerance, impulse control, and social flexibility.

3A.1.4.1.6 Pain- or Fear-Based Touch Responses

Touch from others can feel vastly different depending on internal state.

- When a dog is relaxed, touch produces parasympathetic activation, easing the nervous system.
- When a dog is in pain, touch activates nociceptors and causes stress or defensive reactions.

Humans experience this, too. A gentle shoulder massage feels wonderful, while the exact same pressure on a bruised muscle is unbearable. Understanding this parallel helps caregivers remain empathetic when a dog "overreacts" to being touched where it hurts.

What Touch Does to the Nervous System: Dogs and Humans Share Similar Biochemistry Pleasant, safe touch activates:

- Oxytocin (bonding hormone)
- Lower cortisol levels (stress reduction)
- Parasympathetic nervous system (rest-and-digest)
- Heart-rate variability improvements (sign of emotional regulation)

Researchers at the Human–Animal Bond Research Institute (HABRI) and several veterinary behavior labs have shown that mutual touch between humans and dogs increases oxytocin in both species simultaneously. This is one of the biological foundations of the human–dog bond.

Massage and gentle pressure therapies, such as for example Tellington TTouch® (Toso 2016), can initiate the following:

- Reduce muscle tension
- Improve circulation
- Aid lymphatic flow (Lloyd and Roe 2013)
- Help dogs recover from stress
- Improve proprioception
- Increase calm engagement

Just as massage therapy helps some humans relax or recover from injury, dogs can experience touch as both therapeutic and communicative (Karpiński et al. 2021).

Contextual Variability in Dogs: Tactile Signals Are Not Universal

Touch is interpreted differently based on:

- Social relationship (familiar vs. unfamiliar person/dog)
- Individual preference
- Prior learning (positive or negative associations)
- Pain or undiagnosed medical issues
- Environment (shelter vs. home vs. stressful location)
- Breed tendencies (some are more tactile than others)
- Early socialization experiences

For example:

- A lean from a family dog → affection.
- A lean from an anxious shelter dog → stress-based contact seeking.
- A muzzle nudge from a puppy → play or attention.
- The same nudge from a fearful adult → distance regulation.

Touch is not a universal "language"; it is a dialect, shaped by experience.

Norms surrounding physical contact vary widely across cultures, shaping how people greet, handle, comfort, and control animals. In some cultures, close physical contact such as hugging, face-to-face interaction, or prolonged petting is considered affectionate and reassuring. In others, minimal touch and greater physical distance are signs of respect and restraint.

Examples

- In many Western cultures, hugging dogs is common, but many dogs find hugs restrictive or threatening.
- In other regions, dogs are rarely touched directly and instead communicate primarily through proximity or shared space.
- Some cultures encourage children to engage physically with dogs; others discourage close tactile interaction entirely.
- Professional working dogs (e.g. police and livestock guardians) may not receive the same kind of tactile affection that companion dogs do, but experience touch within the context of partnership and cooperation.

Understanding "*cultural touch norms*" avoids miscommunication and helps prevent negative encounters between people and dogs. Human culture shapes how people expect to touch dogs or be touched by them. In countries where pet dogs are treated as family members and close physical affection is normalized, many people assume that *all* dogs enjoy petting from strangers. This expectation can lead to misunderstandings, stress for the dog and preventable safety incidents. This is why, in cultures where it is common to greet and touch unfamiliar dogs, it is essential to teach both children and adults how to interact appropriately and respectfully. Recognizing that human intentions do not equal canine comfort allows organizations to bridge cultural differences with evidence-based handling practices that prioritize choice, predictability, and the dog's emotional experience. People should always ask the handler *if the dog can be safely approached and petted*, not simply "*Is he friendly?*" That question is unreliable for several reasons:

- Most people hesitate to admit that their dog is uncomfortable with strangers.
- "Friendly" does not necessarily mean "comfortable being touched by unfamiliar hands."
- Many dogs that are otherwise social, still prefer to initiate interactions at their own pace.

A more effective, safety-focused approach is for the handler to offer clear, proactive guidance that sets the dog up for success. For example:

- "He likes to sniff you first."
- "Please let him come to you."
- "You can ask him to sit, he enjoys that before being petted."
- "Scratch him gently on the chest or side, not the top of his head."

These instructions create a structured, predictable interaction that respects the dog's boundaries. They also shift the social pressure away from labeling the dog as "friendly" or "not friendly" and instead create a shared framework for safe, species-appropriate communication. When people know *how* to greet a dog, the dog's comfort and consent become part of the cultural norm and miscommunication becomes far less likely (see Table 3A.4; Siniscalchi et al. 2018; Karpiński et al. 2021).

Table 3A.4 Key Aspects of Canine Tactile Communication (Adapted from Siniscalchi et al. 2018; Karpiński et al. 2021)

Aspect	Description/Purpose	Context/Notes
Whole-Body Communication System	Dogs use paws, muzzle, flanks, tail, head, and full body contact, not just specialized limbs like human hands	Includes playful pawing, leaning, or nudging; whole-body signals convey complex messages
Emotional Transparency	Touch reveals confidence, anxiety, pain, conflict, or desire for connection	Observation of body response helps interpret emotional state
Social Bonding Mechanism	Touch releases oxytocin in both dogs and humans, reinforcing the relationship; being petted increases serotonin in dogs	Includes petting, leaning, or close body contact; strengthens the bond
Context-Dependent Meaning	The same gesture can indicate affection in one moment and distress in another	Requires attention to the situation, timing, and other body signals
Regulatory Function	Touch modulates arousal, decreasing anxiety or increasing excitement depending on how it is applied	Gentle contact can calm; vigorous contact can stimulate
Developmental Significance	Puppies rely heavily on tactile interaction to learn boundaries, social etiquette, warmth, and security	Includes play, grooming, and gentle correction from mother or littermates
Pain-Related Responses	Avoidance, growling, or biting during touch may arise from discomfort, not behavioral problems	Misinterpreting pain as aggression can worsen welfare
Cultural and Individual Variation	Touch expectations differ across households, cultures, and individual dogs	Individual history, past experiences, and environment shape tolerance and preference

3A.1.5 Gustatory (Taste-Based) Communication in Dogs

Gustatory communication refers to information animals gather or convey through taste. While it is not the primary method of communication in dogs, it plays an important supporting role in how they interpret their environment and understand other animals. Dogs, especially puppies, explore the world with their mouths far more than humans realize. For them, taste is intertwined with scent and is part of how they gather social and environmental information. In dogs, gustatory and olfactory communication often complement each other rather than standing alone. It provides additional nuance about identity, environmental clues, reproductive and fitness status of conspecifics, and emotional conditions (see Table 3A.5).

3A.1.6 Body Language – Physical Cues in Dogs

Body language is the core of canine communication and has evolved primarily as a way to prevent conflict. While most people can recognize obvious signals – such as barking, wagging tails, or growling – effective interpretation requires paying close attention to the subtle shifts that make up the true "*language*" of dogs. No single signal carries the full meaning; rather, each cue acts like a *puzzle piece*. When all pieces are observed together, in context, the full message becomes clear.

In social species, where physical conflict can threaten survival, dogs rely heavily on visual communication to defuse tension, negotiate space, and prevent unnecessary fights. Behaviors often mislabeled as "*appeasement*" are more accurately understood as submission or *conflict-avoidance gestures*, indicating a desire to remain safe rather than to pacify another individual. Recognizing

Table 3A.5 Key Aspects of Gustatory Communication in Dogs

Behavior	Description/Purpose	Context/Notes
Licking Objects, Animals, or People	Collects chemical information Adds taste to olfactory exploration	Often exploratory; helps dogs understand their environment
Licking Faces or Mouths of Other Dogs	Social/affiliative behavior Gathers information on diet, location, or emotional state	Can signal submission, bonding, or curiosity
Tasting Urine or Other Secretions	Collects pheromones to learn reproductive status, individual identity, or emotional state	Includes urine, feces, scent markings Often with subtle tongue flicks
Licking Humans	Social gesture, exploratory behavior, or stress response	Multipurpose behavior Context matters in interpreting meaning

these distinctions deepens our understanding of how dogs manage social interactions with dogs as well as humans.

Eyes are one of the most powerful communicators. Direct eye contact can act as a challenge, potentially triggering escalation if mirrored by another dog or a person. Quick blinks, turning the head, or averting the gaze signal uncertainty or submission and are part of a broader suite of behaviors used to reduce social pressure.

Ears amplify this message. Forward-facing or perked ears indicate alertness or potential threat, whereas ears pulled to the side or flattened back against the head signify fear, anxiety, or uncertainty. For floppy-eared dogs, the base of the ear – not the tip – reveals true intent.

Mouth and facial tension provide important additional clues to a dog's emotional state. Tight, retracted commissures typically indicate stress or discomfort, while soft, neutral lips signal relaxation. Lip lifts and snarls function as clear distance-increasing warnings, whereas a so-called "submissive grin" reflects nervousness paired with deference rather than true friendliness. Biting motions – such as extending the jaws or biting without making contact (BSC Level 1; see Chapter 5) – represent a significant escalation in the dog's warning sequence and should be interpreted with caution.

Fur, particularly raised hackles (piloerection), communicates high arousal but not necessarily aggression. This physiological response can reflect fear, excitement, conflict, or uncertainty; its meaning depends entirely on the rest of the dog's body language and the environment and situation.

Tail position and movement are among the most misunderstood signals. A wagging tail does not always indicate friendliness, only readiness to interact. The quality, height, and speed of the wag matter. A stiff, high tail signals risk; a low or tucked tail signals fear; a relaxed, neutral tail reflects comfort.

When humans learn to interpret these signals as a holistic system by integrating posture, movement, facial expression, arousal level, and context, they can understand dogs far more accurately. This ability enhances safety, improves welfare, and strengthens the human–animal bond across all settings: shelters, veterinary clinics, training programs, and homes.

Ultimately, communication is the key to compassion and good relationships. When we learn to listen to dogs on their terms – not ours – we not only prevent misunderstandings and injuries, but also validate their emotional experience and build a foundation of trust.

Body posture in dogs is not a collection of isolated signals from ears, tail, and head position, but a *living, dynamic system* that reflects constant shifts in emotion, intention, and physiological arousal. Dogs communicate through the integration of movement, muscle tension, posture, and facial expression, all of which change moment by moment as their internal state changes. A dog that is confident and comfortable typically carries the head in a neutral, elevated position above the shoulders, with loose muscles and balanced weight distribution (see Figure 3A.20). When the head drops to shoulder height or lower, it often reflects discomfort or uncertainty. This lowering of the head is part of a broader *subordinate display*, a cluster of threat-reducing behaviors designed to prevent conflict. These displays commonly include gaze aversion, blinking, softening of the eyes, ears pulled slightly sideways, and a low or tucked tail.

Conflict-avoiding or subordinate body language is not simply a behavioral choice; it is rooted in neurobiology. When a dog feels threatened or overwhelmed, the autonomic nervous system shifts toward a state of stress activation. Behaviors such as dropping the head, turning the body sideways, or avoiding eye contact reflect this internal shift as the dog attempts to down-regulate tension and communicate non-threatening intent. For example, when a dog yawns in a stressful situation, it is not "*just a calming signal*" but rather part of a physiological self-regulation response, where respiratory patterns and vagal tone interact to ease internal arousal. Hence, these types of body language shifts can be observed in various types of situations and in the presence of other dogs as well as humans. These behaviors serve a critical social function: by displaying deference, the dog helps prevent escalation from another dog or a human who may be uncertain or assertive.

Understanding body language as *fluid* rather than static allows observers to remain objective and avoid over-interpreting single behaviors. A single signal (e.g. a lowered tail) means little without the surrounding context, such as muscle tone, weight shift, facial expression, movement patterns, and environmental triggers. The accompanying body language chart or graph can help observers interpret these signals as part of a continuum, not discrete checkpoints (see Table 3A.6). Dogs developed these nuanced communication strategies over thousands of years to avoid unnecessary physical confrontations. By recognizing the interplay between physiology, emotion, and outward behavior, we gain a more accurate, compassionate understanding of what dogs are truly expressing.

Figure 3A.20 Confident Dog

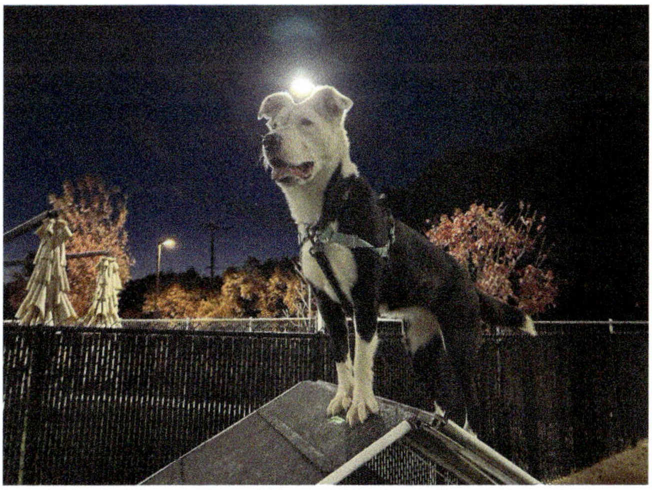

Table 3A.6 Body Language Chart

Category	Relaxed	Ambivalent/ Uncertain	Stressed	Fearful	Defensive	Aggressive
Eyes	Soft, blinking, normal gaze	Slight squint, darting	Wide, frequent blinking	Avoiding gaze, whites visible	Hard stare, dilated pupils	Intense stare, direct gaze, pupils focused
Ears	Neutral, relaxed	Slightly back or rotated	Pulled back, tense	Flattened against head	Erect or angled back	Forward, rigid, alert
Mouth	Closed or relaxed, slight panting	Lips tight, slight licking	Lips pulled back, yawning	Mouth closed, trembling	Lips curled, teeth partially visible	Lips curled, teeth bared, growling
Tail	Neutral or gentle wag	Low wag, uncertain	Tail tucked slightly, rigid	Fully tucked, trembling	Tail raised, stiff	Tail raised, stiff, sometimes bristled
Posture	Loose, balanced	Shifting weight, hesitant	Tense, crouched slightly	Crouched, lowered body	Forward-leaning, rigid	Forward, tense, hackles raised
Overall Behavior	Calm, approachable	Pausing, cautious	Pacing, panting, displacement behaviors	Avoiding, cowering	Lunging, defensive snapping	Biting attempts, lunging, repeated aggression

Communication is separated into **six key categories** (eyes, ears, mouth, tail, posture, and overall behavior) arranged along a continuum from **Relaxed → Ambivalent/Uncertain → Stressed → Fearful → Defensive → Aggressive**.

3A.1.7 Canine Body Language Competency: From Admissions Through Placement

Developing strong skills in reading canine body language is essential for anyone working with shelter dogs, because behavior challenges in this environment are both common and highly context-dependent. Dogs entering a shelter often experience fear, frustration, social deprivation, confusion, or overstimulation, emotions that can rapidly shift and manifest in subtle ways long before they escalate into aggression, panic, or shutdown. Shelter team members who can accurately interpret early warning signs, such as tension around the eyes, changes in breathing, weight shifts, displacement behaviors, or alterations in tail carriage, can intervene proactively rather than reactively. This skill allows shelters to prevent bites, reduce fear, and avoid reinforcing unwanted behavior patterns. It also ensures that every interaction, from admissions and medical handling to daily care, enrichment, and adoption counseling, remains safe and humane for both dogs and people.

When body language is understood with nuance and accuracy, team members gain the ability to match dogs with appropriate housing, enrichment strategies, training plans, and adopters. Subtle indicators of stress or arousal can reveal the comprehensive care trajectory strategy (CTS). In this way, reading body language becomes more than simply recognizing "*fearful*" or "*aggressive*" postures; it becomes the foundation of an entire decision-making system that supports wellbeing, prevents incidents, and improves placement success. Ultimately, the ability to interpret body language empowers shelter teams to meet dogs where they are emotionally, respond in a way that builds trust, and guide them safely from admission to adoption.

3A.1.7.1 Approach and General Observation

When approaching an unfamiliar shelter dog – whether in a kennel, play yard, or on leash – the first seconds of observation are often the most revealing. A dog's initial response offers a snapshot of emotional state, coping style, and comfort with unfamiliar people. The approach should be slow and steady, allowing time to observe. A dog that moves forward with soft eyes, a loose body, and fluid movement is typically showing curiosity and social openness.

In contrast, a dog that stiffens, shifts weight forward, stands tall, or holds ears upright and fixed on the person may be signaling heightened alertness, uncertainty, or a need for space. Equally important are dogs who withdraw rather than advance. Weight shifted backward, a tucked tail, avoided eye contact, or ears held to the side suggest fear or discomfort. Subtle differences in posture, such as leaning away while watching vs. lowering the body and turning the head, convey different emotional states.

By observing these early reactions before interacting, team members can adjust their approach by slowing down, increasing distance, redirecting attention, or offering treats. These initial observations reduce stress, improve safety, and lay the groundwork for respectful, effective, and safe handling.

3A.1.7.2 Dog with Handler Approach

3A.1.7.2.1 Approaching a Dog on Leash When the Pet Owner Is Present (e.g. During Surrender)

Approaching a dog who is still with their owner – especially during a stressful surrender – is very different from approaching a dog alone. The dog in the presence of an owner may feel more confident and comfortable, or he may be conflicted, protective, confused, or overwhelmed. This can make accurate body-language reading challenging and allowing the dog choice and control over the interaction with the unfamiliar person essential.

3A.1.7.3 When Is a Dog Open to Interaction?

A dog receptive to gentle attention will show soft, relaxed body language, including:

- Loose facial muscles
- Soft eyes (no visible sclera/"whale eye")
- Loose lips with a natural "C" shape
- Tail relaxed in a neutral position
- Fluid, forward body movement
- Brief, voluntary eye contact

These signals indicate comfort, curiosity, or social openness.

3A.1.7.3.1 Signs a Dog Does Not Want Contact

Indicators of discomfort or stress include:

- Tucked tail
- Lip licking without food present
- Avoiding eye contact or showing whale eye
- Ears pinned back or held wide to the side
- Weight shifted backward
- Mouth tension or creasing
- Furrowed brows
- Lowered head or crouched posture

When these signs are present, the safest and most respectful response is to pause, create space, and avoid touching the dog.

3A.1.7.4 Time, Space, and Choice

Not every dog welcomes interaction from unfamiliar people, particularly during emotionally charged moments like surrender. Many dogs prefer physical contact only from familiar. Allowing time and space for the dog to assess the handler – even just a few minutes – reduces pressure and significantly improves safety and wellbeing.

3A.1.7.5 Recognizing Different Preferences for Touch

Dogs vary in how they express enjoyment:

- Enthusiastic dogs may nudge the hand, lean in, wag quickly, or wiggle their whole body.
- More reserved dogs may step in quietly, offer the side of their neck, or orient their back toward the person.
- Neutral but accepting dogs may stand still and continue allowing petting without retreating.

All of these can be normal and acceptable as long as the dog remains loose and calm.

3A.1.7.6 When It's Best to Let the Owner Bring the Dog to the Kennel Area First

Not all dogs benefit from immediate interaction with the shelter team during the admission or surrender process. Some dogs arrive emotionally overwhelmed, confused about the environment, stressed by separation from their owner, or highly aroused by new smells, sounds, and movement. In these cases, forcing early engagement can increase anxiety, heighten defensiveness, and create unnecessary risk for both dogs and people.

For these dogs, the safest and most humane option may be to have the owner escort the dog to the kennel area and allow the dog time to settle before any team member interactions occur. This approach should be carried out with special attention to infectious disease control protocols, including appropriate intake separation, use of personal protective equipment as indicated, and adherence to shelter biosecurity procedures to minimize the risk of disease transmission.

Allowing the dog to settle in this way can drastically change the dog's emotional baseline. Once the dog has had time to adjust to the new environment, take in the new smells and sounds and settle into a quieter space, team members can then implement the structured *Initial Safe Introduction to a Dog* protocol (see Table 3A.7). This method reduces social pressure and allows the

Table 3A.7 Initial Safe Introduction to a Dog

Step	What to Do	Why It Matters
1) Use Calm Communication	• Speak softly and quietly • Avoid direct staring; use brief eye contact and look away • Observe using peripheral ("soft") vision	Reduces perceived threat and allows the dog to process safely
2) Body Positioning	• Stand sideways, not head-on • Maintain 5–6 feet of space • Lower into a slight crouch or kneel on one knee • Avoid bending over the dog	Dog-friendly posture minimizes intimidation and pressure

Table 3A.7 (Continued)

Step	What to Do	Why It Matters
3) Allow the Dog to Approach	• Remain still and relaxed • Do not move toward the dog • Let the dog control distance	Choice and control increase safety and confidence
4) Use Treats to Build Trust	• Toss treats gently toward the dog • Offer long treats (e.g. chicken) held near your side • Alternate tossed and hand-delivered treats • Keep hands soft, open, and neutral	Reinforces positive association without overwhelming
5) Begin Touch Thoughtfully	• Wait for the dog to step forward to sniff shoes, pant legs, or hand • Ensure body language remains relaxed before touching • Use slow, deliberate movements	Confirms consent and maintains emotional safety

Table 3A.8 How to Offer Safe, Acceptance-Based Touch

Step	What to Do	What to Watch For/Why It Matters
1) Begin Under the Chin	Reach slowly under the chin, not over the head Keep movements smooth and predictable	Reaching over the head can feel threatening to many dogs Under-chin contact is easier to see and assess
2) Use the Consent Test	Offer 1–2 gentle scratches or soft strokes Withdraw your hand after a brief moment Pause and observe	Allows the dog to choose whether to continue the interaction
3) Read the Response	Acceptance: dog steps closer, stays relaxed, or re-orients toward you Refusal: dog pulls away, freezes, turns head, or stiffens	Continuing only with clear consent reduces stress and bite risk
4) Withdraw Safely	Move your hand away slowly and smoothly Avoid sudden or jerky movements	Some dogs may bite during fast hand withdrawal Slow movement can maintain safety
5) Use Strokes, not Pats	Slow strokes along neck or chest Gentle scratches at the base of the ears	Fast or repetitive patting can be overstimulating or aversive

dog to initiate contact on their own terms, an important welfare-centered principle that increases safety and accuracy for behavioral assessments (see Table 3A.8).

Giving the dog the opportunity for decompression offers several benefits

1) Reduced Emotional Reactivity

   A dog in a heightened state of stress may display barking, lunging, growling, trembling, or avoidance that is not representative of their typical behavior. After settling, many dogs shift into a more neutral emotional state, allowing team members to observe behavior that is more accurate and informative.

2) Increased Safety for Shelter Teams and Volunteers
   A stressed dog experiencing fear or confusion may react defensively toward unfamiliar handlers. Allowing the dog to remain with their owner and transition calmly to the kennel reduces the likelihood of fear-based aggression, leash reactivity, and handling risks.

3A.1.7.7 Dog Exhibits Aggressive Behavior on Approach While on Leash

When a dog displays aggressive behavior on leash – such as growling, barking, hard staring, or lunging – while the owner or Good Samaritan is present, it is essential to approach with caution and professionalism. Dogs may show heightened protective behavior when their owner is nearby, and their reactivity in that moment may not reflect how they behave once separated from the handler.

Always prioritize safety by approaching slowly, maintaining an appropriate distance, and communicating calmly with the person holding the leash (see Table 3A.9).

Table 3A.9 Step-by-Step Approach for a Highly Aroused or Barking Dog

Step	What to Do	What to Watch For/Decision Point
1) Initial Approach	Walk slowly with body angled sideways Stop at a distance where the dog is not lunging Avoid prolonged eye contact; glance and look away Speak softly to the owner/handler Gently toss high-value treats near but not at the dog	Goal: reduce emotional intensity, not rush contact Allow ~2–3 minutes for observation
2) Evaluate Response	Pause and assess before moving closer	Barking slows or stops Dog eats tossed treats Body softens (less facial tension and fewer backward shifts)
3) Test Engagement	Toss a treat directly to the dog If eaten, gently ask for a simple cue (e.g. "sit")	Provides information about tolerance of a stranger voice and direction (cue success not required)
4) Decrease Distance Gradually	Perform a treat scatter/shower 2–5 feet in front of you Allow the dog to move forward voluntarily	Dog should approach with loose body and continued food interest
5) Move Handler Closer	Ask the handler to take one small step toward you Continue tossing treats	Watch for increased relaxation vs. rising tension or reactivity
6) Offer Hand-Fed Treat	Present a long treat with the arm low and neutral	Proceed only if body language remains relaxed
7) Transfer Responsibility	Ask the handler to step fully beside you Take the leash gently while continuing food reinforcement	Smooth handoff prevents sudden pressure

3A.1.7.7.1 Special Considerations for Small Dogs

For small dogs, crouching sideways as they approach can reduce intimidation. However:

- Ensure you have enough space to stand and move away quickly if needed.
- Avoid kneeling near large dogs (>50 lbs), as this places your face at the dog's head level, increasing risk.

3A.1.7.7.2 When Aggressive Behavior Does Not Improve

If the dog continues to display aggression or shows escalating warning signs despite being on leash and your careful approach:

Do not force the interaction.

In these cases, instruct the owner or Good Samaritan to:

1) Walk the dog calmly to a designated holding kennel.
2) Place the dog inside the kennel.
3) Safely remove the leash and collar.
4) Leave the kennel area promptly.

Allow the dog to decompress for a few hours and ensure the dog has water and minimal external stimuli. Stress significantly affects behavior, and the dog's response once separated from the owner may differ greatly.

Later, a team member should reassess the dog's response using the *Initial Safe Introduction to a Dog* protocol (see Table 3A.7), which provides a clearer and more accurate representation of the dog's behavior and emotional baseline.

3A.1.7.8 Dog Without Handler Approach

3A.1.7.8.1 Approaching a Dog While in the Kennel

Approaching a dog in a kennel is similar to approaching a dog on leash: observe body language carefully and allow the dog to initiate interaction. Pause outside the kennel and give the dog time to approach the front voluntarily rather than opening the door or reaching in immediately.

When positioning yourself:

- Avoid leaning forward or reaching toward the dog.
- Speak softly and calmly.
- Turn your body slightly sideways rather than facing the dog head-on.
- If appropriate, gently crouch down to reduce perceived pressure while maintaining a safe distance.

Signs a Dog Is Receptive to Gentle Attention A dog who is open to interaction will display relaxed, soft body language, such as:

- Loose facial muscles.
- Soft eyes with no visible sclera ("whale eye").
- Loose lips.
- Tail held in a relaxed, neutral position.
- Fluid, forward body movement approaching the front of the kennel.
- Brief, voluntary eye contact.

These signals suggest comfort, curiosity, or social openness.

Signs a Dog Does Not Want Contact Indicators of stress, discomfort, or uncertainty include:

- Tucked tail.
- Furrowed brows.
- Weight shifted backward.
- Lip licking in the absence of food.
- Lowered head or crouched posture.
- Remaining in the back of the kennel.
- Ears pinned back or held wide to the side.
- Avoiding eye contact or showing whale eye.
- Tension around the mouth or creasing at the corners.

When these signs are present, the safest and most respectful response is to pause, create distance, and avoid opening the kennel door or reaching through the barrier. Allowing the dog space supports safety, reduces stress, and builds trust over time.

3A.1.7.9 Dog Exhibits Aggressive Behavior on Approach While in the Kennel

When approaching a dog showing aggressive behavior inside a kennel, always prioritize safety and minimize stress for the dog. Dogs in confined spaces often feel trapped, which may intensify defensive or fear-based aggression (see Table 3A.10). Move slowly, avoid cornering the dog, and use positive reinforcement whenever possible. This approach ensures safety and consistency across all shelter teams and volunteers.

Table 3A.10 Dog Exhibits Aggressive Behavior on Approach (While in Kennel)

Situation/Step	Handler Action	Key Observations and Decisions
1) Initial Kennel Approach	Stand 2–3 feet from the kennel, body angled sideways Do not stand directly in front of the door Toss high-value treats into the kennel Avoid prolonged eye contact; use brief glances	If the dog eats treats → indicates some approachability
2) Assess Food Response	Pause and observe	Eating treats = potential to proceed Refusing treats = evaluate alternate strategies
3) Opening Kennel Door (Dog Eating Treats)	Open the door slowly, outward, 1 inch at a time Use the foot at the bottom of the door if the dog pushes or charges	Maintains barrier and prevents sudden escape or escalation
4) Leashing at Kennel Door	If the dog places its head near/through opening, slip the leash calmly over its head Remove the dog to open space before adjusting collar/harness	Open space improves safety and reduces pressure
5) Reduce Environmental Triggers	Set a visual barrier between kennels (X-pen panel, towel, or blanket)	Helpful for dogs reactive to neighboring dogs

Table 3A.10 (Continued)

Situation/Step	Handler Action	Key Observations and Decisions
6) If Dog Will NOT Take Treats	Offer toys (tennis ball, rope tug, squeaky, or crinkle)	Used when food refusal is due to stress, fear, or overarousal
7) Signs You May Proceed	Continue only if body language softens	Relaxed muscles Blinking Head turns Loose tail wag Reduced vocalization
8) Do NOT Approach if Dog Shows	Stop forward movement	Hard staring Stiffening or freezing Head lowered with tension Teeth showing Growling
9) Distance Handling Required	Use a slip leash or snare-style leash on a pole (rigid or flexible)	Maintains safety while minimizing proximity
10) If Dog Refuses to Exit Kennel	Place X-pen panel between you and the dog Slide the panel behind the dog using gentle pressure Guide panel toward the door	Encourages movement without grabbing or cornering
11) Outcome of Panel Method	Dog moves away from the panel toward exit	Prevents escalation and reduces fear-based reactions

3A.2 Breed-Specific Selection of Shelter Dogs

Although the visual appearance of dogs in shelters varies regionally, breed-related behavioral predispositions may still influence assessment and care and must be interpreted with caution. Breed cannot be reliably determined based on phenotype alone (Voith et al. 2009; Gunter et al. 2018). Furthermore, a dog that resembles a Labrador retriever may not enjoy swimming or retrieving. Even among purpose-bred dogs, appearance does not guarantee performance or temperament. There is substantial variation in behavioral expression (Svartberg 2006; Hecht et al. 2019); not every Border Collie will be the next herding champion, and not every Poodle will make the perfect companion.

This distinction is critical in shelter settings, where most dogs are mixed breeds with complex genetic backgrounds. Many adopters select dogs based on appearance or familiarity – choosing a dog that resembles one they grew up with – yet these visual similarities do not predict temperament, trainability, or behavioral needs. Adopter education is critical; physical resemblance does not predict behavior, needs, or suitability for a household. Emphasizing observed behavior, individual history, and ongoing welfare assessment over breed labels supports more realistic expectations and more successful, humane placements.

3A.2.1 Working Breeds vs. Companion Breeds

Not all dogs were originally bred for the same purpose. For centuries, selective breeding emphasized specific traits – such as guarding, herding, hunting, or companionship – that supported particular working roles. While most dogs entering shelters today are mixed breeds rather than purpose-bred working dogs, these historical influences have not disappeared. Behavioral tendencies shaped by generations of selection can still emerge in modern shelter populations, often in complex and unpredictable ways.

Understanding that shelter dogs are predominantly mixed does not negate the relevance of breed history; instead, it underscores the need to view behavior as the result of layered influences, including genetics, early development, environment, and learning. Appreciating these factors provides important context for interpreting behavior, setting realistic expectations, and making ethical placement decisions.

3A.2.2 Working, Herding, and Guardian Breeds

Examples: German Shepherds, Belgian Malinois, Border Collies, Australian Cattle Dogs, Rottweilers, Livestock Guardian Dogs. They may exhibit the following tendencies:

- High mental and physical energy.
- Increased environmental sensitivity.
- Strong bonding to one or few caregivers.
- Intense responses to movement or novelty.
- May display:
  - Barking, pacing, herding behavior.
  - Barrier reactivity.
  - Uncertainty with strangers.

Shelter implications based on these characteristics are:

- Often struggle with noise, confinement, and unpredictable routines.
- Require more advanced enrichment and controlled handling.
- May need targeted pathway planning such as foster, behavior modification, and working-dog rescue partnerships.

3A.2.3 Companion and Toy Breeds

Examples: Cavaliers, Pugs, Shih Tzus, Maltese. They may exhibit the following tendencies:

- Selected mainly for sociability and low conflict.
- Generally human-oriented and tolerant of handling.
- Often display:
  - Attention-seeking behavior.
  - Sensitivity to loud, chaotic environments.
  - Stress vocalizations rather than aggression.

Shelter implications based on these characteristics are:

- Often thrive with increased human contact and foster placement.
- May show hiding behavior or fear reactivity when overwhelmed, especially small dogs.

3A.2.4 Frequently Observed Dog Types in Shelters

Based on shelter population data, commonly represented dogs in many shelters include bully-type breeds, Chihuahuas and other small breeds, German Shepherds and shepherd mixes, Husky-type breeds, and various working and guarding mixes. However, these patterns vary widely by geographic region. Shelter populations largely reflect the dogs of the surrounding community, and breed representation may differ substantially when large-scale transfer programs move dogs between regions, sometimes resulting in shelter populations that differ markedly from local breed demographics.

Behavioral considerations may include:

- Bully breeds: Often highly social with people but may struggle with barrier frustration or dog selectivity.
- Huskies and northern breeds: High prey drive, vocalization, and escape tendencies.
- Shepherds: Increased sensitivity and reactivity when under stress.
- Retrievers: Strong object interest; this is helpful for assessment and training.
- Terriers: High persistence, strong hunting sequences.

3A.2.5 How Breed Differences Impact Wellbeing and Behavioral Assessments

Accurate interpretation supports safer and more effective CTS.

3A.2.5.1 Understanding Baseline Behavior

Understanding breed tendencies can help team members distinguish:

- Fear from frustration.
- Prey drive from aggression.
- Working drive from hyperactivity.
- Stress-related pacing from breed-typical energy.

3A.2.5.2 Predicting Stressors

Working and high-drive breeds may deteriorate faster in shelter environments, lacking exercise and structure.

Cats with high social needs may deteriorate without consistent human contact or predictable territory.

3A.2.5.3 Designing Effective Health and Well-Being Plans

Examples

- Herding breeds: Structured movement outlets, cognitive games.
- Terriers: Digging boxes, scent work.

3A.2.5.4 Improving Safety

Understanding breed-typical responses reduces misinterpretation:

- A shepherd's "freeze and stare" may escalate quickly if mismanaged.
- A terrier's quick, darting movements can trigger handling errors.

3A.2.5.5 Individual Variation Matters

Breed and species tendencies can inform behavior patterns. A "*breed stereotype*" should never overshadow what the specific dog or cat demonstrates through behavior or body language. Shelter team members need to always assess:

- The individual's history.
- Early socialization if information is available.

- Affect status/emotional status.
- Medical status.
- Environmental triggers.
- Learning history.

3A.2.6 Breed and Phenotype Differences – Body Language and Communication

Interpreting canine body language requires an understanding of how breed and phenotype differences shape what signals look like and how clearly they can be expressed. Dogs communicate with the same basic system of posture, facial tension, tail movement, and vocalization, but physical traits can significantly alter the appearance of those cues.

Ear positions can communicate a dog's emotional state, but the same intention can look very different depending on the dog's natural ear type. Erect-eared breeds such as German Shepherds, Huskies, and Dobermans (including dogs with cropped ears) often display alertness, uncertainty, or vigilance with clear, high-contrast signals. In contrast, floppy-eared dogs – such as Labradors, hounds, and many Border Collies – show far subtler shifts, relying on small changes in ear base tension or slight angles that are harder for both humans and other dogs to read. Even among prick-eared breeds, the degree of lift varies: the upright ears of a Cattle Dog and the semi-flopped, side-set ears of a Border Collie can represent similar emotional intensity while appearing very different externally (see Figure 3A.21).

Brachycephalic breeds – Bulldogs, Pugs (see Figure 3A.22), and French Bulldogs – have shortened muzzles, skin folds, and naturally open mouths, which can obscure normal expressions such as lip tension, snarling, or panting. Their restricted airways also create snorting, gasping, or wheezing sounds that may be misread as growling or distress by people unfamiliar with the breed. Dogs with underbites or prominent teeth – Boxers, Shih Tzus – may appear to "show teeth" even when relaxed, creating further potential for misinterpretation.

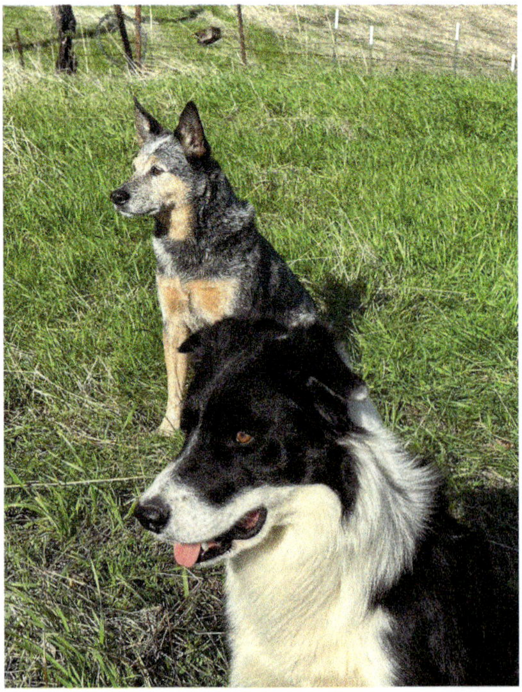

Figure 3A.21 Erect Ears vs. Floppy Ears

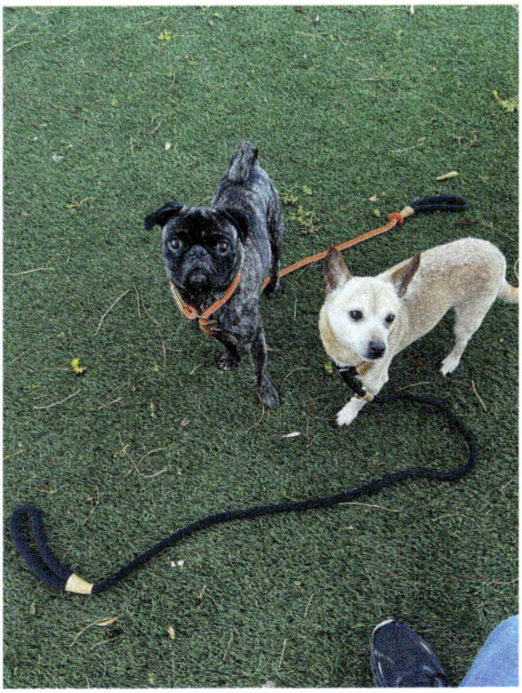

Figure 3A.22 Brachycephalic vs. Mesocephalic Face

Tail variation also plays a major role. Dogs with long, expressive tails can communicate subtle shifts in arousal or uncertainty, while stub tails or docked tails remove an entire communication channel. These dogs may compensate with more whole-body signaling such as torso shifts, weight distribution, or exaggerated facial displays, which other dogs may misread. Similarly, heavily coated breeds or "curly-tailed" breeds may obscure the usual low-vs.-high tail indicators used to signal confidence, fear, or threat.

Breed differences extend beyond appearance to behavioral tendencies and play styles, which shape how well dogs understand one another (Asp et al. 2015). Herding breeds tend to engage in stalking, eye contact, and heel-biting, bully breeds may prefer full-body wrestling and pressure play, sighthounds favor chase, and guardian breeds may engage less in play overall. When dogs with drastically different styles are paired, their signals may be misinterpreted. For example, a herding dog's fixed stare may be perceived as threatening by a more sensitive breed, while a rough-and-tumble wrestler may overwhelm a dog that prefers chase or parallel play. In shelters, monitoring body language carefully and matching compatible play styles helps reduce conflict, improve wellbeing, and allow for safer, more satisfying social interactions.

In summary, these differences highlight the importance of considering phenotype, breed-related tendencies, and individual variation when conducting behavior observations, organizing playgroups, or interpreting kennel behavior. Understanding how a dog's physical design influences communication – both in how signals are expressed and perceived – reduces misinterpretation, minimizes unnecessary stress, and supports more accurate, humane, and effective case trajectory strategy. These considerations are equally essential for adopter education and ethical placement, helping ensure realistic expectations and better long-term outcomes for both dogs and families.

References

Asp, H.E., Ikse, W.F., Nilsson, K., and Strandberg, E. (2015). Breed differences in everyday behavior of dogs. *Applied Animal Behaviour Science* 169: 69–77. https://doi.org/10.1016/j.applanim.2015.04.020.

Beaver, B.V. (2009). *Canine Behavior Insights and Answers*, 2e. St. Louis: Saunders.

Buzek, A., Serwańska-Leja, K., Zaworska-Zakrzewska, A., and Kasprowicz-Potocka, M. (2022). The shape of the nasal cavity and adaptations to sniffing in the dog (*Canis familiaris*) compared to other domesticated mammals: a review article. *Animals* 12 (4): 1–18. https://doi.org/10.3390/ani12040517.

Gunter, L.M., Barber, R.T., and Wynne, C.D.L. (2018). A canine identity crisis : genetic breed heritage testing of shelter dogs. *PLoS One* 13 (8): e0202633. https://doi.org/10.1371/journal.pone.0202633.

Hecht, E.E., Smaers, J.B., Dunn, W.D. et al. (2019). Significant neuroanatomical variation among domestic dog breeds. *Journal of Neuroscience* 39 (39): 7748–7758. https://doi.org/10.1523/JNEUROSCI.0303-19.2019.

Karpiński, M., Ognik, K., Garbiec, A. et al. (2021). Effect of stroking on serotonin, noradrenaline, and cortisol levels in the blood of right-and left-pawed dogs. *Animals* 11 (2): 1–11. https://doi.org/10.3390/ani11020331.

Lee, S.W., Kim, B.H., and Seo, Y.H. (2023). Olfactory system-inspired electronic nose system using numerous low-cost homogenous and heterogeneous sensors. *PLoS One* 18 (12 December): 1–18. https://doi.org/10.1371/journal.pone.0295703.

Lloyd, J. and Roe, E. (Lib)(2013). Using TTouch to reduce stress and enhance learning when training guide dogs. *International Journal of Orientation and Mobility* 6 (1): 8–20. https://doi.org/10.21307/ijom-2013-002.

McGlone, J.J., Archer, C., and Henderson, M. (2022). Interpretive review: semiochemicals in domestic pigs and dogs. *Frontiers in Veterinary Science* 9: https://doi.org/10.3389/fvets.2022.967980.

Mills, D., Dube, M.B., and Zulch, H. (2013). Principles of pheromonatherapy. In: *Stress and Pheromonatherapy in Small Animal Clinical Behaviour*, 127–145. Wiley https://doi.org/10.1002/9781118702642.ch6.

Simpson, B.S. (1997). Canine communication. *Veterinary Clinics of North America: Small Animal Practice* 27 (3): 445–464.

Siniscalchi, M., d'Ingeo, S., Minunno, M., and Quaranta, A. (2018). Communication in dogs. *Animals* 8 (8): https://doi.org/10.3390/ani8080131.

Svartberg, K. (2006). Breed-typical behaviour in dogs — historical remnants or recent constructs? *Applied Animal Behaviour Science* 96: 293–313. https://doi.org/10.1016/j.applanim.2005.06.014.

Toso, A.D. (2016). Is Tellington-touch a relaxation technique for dogs? *Dog Behavior* 2 (3): 21–25. https://doi.org/10.4454/db.v2i3.35.

Voith, V.L., Ingram, E., Mitsouras, K., and Irizarry, K. (2009). Comparison of adoption agency breed identification and DNA breed identification of dogs. *Journal of Applied Animal Welfare Science* 12 (3): 253–262. https://doi.org/10.1080/10888700902956151.

Yeon, S.C. (2007). The vocal communication of canines. *Journal of Veterinary Behavior: Clinical Applications and Research* 2 (4): 141–144. https://doi.org/10.1016/j.jveb.2007.07.006.

Yin, S. and McCowan, B. (2004). Barking in domestic dogs: context specificity and individual identification. *Animal Behaviour* 68 (2): 343–355. https://doi.org/10.1016/j.anbehav.2003.07.016.

3B

Understanding Feline Behavior and Communication

3B.1 Basics of Feline Behavior

Understanding feline communication requires far more than recognizing isolated cues. It demands appreciating behavior as a dynamic, integrated system, shaped by predatory ancestry, solitary hunting ecology, and a strong instinct for self-preservation. Cats communicate through a sophisticated tapestry of visual, auditory, olfactory, tactile, and gustatory signals. Each signal is influenced by context: who are they communicating with, where does the interaction occur, and what their emotional and physiological state is at that moment.

Cats communicate both with each other and with humans through vocalizations, body posture, facial expressions, scent marking, and physical contact. However, compared to dogs, cats often display more subtle signals, owing to their smaller facial features, rapid micro-movements, and a communication system designed to prevent conflict rather than escalate it. From an evolutionary standpoint, cats evolved many of their visual and auditory behaviors to avoid physical confrontations, since even minor injuries could be life-threatening for a solitary hunter.

3B.1.1 Key Aspects of Visual Communication

Interpreting feline body language requires looking at the *entire* animal rather than focusing on a single signal in isolation. Cats communicate through a constellation of micro-movements including ear rotations, tail carriage, whisker tension, pupil size, and posture. Only when we "assemble all the pieces," can we understand the true emotional message. Because cats evolved as solitary hunters whose survival depended on avoiding injury, their visual signals tend to be subtle, fleeting, and highly context-dependent.

3B.1.1.1 Eyes

In the animal world, direct, unblinking eye contact signals confrontation. When a cat delivers a hard stare accompanied by a stiff posture or piloerection along the back and tail, the message is clear: *increase distance or risk escalation*. Cats offering an offensive threat often lean their bodies forward, stiffen their hind limbs, or arc their backs at the base of the tail. Ear bases may rotate sideways; tomcats have been observed moving their heads slowly from side to side as a threat display (Beaver 2003; Crowell-Davis 2007). In contrast, cats in a defensive posture typically crouch, avoid eye contact, and flatten their ears (Crowell-Davis 2007; Brown and Bradshaw 2014).

Positive visual communication is equally significant: a cat that meets your gaze with soft eyes and performs a slow blink signals trust and amicability. Research shows cats are more likely to approach humans who slow blink at them, and cats who slow blink at adopters may be adopted at higher rates (Humphrey et al. 2020a,b).

3B.1.1.2 Ears

Cats' ears act like high-resolution emotional antennas.

- Forward, upright ears → interest, curiosity, or confidence (see Figure 3B.1).
- Ears turned sideways → neutrality, hesitation, or uncertainty (see Figure 3B.2).
- Ears flattened or pulled laterally → fear, anxiety, or defensive aggression.

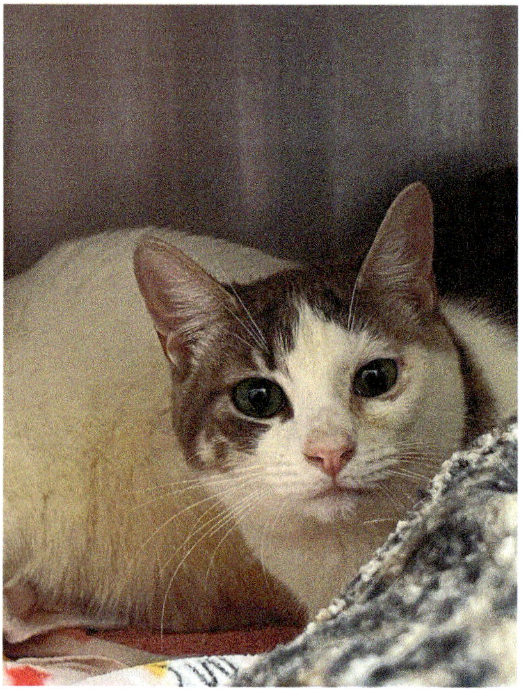

Figure 3B.1 Ears Forward

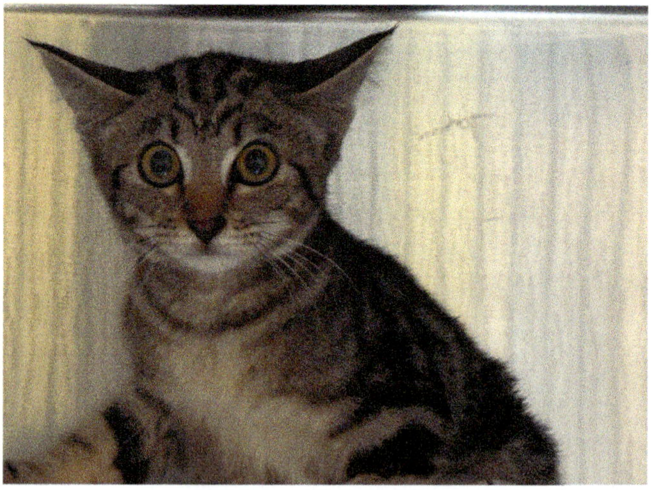

Figure 3B.2 Ears Sideways

Ear movement often precedes shifts in body posture and is therefore an excellent early indicator of mood.

3B.1.1.3 Mouth and Whiskers

Lip-licking in the absence of food is a strong indicator of stress or conflict. Severe stress can provoke open-mouth panting, which in cats is unusual and always significant.

Whiskers should be assessed along with the mouth. Cats are farsighted, relying on their whiskers for close-range spatial and tactile information.

- Forward, splayed whiskers → arousal, excitement, or offensive threat (see Figure 3B.3).
- Whiskers pulled back → fear or avoidance (see Figure 3B.4).

Figure 3B.3 Whiskers Forward

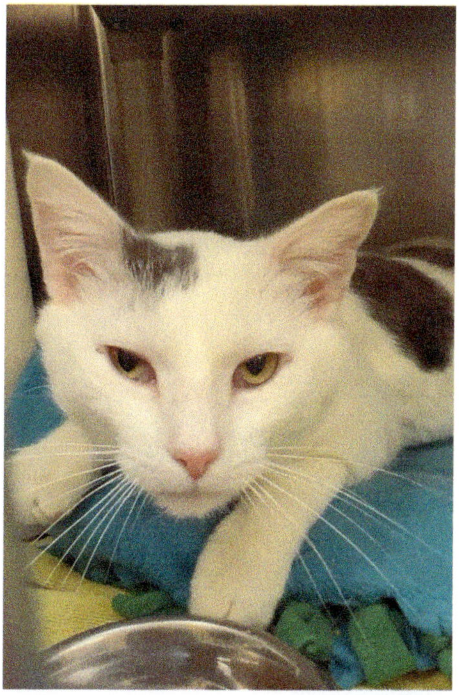

Figure 3B.4 Whiskers Pulled Back

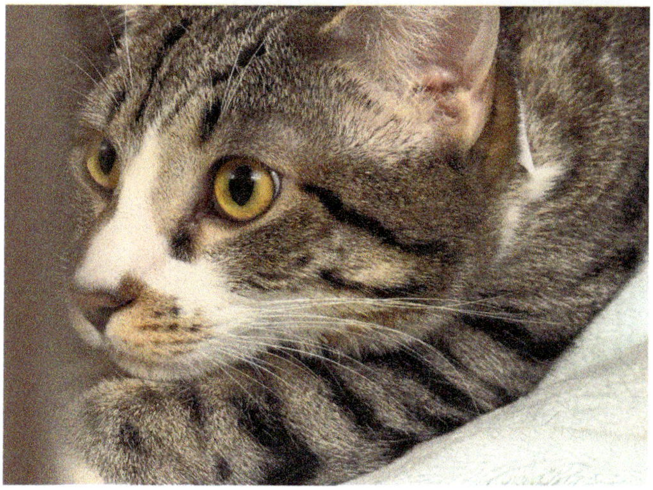

3B.1.1.4 Fur

Piloerection, when the fur stands upright along the back or shoulders, is a clear sign of heightened arousal and increased emotional intensity. The response may be triggered by fear, excitement, play, or uncertainty. Piloerection that runs from the head along the spine to the tail generally signals significant emotional activation.

3B.1.1.5 Tail

Tail posture offers some of the most recognizable feline signals:

- Upright tail ("flagpole tail") signals a friendly greeting (see Figure 3B.5). Cats often pair this with nose touches or allorubbing. Studies show cats approach tail-upright silhouettes more quickly, suggesting this posture is deeply ingrained as a social cue (Brown and Bradshaw 2014). This behavior may originate from kittens approaching their mothers with upright tails (Beaver 2003; Cafazzo and Natoli 2009).
- A tucked tail indicates fear or defensive posturing (see Figure 3B.6).

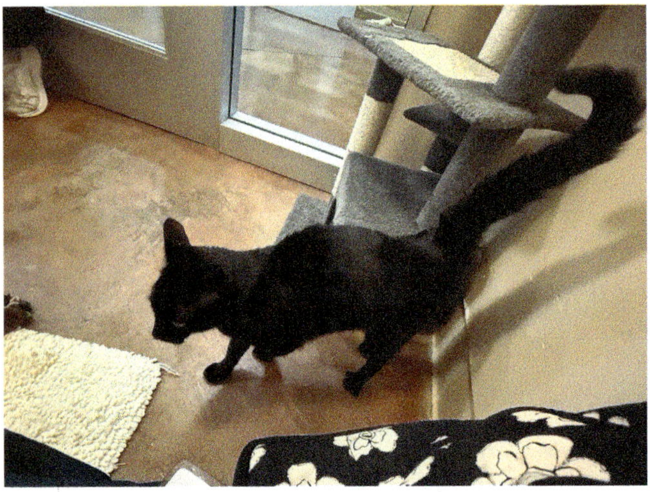

Figure 3B.5 Flagpole Tail

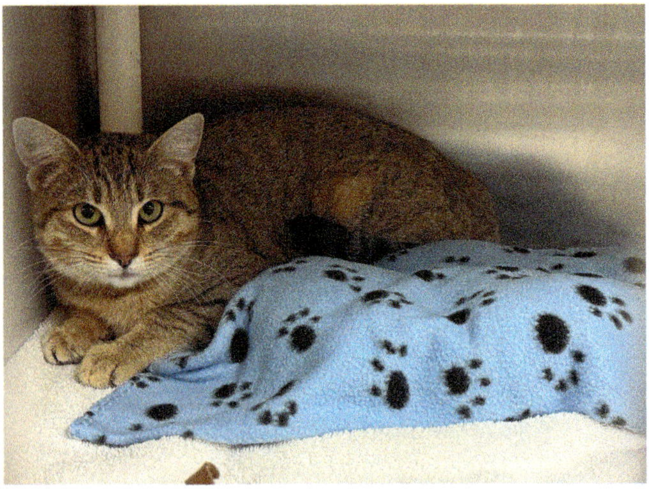

Figure 3B.6 Tail Tucked

- Tail lashing/flagging – rapid, forceful back-and-forth movement – signals agitation or conflict and often precedes an aggressive display.
- Concave tuck associated with arched back and piloerection is a classic defensive threat posture (Bradshaw et al. 2012).

3B.1.1.6 Body Roll

Rolling onto the back or side can serve multiple functions depending on context: it may be a play solicitation in kittens (Beaver 2003), a relaxed greeting behavior in adult cats (see Figure 3B.7), a subordinate signal from younger males toward mature males (Brown and Bradshaw 2014) or part of pro-estrus behavior in females accompanied by purring, rubbing, stretching, and kneading. Context determines whether this posture is affiliative or defensive. In cats, some visual signals also convey chemical information, as body postures and movements can facilitate the release and detection of scent cues.

3B.1.1.7 Fecal Marking

Outdoor and free-roaming cats typically bury feces within the core area of their territory (Feldman 1994). Exposed feces may result from incomplete burying or excavation by other cats, and while some researchers have proposed a territorial signaling function, evidence remains mixed. Cats commonly investigate buried feces but rarely sniff exposed feces. They spend more time examining feces from unfamiliar cats than from themselves or familiar individuals (Nakabayashi et al. 2012). Although feces likely convey information related to identity or health, consistent or intentional "fecal marking", also known as middening, is not well supported in domestic cats.

3B.1.1.8 Scratch Marking

Scratching serves both visual and chemical signaling functions (see Figure 3B.8). Visually, it leaves gouges, shredded material, or grooves, while chemically it deposits scent from the digital and interdigital glands (Bradshaw et al. 2012). Outdoor cats typically scratch trees, logs, or shed siding, whereas indoor cats use furniture or scratching posts, often developing strong preferences for specific surfaces. Scratching is usually concentrated along high-traffic pathways rather than territorial boundaries, and feral cats increase scratching in the presence of conspecifics, suggesting a social component to the behavior.

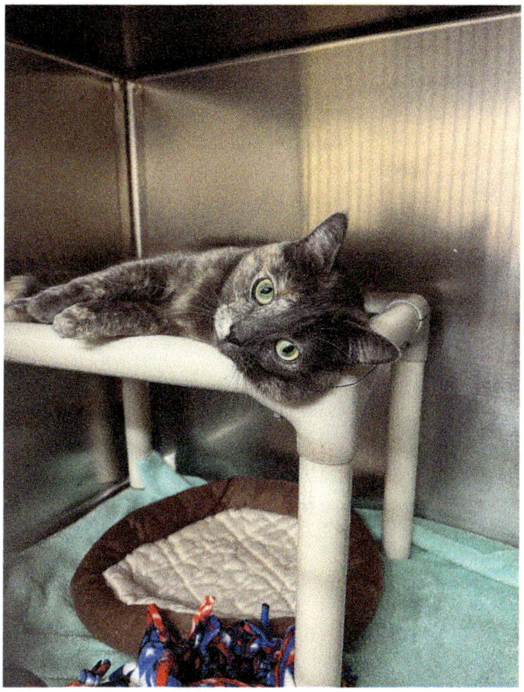

Figure 3B.7 Body Roll

3B.1.2 Auditory Communication – Expanded Key Vocalizations

Auditory communication in cats is far more complex than many people realize. While most owned cats frequently vocalize to people

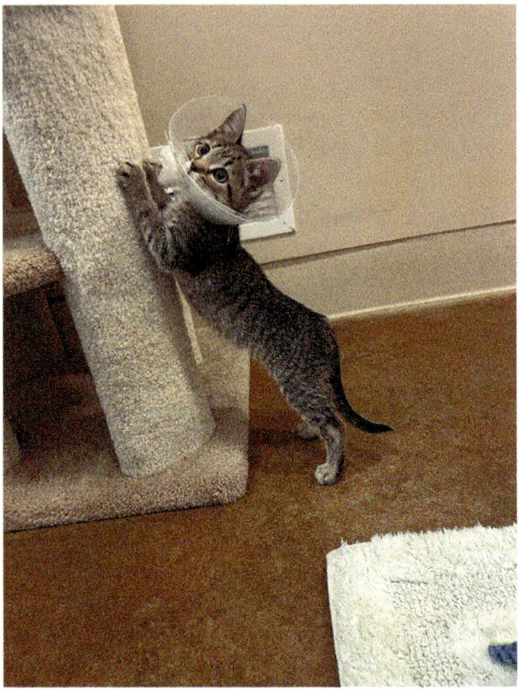

Figure 3B.8 Scratching on Post

and often to other cats, feral or free-ranging cats tend to be significantly quieter. Vocal silence is adaptive in the wild, where avoiding predators and not revealing one's position during hunting are essential to survival. In contrast, the proximity to and daily interaction with people in domestic homes have shaped a richer and more frequent vocal repertoire in owned and shelter cats. Some breeds, such as Siamese and Oriental breeds, are recognized for especially high vocal output.

Cats use vocalizations strategically. They communicate during conflict, mating, and maternal care. However, many of the sounds most familiar to humans, such as meows or solicitive purrs, are used primarily in cat–human communication, not cat–cat communication (see Table 3B.1).

Table 3B.1 Common Feline Vocalizations and Meanings Relevant to Behavior and Welfare Assessments

Vocalization	Description	Primary Function/Context
Call	Attention-seeking vocalization directed at people or other cats	Encourages approach Queens use variations to retrieve kittens (Moelk 1944; Beaver 2003)
Purr	Continuous low-frequency vibration during inhalation and exhalation	Occurs in pleasure and bonding, but also in pain, illness, stress, and near death May function as self-soothing or care solicitation (Beaver 2003)
Trill/Chirr/Chirrup	Short, melodic sounds	Friendly greeting toward familiar cats or humans Signals affiliative intent
Mating Cry/Yowl	Loud, prolonged vocalization	Mate attraction and long-distance advertisement, especially in females in estrus
Growl	Low, harsh, guttural sound	Distance-increasing warning when threatened
Hiss/Spit	Sudden, forceful exhalation; spit is more explosive	Defensive warning Used when startled, fearful, or deterring approach
Snarl	Intense, harsh vocalization with bared teeth	Escalated aggression Commonly during fights between adult males
Chatter	Rapid teeth clicking while watching inaccessible prey	Predatory arousal, excitement, or frustration (Schötz 2015)
Wail/Anger Wail	Loud, distressed vocalization	Kitten distress (separation, cold, and restraint) Adults: pain, fear, or severe discomfort
Meow	Variable-pitch vocalization rarely used cat-to-cat	Primarily human-directed Used to solicit food, attention, or access Highly adaptable based on caregiver response (Tavernier et al. 2020)

Cats produce vocalizations in three general categories based on mouth position:

1) Mouth closed: Purr, trill, chirrup, grunt, murmur.
2) Mouth open: Growl, hiss, spit, snarl, mating call/cry, chatter.
3) Mouth open then gradually closing: Meow, wail, demand calls, complaint calls.

3B.1.3 Forms of Olfactory Communication

Cats inhabit a world structured by scent. Unlike humans, who rely primarily on vision and sound, cats use olfaction to map territory, regulate social relationships, avoid conflict, and assess the identity and emotional state of other cats. Scent marks function as invisible messages that continue to shape feline interactions long after the cat has left. Understanding these behaviors is essential for interpreting stress, territoriality, and social compatibility in both home and shelter settings.

3B.1.3.1 Urine Marking: The Scent "Bulletin Board"

Urine spraying is a powerful form of feline communication, not a toileting behavior. A spray mark conveys presence, identity, and territorial status, essentially announcing "*I was here.*" Spraying typically occurs on vertical surfaces: the cat turns away, raises a quivering tail, and forcefully directs urine backward and upward, often 1–2 feet above the ground (Beaver 2003). Outdoors, common targets include trees, fence posts, and corners; indoors, cats often spray doorways, windows, or items carrying salient human or animal scent (Herron 2010).

Sprayed urine contains rich chemical information about sex, health, reproductive status, and recency of presence. Because fresh spray includes more volatile compounds, cats spend more time investigating vertical spray marks than horizontal urine deposits (Bradshaw et al. 2012). Although problematic in managed environments, spraying is a normal communication strategy that increases when cats feel socially conflicted, threatened, or uncertain, particularly in multi-cat households.

3B.1.3.2 The Flehmen Response

After encountering urine, pheromones, or strong scent marks, cats may pause, lift the head, part the mouth, curl the upper lip, and draw air across the vomeronasal organ. This flehmen response enables cats to decode detailed chemical information, including reproductive status, territorial boundaries, emotional state, and individual identity. In shelters, it is commonly seen when cats investigate bedding, carriers, or unfamiliar animals.

3B.1.3.3 Rubbing and Shared Scent

When cats rub against people, objects, or other cats, they are actively depositing scent from sebaceous glands located on the face, chin, lips, forehead, tail base, perianal region, and paws (Mills 2005; Crowell-Davis 2007). Head rubbing typically begins at the nose and cheek and extends toward the eye region (Beaver 2003). When directed on objects, this behavior is called bunting; when directed at other cats, it is known as allorubbing.

Allorubbing helps establish a shared "*colony scent*," allowing familiar cats to recognize one another as safe and reducing social friction. These interactions often include body rubbing, tail intertwining, and purring. Allogrooming – licking the head or neck of another cat – further reinforces social bonds and blends saliva-based scent cues. It occurs primarily between affiliative cats and is often solicited by a lowered head posture (Crowell-Davis 2007; Brown and Bradshaw 2014).

3B.1.3.4 Pheromones: Chemical Communication

Pheromones represent the most specialized layer of feline scent signaling, conveying emotional, and social information. Five facial pheromone fractions (F1–F5) have been identified. Pheromone fraction F3 is associated with facial marking and environmental security, while F4 functions as a

Table 3B.2 Human–Cat Touch as Communication

Tactile Behavior	What the Cat Is Doing	What It Communicates
Rubbing/leaning	Rubs against legs, hands, or objects Repeated gentle contact	Solicits interaction, mixes scent, marks person as familiar and safe, often a greeting
Preferred touch zones	Accepts touch on cheeks, base of ears, under chin, forehead, shoulders	Indicates comfort and consent to continue interaction
Sensitive/ overstimulation zones	Reacts to touch on belly, lower back, tail base, hindquarters, or fast full-body strokes	Signals rising discomfort Risk of swatting or biting
Early "stop" signals	Skin twitching, tail flicking, ears rotating back, head turns, pupil dilation, stiffening	Requests reduction or cessation of touch before escalation
Head-butting (bunting)	Gently bumps head into person	Affiliative gesture Invites soft contact Indicates trust or bonding
Kneading	Alternating paw pressure on lap, blanket, or arm	Comfort, emotional security, positive arousal (not aggression)
Grooming-like licking	Brief licking of hand or arm	Bonding or calming behavior Excessive licking may indicate stress
Mutual petting interaction	Cat leans in, repositions, or returns for more touch	Two-way consent Staying close = continue Moving away = stop

social, affiliative signal that helps reduce tension between familiar cats. The roles of F1 and F5 remain unclear, and F2 is linked to sexual signaling in tomcats.

Synthetic analogues of these pheromones have practical applications. Pheromone F3 analogues (e.g. Feliway™) reduce urine marking, scratching, and anxiety-related behaviors, while supporting feeding, play, and relaxation (Pageat and Gaultier 2003). The synthetic version of F4 analogues to F4 (Feliway Friends/Multicat) helps decrease inter-cat conflict during introductions or in socially strained households (DePorter et al. 2019).

3B.1.4 Forms and Functions of Tactile Communication

Tactile communication – physical contact that conveys information – is more limited in cats than in many social species, but it plays an important role in secure attachment, affiliative behavior, and emotional regulation. Cats use touch selectively, and their preferences can vary widely. Understanding how cats communicate through human-directed touch is essential for safe handling and accurate behavior assessments (see Table 3B.2). Understanding these micro-signals is particularly important in the shelter environment, where cats may be stressed, over-stimulated, or touch-averse.

3B.1.5 Relevance for Shelter Team and Behavioral Assessments

In a shelter setting, tactile communication helps determine:

- Approachability: Does the cat seek or avoid touch?
- Stress level: Does the cat stiffen, flinch, or retreat when gently touched?

- Handling tolerance: Is the cat comfortable being petted, lifted, or examined?
- Arousal/overstimulation: How quickly does the cat escalate during petting?
- Matchmaking: Which adopters are appropriate for this cat's touch preferences?

Proper interpretation of tactile cues reduces bites and scratches, supports well-being, and improves placement outcomes.

Tactile experiences play a central role in how cats interact with their environment and are especially influential in two areas that commonly create conflict in homes and shelters: scratching and elimination. Cats often have strong tactile preferences for the texture, firmness, and "give" of the surfaces they touch with their paws.

Scratching surfaces vary widely in tactile feedback. Carpeted posts, sisal rope, corrugated cardboard, wood, and vertical vs. horizontal orientations each feel different to the cat. Some cats prefer firm, resistant surfaces that allow for a strong pull and full claw extension, while others seek softer materials that shred and provide immediate tactile feedback. When a cat's preferred texture is not available, scratching behavior often shifts to household items such as couches, rugs, or doorframes – not as misbehavior, but because those surfaces provide the desired sensory experience.

The same tactile principles apply to elimination behavior. Litter substrates differ dramatically in texture and sensation, ranging from fine clay or sand-like litters to coarse granules, pellets, crystals, or natural fiber products. Most cats prefer soft, fine-grained substrates that resemble natural soil and allow comfortable digging and covering. Sharp, hard, or unfamiliar textures are commonly avoided. When the tactile quality of the litter does not match a cat's preference – or when changes occur suddenly – cats may begin eliminating outside the litter box. This sensory mismatch is a well-recognized contributor to undesirable elimination and remains a common reason why cats are relinquished to shelters.

Understanding and accommodating feline tactile preferences is therefore not a luxury but a critical component of behavioral wellness, environmental design, and successful long-term placement.

Respecting tactile preferences helps prevent two major behavior problems linked to relinquishment:

1) Destructive scratching of household items, when preferred scratching outlets are absent.
2) Litter box avoidance, when the substrate feels uncomfortable or aversive.

Providing a variety of scratching textures and offering soft, fine-grained unscented litter options allows cats to meet their tactile needs in appropriate ways, protects the home, and significantly improves feline welfare and shelter placement success.

3B.1.6 Key Aspects of Gustatory (Taste-Based) Communication

Although less obvious than visual, auditory, or olfactory cues, gustatory communication plays a subtle but important role in how cats gather information about their environment, other animals, and people. Taste is closely integrated with scent through the vomeronasal (also known as Jacobson's organ) organ, allowing cats to process chemical information as a combined sensory system rather than in isolation.

3B.1.6.1 Licking and Mouthing Objects

Cats may lick or mouth unfamiliar objects to confirm identity, assess novelty, or threat and gather chemical cues from new environments. These behaviors are part of information gathering rather than misbehavior, particularly in multi-cat settings.

3B.1.6.2 Why This Matters

Gustatory cues help cats assess territory, familiarity, group membership, and stress levels, contributing to a multisensory understanding of their environment. Recognizing these behaviors helps caregivers interpret licking or mouthing accurately, avoid mislabeling them as problematic and prioritize scent and hygiene management in home and shelter environments.

3B.1.7 A Multisensory Communication System

For cats, the world is experienced in overlapping layers of smell, taste, touch, sight, and sound. These various forms of communication can be subtle, but they play an important role in how cats interpret spaces, understand social relationships, and respond to change. Recognizing this helps us create more cat-friendly environments and improves both welfare and behavioral outcomes in shelters and homes.

3B.1.8 Body Language – Physical Cues in Cats

Interpreting feline body language requires assessing the whole cat rather than a single feature. Eyes, ears, tail, whiskers, body posture, and movement patterns must be read together to understand a cat's emotional state and predict how they may respond to handling or approach. Because cats communicate subtly and can shift rapidly between comfort and fear, careful observation is essential for safety and well-being, especially in a shelter setting.

3B.1.9 Feline Body Language Competency: From Admissions Through Placement

Accurately reading feline body language is essential at every stage of a cat's shelter journey. Cats communicate through subtle shifts in posture, facial expression, and movement. Misinterpreting these cues can quickly increase fear or lead to defensive aggression. From the moment a cat arrives, body language helps team members choose the safest approach, reduce stress, and guide handling and housing decisions. Throughout evaluation, daily care, and adoption, these skills help identify behavior challenges early and support each cat's well-being. Reading cats well sets the tone for positive, safe interactions, and ultimately helps them move successfully from admissions to placement.

3B.1.9.1 Approach and General Observations

When approaching a cat in a kennel, move slowly with your body angled sideways to appear less threatening (see Table 3B.3). Avoid bending over the cat or reaching directly toward the face. Brief, soft eye contact followed by looking away signal friendliness without intimidation.

3B.1.9.1.1 Piloerection

Raised fur, arched back, and puffed tail indicate high emotional arousal, which can be linked to either:

- Intense fear
- Threatening/offensive posture
- Startle response
- Overstimulation during interaction

Regardless of cause, piloerection always means the cat's arousal level is elevated. Caution is required.

Table 3B.3 Feline Body Language: Emotional State at a Glance

Emotional State	Key Body Language Signs	What It Means/How to Respond
Confident and Friendly	Tail held high (may have a slight forward "hook") Ears forward or neutral Upright posture with loose muscles Soft eyes, slow blinking Approaches front of kennel, rubs, sniffs	Cat is relaxed, social, and receptive Proceed calmly Allow the cat to initiate interaction
Note on Rolling	Rolls onto side or back, exposing belly	Indicates trust, not an invitation for belly touching Avoid abdominal contact to prevent defensive reactions
Uncertain/Mildly Uncomfortable	Crouched posture Tail tucked or wrapped close to body Averted gaze or half-lidded looks Ears slightly to the side Lip licking, yawning, or grooming out of context Hesitant movement or staying toward back of kennel	The cat is conflicted or cautious Slow down, reduce pressure, give time, and space Allow cat to choose whether to approach
Fearful/ Threat-Perceiving	Ears pinned flat ("airplane ears") Body pressed low, limbs tucked Head withdrawn Tail tightly tucked or curled, tip flicking Dilated pupils, freezing Hissing or growling	The cat feels unsafe and may escalate Increase distance; do not force interaction
Offensive Aggression	Tall, stiff posture Leaning forward, weight on forelimbs Direct, unblinking stare Ears rotated outward Piloerection along back or tail	The cat is actively trying to drive the threat away Pause, increase distance, reassess handling plan
Defensive Aggression	Crouched body with curved spine Head lowered Ears flattened sideways or back Tail tightly tucked Teeth displayed, hissing, or spitting Attempting to retreat or cornered	Fear-based aggression High risk if pressured Provide escape routes and minimize handling

3B.1.9.2 Assessing a Cat in the Kennel

Use a pompom tool to gauge how the cat responds to approach (see Figure 3B.9). Gently extend the pompom and rub it along the cat's cheek. Watch for relaxed signs such as closing eyes, leaning in or soft facial muscles. If receptive, continue lightly petting the cheek, under the chin, the neck, and the top of the head.

If the cat remains comfortable, slowly withdraw the pompom, and offer your hand by approaching from below the chin, not over the head. When a few inches away, extend your index finger toward the cat's nose. A nose touch indicates readiness for gentle chin and neck petting

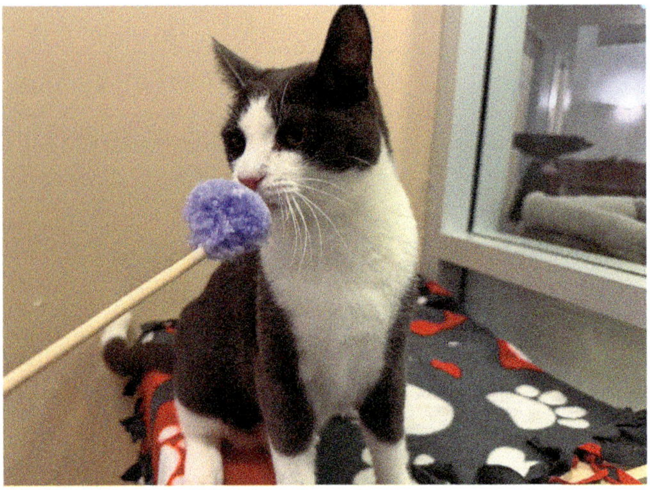

Figure 3B.9 PomPom Touch

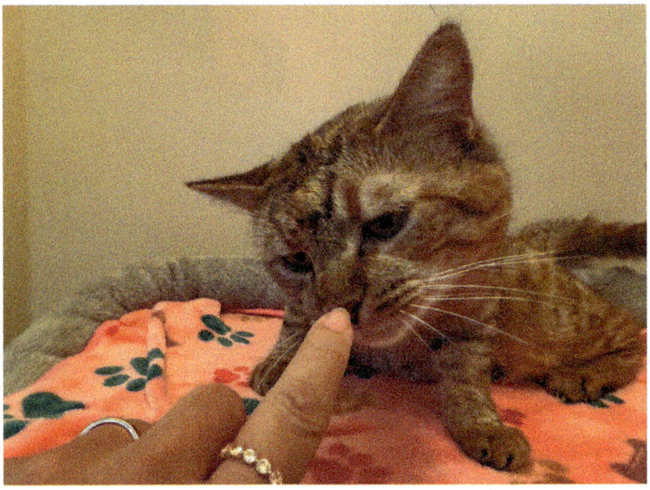

Figure 3B.10 Nose Touch

(see Figure 3B.10). Spend a moment building rapport and then offer a small treat. If the cat eats and remains relaxed, you may carefully slide your hand under the chest and lift the cat toward you.

If body language is uncertain or defensive, use a towel wrap instead of handling directly. Drape the towel over the cat, tuck one end underneath, fold the second end over securely, and tuck the rear of the towel so that the cat cannot back out (see Figure 3B.11). Lift with the cat's head facing away, keeping one arm under the body for support and one hand holding the towel snugly at the neck opening. This method avoids scruffing, which increases fear and anxiety, especially with unfamiliar handlers.

3B.1.9.3 Assessing a Cat in the Carrier

Assessing a cat while it is still in a carrier is difficult, so it's best to let the cat move into a cage or small room before evaluating behavior. If the cat is hissing, growling, or spit-stomping when approached in the carrier, follow your organization's specific handling policy. For owned cats with current vaccines, place the cat in a cage with a hide box, litter box, food, and water, and allow 24–48 hours of quiet recovery time. Add a visual barrier – for example plastic, plexiglass, sheet, or towel – if the cat appears highly stressed.

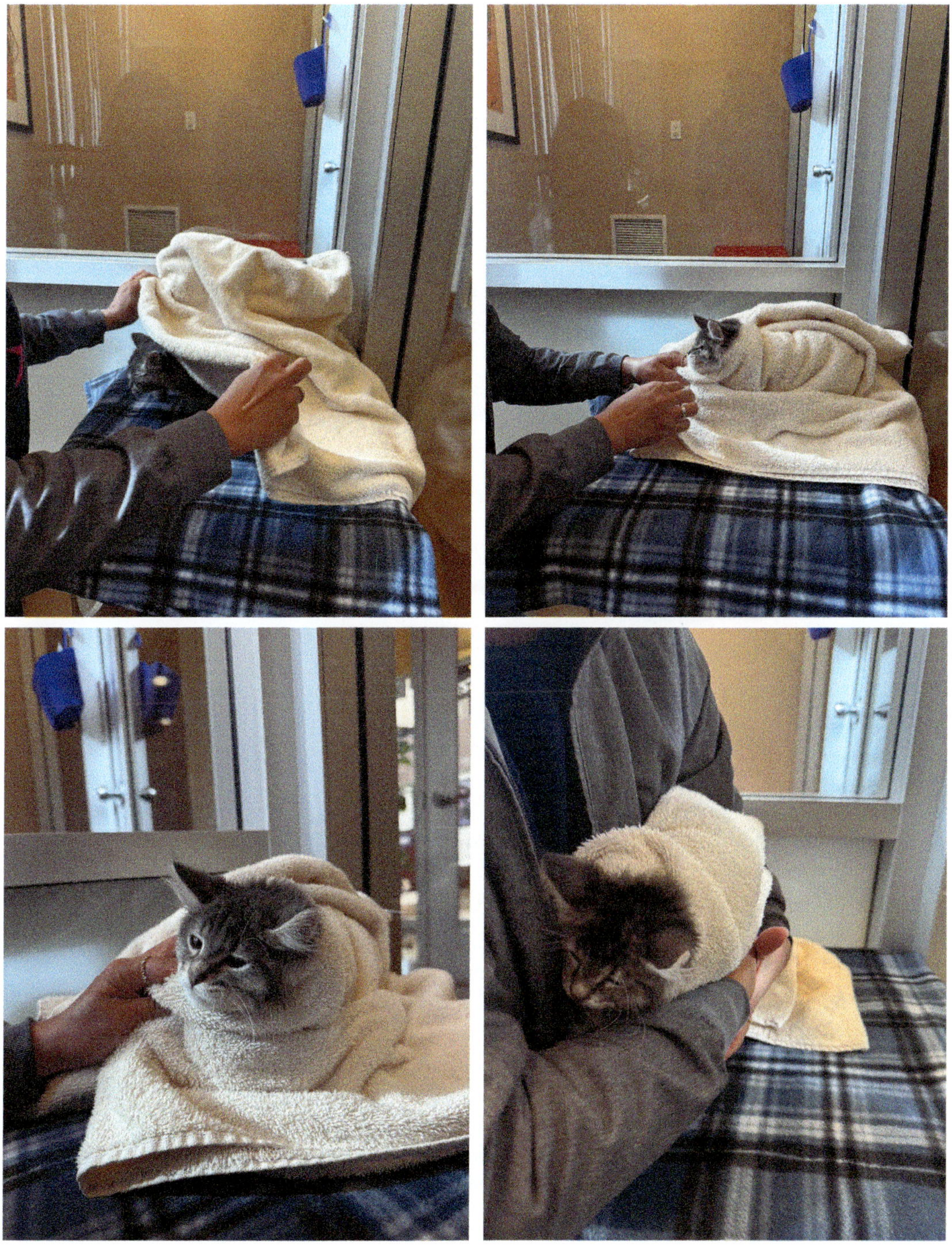

Figure 3B.11 Cat Toweling Sequence

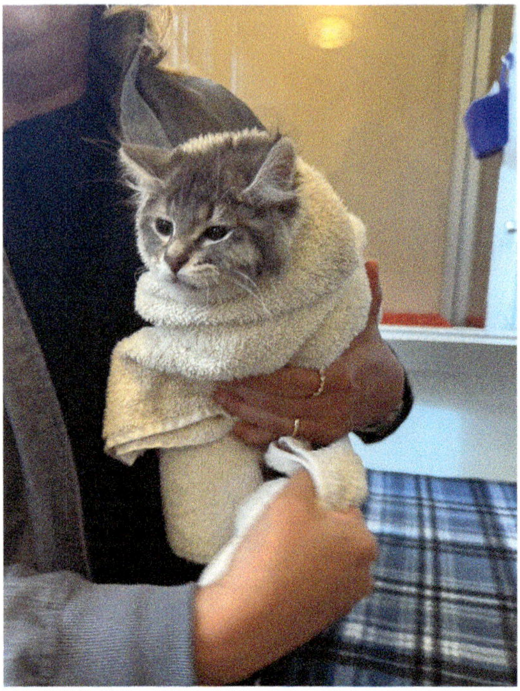

Figure 3B.11 (Continued)

Most resilient cats settle within 24 hours, though some may need up to 72 hours to acclimate. Once the cat is calm, you can proceed with the veterinary exam and behavioral assessment.

3B.1.9.4 Managing Cats with Continued Aggressive Behavior and No Vaccination History

For cats that remain aggressive and lack vaccination history, begin by offering anxiolytic medication hidden in food. After the cat eats, reassess to determine whether the medication has reduced arousal enough to allow safe handling and examination.

If the cat does not eat the medicated food or the dose is insufficient, proceed with injectable sedation so a full physical exam and core vaccinations – rabies and feline viral rhinotracheitis, calicivirus, and panleukopenia vaccine (FVRCP) – can be completed.

Depending on handler skills and available resources, sedation may be delivered using the following methods:

- Thick towel or blanket toss to safely restrain long enough for an intramuscular (IM) injection.
- Injection pole: Syringe attached to a pole to allow distance while administering the sedative.
- Feral den that allows safe injection through built-in ports.
- EZ Nabber/cat-catcher clamp net.
- Animal net on a pole.

3B.1.9.5 Sedation for Examination

Sedation can greatly reduce fear, anxiety, and stress in cats who are unable to tolerate handling. By lowering arousal and muscle tension, sedation allows the veterinary team to work calmly and efficiently while preventing escalation, defensive aggression, or injury. It also helps avoid repeated attempts at restraint, which can increase distress and worsen future handling and veterinary visits. Once sedation has taken effect, a complete physical examination can be performed with minimal stress to the cat.

This is the safest method for:

- Cats who show fear-based aggression or defensive behaviors.
- Cats who cannot be safely or thoroughly examined when awake.
- Preventing fear-learning and negative associations during veterinary care.
- Patients that require procedures that would be painful, frightening, or prolonged.
- Reducing the risk of handler injury when attempting to restrain a distressed cat.
- Cats with underlying medical conditions where stress could worsen clinical status.

This is the safest method for:

- Updating rabies and FVRCP vaccines.
- Obtaining diagnostics (e.g. blood draw, microchip placement, and parasite screening).
- Conducting a thorough medical assessment without triggering fear or aggression.
- Minimizing risk of injury to team members while ensuring the cat receives appropriate medical care.

After the exam, place the cat in a quiet, climate-controlled recovery area with dim lighting and a soft surface and observe with minimal disturbance until fully awake.

3B.2 Breed-Specific Selection in Shelter Cats

3B.2.1 Representative Cat Selection in the Shelter Population

Unlike dogs, shelter cats do not represent a wide variety of distinct breeds. The vast majority of cats entering shelters are domestic shorthair or domestic longhair cats, reflecting the general pet cat population rather than purpose-bred animals. While breed-specific cat rescues do exist, they account for only a small proportion of cats entering municipal and nonprofit shelters.

Breeding in cats has historically been far less behaviorally specialized than in dogs. Most cat breeds were selected primarily for physical traits rather than working function, resulting in fewer predictable, breed-linked behavioral patterns. Consequently, early socialization, life experience, and environment are far more influential than breed in shaping behavior for most shelter cats, a finding supported by shelter medicine and feline behavior literature.

3B.2.2 How Breed Differences Impact Well-Being and Behavioral Assessments

That said, shelter professionals should still be aware of certain tendencies observed in specific breed types when they do appear in shelter populations:

- Oriental-type breeds (e.g. Siamese and Oriental Shorthairs). Often highly vocal, socially oriented, and prone to forming strong attachments to specific people. These cats may experience heightened stress in confinement and benefit from early placement and increased human interaction.
- Persian and other longhair breeds. Typically, lower in activity and arousal, but more likely to shut down or mask stress-related behaviors in the shelter environment, which can complicate behavioral assessment.

- Bengals and other hybrid or high-drive breeds. Often exhibit high energy, low frustration tolerance, and increased environmental needs. Without adequate enrichment and stimulation, these cats may develop stress-related behaviors rapidly.

Despite these tendencies, breed alone should never be used to predict behavior, suitability, or adoptability. For most shelter cats, understanding socialization history, observed behavior over time and response to the shelter environment provides a far more accurate foundation for assessment and placement. Recognizing breed tendencies as one contextual factor – rather than a determining one – supports more humane handling, better welfare outcomes, and more realistic adopter education.

3B.3 Behavioral Differences Across Species

Understanding how behavior and body language vary between species – and within dogs and cats – is essential for accurate welfare assessment and effective CTS in shelter environments. Recognizing inherited behavioral tendencies, species-specific needs, and historical selection pressures allows shelter teams to interpret behavior more accurately, set realistic expectations, and design care plans that support both welfare and safety.

In some shelters, teams, and volunteers are species-specific in their experience or preference. Some individuals feel more comfortable working with dogs, others with cats, and some organizations may rely heavily on volunteers whose exposure is limited to one species. While specialization can be valuable, it also increases the risk of misinterpretation when knowledge from one species is unintentionally applied to another. Unless an organization focuses exclusively on a single species, it is critical that shelter teams understand the fundamental behavioral, medical, and evolutionary differences between dogs and cats.

Dogs and cats evolved under very different selective pressures. Dogs are social, cooperative animals shaped by thousands of years of close partnership with humans, often selected for working roles that emphasize communication, responsiveness, and tolerance of proximity and handling. As a result, many canine behaviors – such as overt signaling, appeasement gestures, and social play – are relatively easy for humans to observe and interpret.

Cats, by contrast, evolved as solitary hunters with a strong emphasis on self-preservation, environmental control, and subtle communication. Feline stress responses are often quiet and easily overlooked, and cats may mask distress by withdrawing, freezing, or appearing "calm." Behaviors that might be interpreted as compliance or relaxation by dog-oriented observers may, in cats, reflect fear, shutdown, or learned helplessness. This distinction is so fundamental that it is often emphasized in veterinary education with the reminder that *cats are not small dogs*.

These differences have direct implications in shelters. Housing design, handling protocols, enrichment strategies, medical care, and behavioral assessments must be species-specific. For example, frequent handling, high noise levels, and constant visual exposure – often tolerated or even enriching for some dogs – can be profoundly stressful for cats. Similarly, canine play styles, arousal patterns, and social needs differ markedly from feline interaction preferences and stress thresholds.

Failure to account for these differences can lead to mislabeling behavior, unnecessary restrictions, inappropriate interventions, or flawed placement decisions. Conversely, when shelter teams are trained to recognize species-specific communication and needs, they are better equipped to reduce stress, prevent escalation of behavioral concerns, and create realistic, humane CTS.

Table 3B.4 Relevant Species Comparison

Dogs	Cats
Generally social animals that co-evolved with humans for cooperative living	Evolved primarily as solitary hunters with flexible social structures
Often look to humans for guidance, reassurance, and problem-solving	Rely heavily on environmental control, territorial security, and predictability
Communicate overtly through body language, vocalizations, and scent	Communicate more subtly Stress signals are often quiet and easily missed
Stress is commonly expressed through vocalization, agitation, or increased activity	Stress often manifests as hiding, reduced appetite, avoidance, or sudden defensive aggression
Typically benefit from predictable routines and frequent social interaction	Typically benefit from environmental stability and control rather than social engagement
Welfare improves with physical activity, cognitive enrichment, and positive reinforcement training	Welfare improves with hiding spaces, vertical territory, minimal forced interaction, and scent continuity

In short, effective sheltering requires an intentional, informed approach to species differences. Understanding that dogs and cats communicate, cope, and respond to stress in fundamentally different ways is not only a matter of best practice – it is a cornerstone of ethical, welfare-centered shelter care (see Table 3B.4).

In summary, individual variation matters. While species differences and breed-related tendencies provide valuable context, they should never override what an individual dog or cat is actually communicating. Behavior is shaped by a complex interaction of genetics, early socialization, learning history, health, emotional state, and environment. Relying on breed stereotypes risks misinterpretation and inappropriate care decisions.

Effective shelter assessment requires teams to evaluate each animal as an individual by considering available history, socialization experiences, current affective and medical status, environmental triggers, and learned responses. Integrating this individualized information with species-informed knowledge supports more accurate welfare assessments, safer handling, and ethical, humane care trajectory strategy from admission through placement.

References

Beaver, B.V. (2003). *Feline Behavior: A Guide for Veterinarians*, 2e. St. Louis, MO: Saunders.

Bradshaw, J.W.S., Casey, R.A., and Brown, S.L. (2012). *The Behaviour of the Domestic Cat*, 2e. Wallingford: CABI.

Brown, S.L. and Bradshaw, J.W.S. (2014). Communication in domestic cats. *Behavioural Processes* 106: 1–12.

Cafazzo, S. and Natoli, E. (2009). The social function of tail up in the domestic cat (*Felis silvestris catus*). *Behavioural Processes* 80 (1): 60–66.

Crowell-Davis, S.L. (2007). Cat behaviour. In: *BSAVA Manual of Canine and Feline Behavioural Medicine*, 2e (ed. D.F. Horwitz and D.S. Mills), 47–64. Gloucester: BSAVA.

DePorter, T., Bledsoe, D.L., Beck, A. et al. (2019). Evaluation of a synthetic feline pheromone analogue for reducing inter-cat conflict in multicat households. *Journal of Feline Medicine and Surgery* 21 (6): 517–525.

Feldman, H.N. (1994). Methods of scent marking in the domestic cat. *Journal of Mammalogy* 75 (2): 392–401.

Herron, M.E. (2010). Advances in understanding and treatment of feline elimination disorders. *Topics in Companion Animal Medicine* 25 (4): 195–202.

Humphrey, T., Proops, L., Forman, J. et al. (2020a). The role of slow blinking in cat–human communication. *Scientific Reports* 10: 16503.

Humphrey, T., Stringer, M., Proops, L. et al. (2020b). Slow blinking promotes positive cat–human interactions in a shelter environment. *Applied Animal Behaviour Science* 230: 105071.

Mills, D.S. (2005). Pheromonal communication in cats. *Veterinary Clinics of North America: Small Animal Practice* 35 (1): 41–54.

Moelk, M. (1944). Vocalizing in the house cat; a phonetic and functional study. *American Journal of Psychology* 57 (2): 184–205.

Nakabayashi, M., Yamaoka, R., and Nakashima, Y. (2012). Chemical communication in feces of domestic cats. *Journal of Ethology* 30 (1): 51–58.

Pageat, P. and Gaultier, E. (2003). Current research in canine and feline pheromones. *Veterinary Clinics of North America: Small Animal Practice* 33 (2): 187–211.

Schötz, S. (2015). Agonistic vocalisations in domestic cats: a case study. In: *Working Papers*, vol. 55 (ed. M.S. Lundmark, G. Ambrazaitis, and J.V.D. Weijer), 85–90. Lund University.

Tavernier, M., Ahmed, R., Houpt, K.A., and Erb, H.N. (2020). Human-directed vocalizations in domestic cats. *Journal of Veterinary Behavior* 37: 1–8.

4

Normal Behavior (Neurotypical) vs. Behavioral Disorders (Behavioral Dysregulation)

Recognizing the difference between species-typical (neurotypical) behavior and behavior problems is essential for accurate assessment, humane care, and ethical decision-making in shelter environments.

Both genetics and environment – including early socialization and broader influences such as the COVID-19 pandemic – play a significant role in shaping an animal's behavioral responses to the environment. When addressing a shelter pet's behavioral needs, it is essential that team members can distinguish between species-typical (neurotypical) behaviors and behaviors that indicate dysregulated behaviors or clinically significant distress.

In this context, *neurotypical* refers to behaviors that fall within the expected range for a species when responding to stress, novelty, or confinement. For example, dogs may bark, pace, seek human interaction, or show heightened arousal in a shelter environment. While cats may hide, reduce activity, limit social engagement, or display subtle defensive behaviors. These types of behaviors often reflect normal coping strategies shaped by a species' evolutionary history and sensory priorities. Mislabeling these behaviors as "*abnormal*" can lead to unnecessary restriction, inappropriate intervention, or flawed placement decisions.

Applying **a Five Domains** framework helps clarify this distinction (see Chapter 1):

- In the **Environment** and **Behavior** domains, species-typical responses signal how well the animal can cope with housing, handling, and enrichment.
- The **Nutrition** domain may be affected differently across species, as stress-related appetite changes are common and often more pronounced in cats.
- The **Health** domain reminds teams that pain or illness can alter behavior and must be ruled out before attributing responses to temperament.
- The **Mental State** domain integrates these observations, helping determine whether behaviors reflect adaptive coping or ongoing distress.

By grounding behavioral assessment in species biology and neurotypical response patterns, shelter teams can more accurately identify when a pet is coping within expected limits vs. when wellbeing is compromised. This approach supports humane care trajectory strategies (CTS) and treatment planning. It reduces misinterpretation and ensures interventions are targeted toward improving wellbeing across all five domains.

Fear, stress, anxiety, and frustration can have profound effects on both physiological and psychological health (see Chapter 7). When these states are chronic or unmanaged, they may contribute to behavioral dysregulation and lead to maladaptive patterns. Dysregulated behaviors refer to responses that differ from what is considered typical or expected for the species (neurotypical behavior) and arise from differences or disruptions in how an animal's nervous system processes stress, stimuli, learning, or emotion. These patterns are especially likely to develop in environments marked by confinement, unpredictability, and either sensory deprivation or sensory overload. Recognizing how both inherited traits and environmental pressures shape behavior allows shelters to respond more accurately, compassionately, and effectively to each animal's presentation.

In pets – particularly in shelter settings – dysregulated behaviors are not diagnoses and should never be interpreted as character flaws or intentional misconduct. Instead, they often represent maladaptive coping strategies formed in response to chronic fear, stress, anxiety, frustration, pain, or limited control over the environment. Understanding behavior through this lens supports humane handling, appropriate intervention, and more ethical decision-making.

Examples of **dysregulation** may include:

- Extreme or persistent hypervigilance.
- Repetitive or compulsive behaviors (e.g. pacing, spinning, or self-directed behaviors).
- Disproportionate fear responses to routine or low-level stimuli or repeated stimuli.
- Difficulty recovering or returning to baseline after stressors.
- Atypical learning responses or reduced behavioral flexibility.

4.1 Development of Behavioral Disorders (Behavioral Dysregulation)

Fear, stress, anxiety, and frustration have significant effects on both the medical and emotional wellbeing of shelter pets, influencing immune function, learning capacity, emotional regulation, and behavioral expression. For this reason, when addressing a shelter pet's behavioral needs, it is essential that team members can distinguish between normal, species-typical behavior and behavior that is maladaptive or dysregulated. Some behaviors are developmentally normal yet may still be perceived as nuisance or problematic depending on context, intensity, or associated risk. For example, many dogs jump up when greeting people – a behavior rooted in normal canine social interaction, as dogs naturally greet one another face-to-face. This behavior is common in puppies and adolescent dogs and may persist into adulthood. While biologically normal, jumping up is often classified as a nuisance behavior because it may result in scratching, accidental injury, or soiling of clothing. In larger or more mature dogs, however, jumping up may signal a more serious behavioral concern when accompanied by barking, growling, snarling, or biting.

While *nuisance behaviors* generally fall under neurotypical, species-typical, and normal behaviors, they are often perceived by people as undesirable behaviors, particularly when they conflict with human expectations or living environments (Berger and Haug 2014). These behaviors are not inherently abnormal or pathological, but may require management, training, or environmental modification to ensure successful cohabitation.

Behaviors such as pulling back, cowering, or flattening the ears when an unfamiliar person reaches over a dog's head are frequently misinterpreted as signs of past abuse. The pet's response to stimuli – including people, other animals, noises, and environmental changes – is shaped by early socialization during puppyhood or kittenhood, prior learning experiences, and exposure to stressful or traumatic events. The perception of trauma is highly individualized; what one pet experiences as traumatic may be tolerated or quickly recovered from by another.

Furthermore, in many cases, such avoidance reflects normal fear-based or appeasement responses to a perceived threatening gesture, with the dog simply attempting to increase distance, reduce conflict, or avoid harm. For example, a dog who cowers or avoids when a person reaches to clip the leash to its collar may be displaying developmentally normal fear or appeasement behavior. Although some people perceive this as a nuisance, it is a more concerning issue when the fear is debilitating or when the dog's response intensifies over time. Routine activities such as placing a leash – a task that occurs multiple times a day in both homes and shelters – can become a significant stressor. When a dog consistently pulls away, hides under furniture, or shows escalating avoidance, the behavior may be classified as maladaptive or dysregulated. Accurately interpreting these responses within their environmental and developmental context is essential for humane handling, appropriate intervention, and informed decision-making.

Common canine behaviors that may be considered neurotypical but have the potential to escalate to nuisance or develop into behavioral disorders, include (see Chapter 11 for specific behavior conditions):

- Jumping up on people
- Pulling on the leash
- Chasing small prey animals
- Barking at people or other dogs
- Biting or grabbing the leash
- Urinating inside the home or kennel

Common feline behaviors that may be considered neurotypical but may have the potential to escalate to nuisance or develop into behavioral disorders, include (see Chapter 11 for specific behavior conditions):

- Scratching people's hands or feet during play
- Climbing up people's pant legs
- Grabbing and biting hands or feet during play
- Pouncing on moving hands or feet
- Urinating outside the litterbox

Nuisance behaviors can have the potential to escalate in some pets, depending on their level of emotional arousal, the intensity and frequency of the behavior, and the pet's ability to recover and regain emotional regulation afterward. When behaviors escalate or worsen, they are often associated with an underlying behavioral pathology that includes a significant emotional component – such as fear, anxiety, frustration, or aggression. These pets have a decreased resilience and coping strategies. Their interpretation and response to interactions and environmental challenges are exaggerated, resulting in behavioral outcomes at the far end of the spectrum, indicative of behavioral dysregulation.

Examples of *dysregulated behavioral disorders* may include:

- A dog that consistently flees to the back of the kennel or urinates when team members approach to take them for a walk, indicating a fear-based response that interferes with routine care.
- A cat that hisses, swats, or displays defensive aggression when team members open the kennel door to provide meals, suggesting heightened fear or anxiety associated with human approach.

4.2 The Role of Genetics and Environment in Behavior

4.2.1 Epigenesis

Epigenesis refers to the process by which a pet's behavior and temperament develop through the continuous interaction between genetic predispositions and environmental experiences across the lifespan. Rather than being fixed at birth, behavior emerges as genes are expressed, modified, or suppressed in response to developmental conditions, learning, and experience.

The theory of behavioral epigenesis was proposed by Zing-Yang Kuo, a Chinese psychologist associated with the behaviorist tradition (Qian et al. 2020). Kuo described behavioral epigenesis as the idea that every animal is shaped by its unique developmental history and will respond to a given stimulus in a particular way depending on the environmental context in which it occurs. In other words, behavior cannot be understood by genetics alone but must be viewed as the product of both inherited traits and lived experience.

Kuo conducted experimental work across multiple species to demonstrate this concept. In one well-known study, kittens raised in close contact with rats did not exhibit predatory behavior toward them as adults, illustrating how early experience can alter the expression of species-typical behaviors (Qian et al. 2020). As animals progress through different developmental stages, certain behavior-related genes may be activated or suppressed depending on exposure to specific stimuli – or the absence of such exposure.

Small genetic differences between individuals, combined with variation in environmental experiences, can result in markedly different behavioral outcomes. An individual pet's behavior therefore develops through a complex interplay between genetics and both positive and negative interactions encountered during development.

In summary, epigenesis describes the ongoing interaction between genes and environment throughout an animal's life, shaping behavior, temperament, and coping capacity as the animal matures into adulthood.

4.2.2 Socialization

Socialization is an *epigenetic process* through which animals learn to function as social members of their species via repeated exposure and interaction with conspecifics. Early interactions with parents, littermates, and other group members teach puppies and kittens how to interpret body language, regulate arousal, and engage in appropriate social behavior. In dogs, the primary socialization period typically occurs between approximately 3 and 12 weeks of age and in cats between 2 and 7 weeks. However, social development does not cease abruptly at the end of these windows; fixed developmental cutoffs are overly simplistic, and in some breeds and individuals, meaningful social learning continues well beyond these timeframes.

As puppies and kittens progress through development, behavioral changes occur simultaneously across multiple organizational levels – neurological, emotional, and social. These changes are not strictly linear and are often conditional on experience. Animals that receive little or inadequate social exposure may demonstrate impaired learning, heightened fear of people or other animals, exaggerated reactivity to stimuli, neophobia, and poor arousal regulation. Such responses may include barking and lunging at novel objects or people, hissing, swatting, freezing, avoidance, or escalated attempts to flee perceived threats.

Socialization should therefore be understood as an *ongoing process* rather than a finite developmental event. Research has shown that experiences occurring during juvenile and adolescent periods – after the primary socialization window – can have lasting behavioral effects. Serpell and Duffy found that prospective guide dogs raised by more experienced puppy raisers and in households with at least one other well-socialized, emotionally stable dog demonstrated lower levels of fear and aggression toward people and unfamiliar dogs (Serpell and Duffy 2016). Conversely, puppies exposed to frightening or threatening interactions showed significantly higher fear responses toward strangers and conspecifics. The study also identified breed-related differences in developmental sensitivity, with German Shepherd Dogs exhibiting increased stranger-directed aggression between 6 and 12 months of age, a pattern not observed in Golden Retrievers, Labrador Retrievers, or their crosses.

These findings underscore that behavioral sensitivity extends beyond early socialization and that negative experiences at any stage of development can have enduring consequences. Like humans, animals learn through association; when interactions with people or other animals are perceived as threatening, avoidance, fear-based responses, or aggression may emerge as coping strategies. While these responses may initially be directed toward a specific individual, they can generalize over time to broader categories, such as unfamiliar people or animals, shaping long-term temperament and behavior.

4.2.3 Prevalence and Patterns of Behavioral Disorders

Tiira et al. examined the prevalence and co-occurrence of behavior problems in dogs and found that anxiety-related conditions were common within the population (Tiira et al. 2016). Noise sensitivity was reported in 39.2% of dogs, general fearfulness in 26.2%, and separation anxiety in 17.2%. Significant comorbidity was observed, with fearful dogs showing higher rates of noise sensitivity and separation anxiety, as well as increased aggression, compared to nonfearful dogs. Noise sensitivity most commonly emerged around a median age of two years but showed a wide range of onset from 8 weeks to 10 years. Sensitivity to one type of loud noise was strongly correlated with similar responses to other loud stimuli, such as thunder, fireworks, and gunshots, highlighting the interconnected nature of anxiety-related behaviors.

Comparable patterns have been reported in cats, although prevalence estimates vary due to differences in study design and caregiver reporting. Feline behavior research consistently identifies fearfulness, anxiety-related behaviors, and aggression as among the most common concerns presented to veterinarians and behavior specialists (Amat et al. 2009). Cats frequently exhibit comorbidity between fear, stress-related behaviors, and elimination or aggression problems, particularly in environments with high unpredictability or limited perceived control. Noise sensitivity and startle responses have also been documented in cats, often co-occurring with generalized anxiety and environmental stress (Stella et al. 2013). As in dogs, early life experience, environmental stability, and individual temperament play a significant role in the development and expression of these behaviors, underscoring that anxiety-related disorders in cats are similarly multifactorial and interconnected.

4.2.4 How COVID Affected the Pet Population and Pet Owners

The COVID-19 pandemic had a profound and multifaceted impact on the pet population, both within shelters and in the broader community, while simultaneously altering the human–animal bond. Widespread lockdowns, remote work, and social restrictions reshaped how people acquired, cared for, and interacted with companion animals.

The behavioral effects observed in the pet population during and after the COVID-19 pandemic can be understood through the lenses of epigenesis and socialization. Pandemic-related changes – such as prolonged confinement; reduced exposure to unfamiliar people, animals, and environments; disrupted routines; and increased human presence – created atypical developmental conditions for many puppies and kittens during sensitive learning periods. From an epigenetic perspective, these environmental factors likely influenced the expression of behavior-related genes, shaping stress responses, emotional regulation, and coping strategies without altering genetic makeup. Limited or altered social experiences during early development reduced opportunities for pets to learn appropriate social cues, tolerance to novelty, and recovery from mild stressors. As a result, many animals entered adolescence or adulthood with diminished behavioral flexibility, heightened fear, or frustration responses and increased vulnerability to anxiety-related behaviors. These pandemic-driven developmental influences help explain the rise in behavior challenges observed in shelters, veterinary offices, and homes post-COVID and underscore the importance of interpreting behavior within the context of an animal's developmental history rather than viewing it as fixed or purely temperament-based.

The COVID-19 pandemic also had a complex impact on the shelter pet population, reshaping shelter intake patterns, daily animal care, and the human–animal bond across different regions. Widespread lockdowns, remote work, and social restrictions altered how people acquired and interacted with companion animals, leading many shelters to experience increased adoptions and foster placements while overall intake and owner relinquishment declined. In the United States, shelter intake dropped by approximately 23% in 2020 and owner surrenders decreased by roughly 20–24%, largely due to reduced public movement, limited access to services, and increased time spent at home (Powell et al. 2021). Similar trends were observed in the United Kingdom, where 4.6% of survey respondents reported adding a pet to their household during lockdown (Ratschen et al. 2020). Contrary to widespread concerns and some media narratives, intake did not surge above pre-pandemic levels once restrictions eased; instead, intake and relinquishment gradually returned toward, but generally remained below, 2019 baselines, and national surveys showed that most pandemic-acquired pets remained in their homes rather than being relinquished en masse.

Responses to the pandemic, however, were not uniform across countries. In Serbia, for example, the total pet acquisition in 2020 decreased by a factor of 2.67 compared with 2019 (Vučinić et al. 2022). Although adoption rates increased (61% in 2020 vs. 49% in 2019), pet purchases declined by approximately 1.5 times, likely reflecting reduced access to breeders and sellers, economic instability, and concerns about disease transmission. Across regions, lockdown conditions significantly altered pets' daily routines. Increased human presence was accompanied by reduced exposure to unfamiliar people, animals, and environments; fewer dog–dog interactions; and disrupted opportunities for social learning.

4.2.4.1 Separation-Related Behavior (SRB)

Media coverage widely predicted a surge in SRB once COVID-19 restrictions were lifted; however, available data present a more nuanced picture. In the United Kingdom, the proportion of dogs left alone for more than five minutes per day dropped markedly during lockdown, from 14.6% pre-pandemic to 58% during restrictions (Christley et al. 2021). Longitudinal studies found that the overall prevalence of SRB signs in the pet dog population actually decreased during lockdown, from 22.1% to 17.2% (Harvey et al. 2022). Nevertheless, approximately 9.9% of dogs developed new SRB signs by October 2020, with risks strongly associated with changes in time spent alone. Dogs whose alone time decreased the most during lockdown were at a greatest risk of developing SRB when left alone again, highlighting the role of routine disruption rather than the pandemic itself as the primary driver.

4.2.4.2 Impact on Puppies

Pandemic-related closures of dog-training facilities and restrictions on social interaction limited access to in-person guidance and early learning opportunities for many puppies. As a result, dogs acquired during the pandemic have been shown to exhibit higher rates of fear- and aggression-related behaviors in adulthood compared with dogs born after restrictions eased (Sacchettino et al. 2023). These findings support long-standing concerns among behavior professionals that reduced exposure to novel environments, visitors, other dogs, and routine veterinary handling during critical socialization periods negatively affected behavioral development.

4.2.4.3 Shelter Impacts

Analyses of shelter dogs during the COVID-19 quarantine period found increased kennel activity and movement compared to pre-pandemic observations, suggesting heightened arousal or frustration (Byosiere et al. 2022). This change was hypothesized to result from reduced enrichment opportunities, including limited walks, playgroups, and volunteer interaction due to staffing and safety restrictions.

In parallel, disruptions to routine veterinary services – particularly spay and neuter surgeries – caused by medical supply shortages, staffing limitations, and public health restrictions during COVID-19 further strained animal shelters. These interruptions led to increased intake pressure, delayed surgeries, prolonged length of stay, and growing backlogs that many communities are still working to recover from.

4.2.4.4 Injury Risk

Research conducted during the COVID-19 pandemic reported a significant increase in dog bite incidents directed toward children, with one study documenting an almost threefold rise in mean monthly cases compared to previous years (Tulloch et al. 2021). The authors suggested that this increase was likely associated with children spending substantially more time at home due to school closures, combined with increased opportunities for unsupervised interactions with dogs while caregivers were engaged in remote work. These findings highlight how changes in household structure and supervision can elevate injury risk, even in otherwise stable home environments.

4.2.4.5 Owner Well-Being and Pet-Related Effects

During COVID-19 lockdowns, many owners perceived their pets as an important source of emotional support. In the United Kingdom, pet ownership was associated with smaller declines in mental health scores and smaller increases in loneliness compared with non-pet owners. However, longitudinal studies reveal more complex findings. Research conducted in Hungary found that while acquiring a pet initially increased cheerfulness, this effect was short-lived – lasting approximately one to four months – and dog ownership was subsequently associated with declines in calmness, activity, cheerfulness, and overall life satisfaction (Mokos et al. 2025). Although some studies report positive mental and physical health benefits of pet ownership, others document increased stress related to caregiver burden, highlighting that the impact of pet ownership during the pandemic varied widely depending on individual circumstances, resources, and support systems (Applebaum et al. 2020).

In summary, understanding shelter pet behavior is much like examining a *layered cake*: At the base lies the pet's genetic predisposition, which sets the foundation for temperament and resilience; the middle layer reflects early experiences and socialization – both positive exposure and the absence of it – which shape how the pet interprets the world; and the top layer consists of

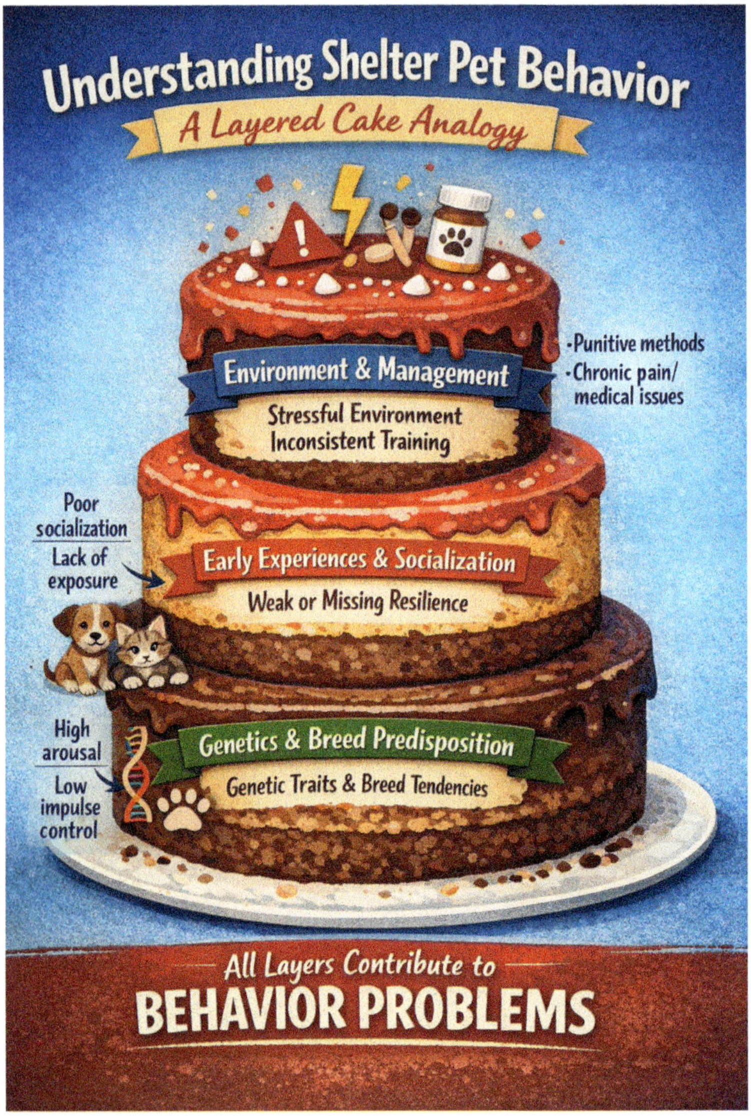

Figure 4.1 Layered Cake Analogy of Shelter Pet Behavior

the current environment, management practices, stressors, punitive handling, and chronic pain (see Figure 4.1). Together, these layers interact continuously, creating the behavior we observe and helping explain why each pet responds differently in a shelter setting.

References

Amat, M., de la Torre, J.L.R., Fatjó, J. et al. (2009). Potential risk factors associated with feline behaviour problems. *Applied Animal Behaviour Science* 121: 134–139. https://doi.org/10.1016/j.applanim.2009.09.012.

Applebaum, J.W., Tomlinson, C.A., Matijczak, A. et al. (2020). The concerns, difficulties, and stressors of caring for pets during covid-19: results from a large survey of U.S. pet owners. *Animals* 10 (10): 1–14. https://doi.org/10.3390/ani10101882.

Berger, J. and Haug, L.I. (2014). I know they're normal behaviors, but how do I fix them? In: *Decoding Your Dog* (ed. D.F. Horwitz, J. Ciribassi, and S. Dale), 127–149. New York: Houghton Mifflin Harcourt Publishing Company.

Byosiere, S.-E., Feighelstein, M., Wilson, K. et al. (2022). Evaluation of shelter dog activity levels before and during COVID-19 using automated analysis. *Applied Animal Behaviour Science*. Elsevier B.V. 250 (January): 105614. https://doi.org/10.1016/j.applanim.2022.105614.

Christley, R.M., Murray, J.K., Anderson, K.L. et al. (2021). Impact of the first COVID-19 lockdown on management of pet dogs in the UK. *Animals* 11 (1): 1–25. https://doi.org/10.3390/ani11010005.

Harvey, N.D., Christley, R.M., Giragosian, K. et al. (2022). Impact of changes in time left alone on separation-related behaviour in UK pet dogs. *Animals* 12 (4): https://doi.org/10.3390/ani12040482.

Mokos, J., Kubinyi, E., Ujfalussy, D.J. et al. (2025). Short-term effects of pet acquisition and loss on well-being in an unbiased sample during the COVID-19 pandemic. *Scientific Reports* 15 (1): 1–17. https://doi.org/10.1038/s41598-025-06987-7.

Powell, L., Houlihan, C., Stone, M. et al. (2021). Animal shelters' response to the COVID-19 pandemic: a pilot survey of 14 shelters in the Northeastern United States. *Animals* 11 (9): 1–13. https://doi.org/10.3390/ani11092669.

Qian, Y., Chen, W., and Guo, B. (2020). Zing-Yang Kuo and behavior epigenesis based on animal experiments. *Protein & Cell*. Higher Education Press 11 (6): 387–390. https://doi.org/10.1007/s13238-018-0516-9.

Ratschen, E., Shoesmith, E., Shahab, L. et al. (2020). Human-animal relationships and interactions during the Covid-19 lockdown phase in the UK: investigating links with mental health and loneliness. *PLoS One* 15 (9): e0239397. https://doi.org/10.1371/journal.pone.0239397.

Sacchettino, L., Gatta, C., Chirico, A. et al. (2023). Puppies raised during the COVID-19 lockdown showed fearful and aggressive behaviors in adulthood: an Italian survey. *Veterinary Sciences* 10 (3): 198. https://doi.org/10.3390/vetsci10030198.

Serpell, J.A. and Duffy, D.L. (2016). Aspects of juvenile and adolescent environment predict aggression and fear in 12-month-old guide dogs. *Frontiers in Veterinary Science* 3 (JUN): 1–8. https://doi.org/10.3389/fvets.2016.00049.

Stella, J., Croney, C., and Buffington, T. (2013). Effects of stressors on the behavior and physiology of domestic cats. *Applied Animal Behaviour Science*. Elsevier B.V. 143 (2–4): 157–163. https://doi.org/10.1016/j.applanim.2012.10.014.

Tiira, K., Sulkama, S., and Lohi, H. (2016). Prevalence, comorbidity, and behavioral variation in canine anxiety. *Journal of Veterinary Behavior: Clinical Applications and Research* 16: 36–44. https://doi.org/10.1016/j.jveb.2016.06.008.

Tulloch JSP, Minford S, Pimblett V, Rotheram M, Christley RM, Westgarth C. Paediatric emergency department dog bite attendance during the COVID-19 pandemic: an audit at a tertiary children's hospital. *BMJ Paediatrics Open*. 2021;5:e001040. https://doi.org/https://doi.org/10.1136/bmjpo-2021-001040

Vučinić, M., Nenadović, K., and Vučićević, M. (2022). Type and manner of pet acquisition during covid 19 in Serbia. *Journal of Veterinary Behavior*. Elsevier Inc. 48: 49–55. https://doi.org/10.1016/j.jveb.2021.07.004.

5

Behavioral Assessment in Shelters

5.1 Importance of Behavioral and Welfare Assessments

Animal shelters face immense pressure because most pets arrive with little to no medical or behavioral history. It is therefore essential to gather as much information as possible upon admissions to ensure that each animal has the best chance for a positive shelter journey. Within hours of arrival, shelters are often tasked with determining key details such as species, breed, age, and even reproductive status. Equally important is assessing each pet's physical and mental health, identifying any concerns that require treatment or management, and documenting these findings accurately before the pet becomes available for adoption.

These initial evaluations are critical – not only for safeguarding the pet's immediate wellbeing within its new and often stressful environment but also for helping predict potential outcomes. Medical and behavioral findings must be triaged promptly so that care decisions can be made efficiently. Admission assessments influence how pets are housed, the level of husbandry and enrichment they require, and whether medical or behavioral treatment is necessary. Ultimately, these early decisions shape resource allocation across the organization and directly impact both individual wellbeing and the overall scope of sustainability (SoS).

Animal shelter teams face numerous challenges, one of the most difficult being the need to make quick yet rational decisions regarding an animal's fate. Decision-making is the process of selecting the best course of action among several possible alternatives. In the shelter environment, this process often requires a delicate balance between rational thinking informed by limited data, intuition shaped by years of experience, and emotional considerations that inevitably accompany working with vulnerable animals. At its core, effective decision-making involves recognizing a problem or situation, evaluating available options, and choosing the most appropriate path forward – always with the wellbeing of the animal, team members, and the mission of the organization in mind.

Many factors contribute to the difficulty of making decisions for animals in shelters, including:

1) Time pressure: In animal shelters, constant time pressure often forces rapid decisions based on limited information. Balancing the need for quick action with thoughtful consideration is one of the greatest challenges faced by shelter professionals. These high-stress situations can increase the risk of impulsive or less optimal choices, highlighting the need for clear protocols and structured decision-making frameworks.
2) Emotions: Emotions can cloud judgment or, conversely, provide valuable insights. In particular, animal sheltering is a very emotional business at its core, and while fear-based emotions may lead to overly cautious decisions, excitement may lead to taking unnecessary chances.

3) Cognitive biases: These biases are mental shortcuts or heuristics that can simplify decision-making but also can lead to errors in thinking. Examples include favoring information that confirms existing beliefs (confirmation bias), relying too heavily on the first piece of information (anchoring bias), and basing judgments on readily available information (availability bias). We all fall victim to our own biases, and it is critical to be self-aware in order to make more informed and rational choices, especially under pressure.
4) Social pressure: Decisions can be influenced by others, whether it's colleagues, leadership, volunteers, donors, board members, or the society at large. Animal shelter settings are subject to social pressures that cannot be underestimated. It is easy to burn out in this field if we have to make decisions that don't align with our values or true desires.
5) Personal values and beliefs strongly influence decision-making. For an organization to be successful, it must clearly communicate and consistently operate according to its mission, vision, and values. Likewise, individuals should understand their own values and honestly assess whether they align with the organization's. When alignment is lacking, it may be necessary for the individual to seek a different role or cause that better fits their personal principles.

Ultimately, effective decision-making about the shelter pet's wellbeing isn't about making the perfect choice all the time; it's about making the best choice with the information available and learning from the results. This involves a logical and systematic approach, documentation and collection of facts, analysis, and clear set of criteria.

5.2 Formal Behavioral Evaluation Protocols – Science Behind It

A vital part of decision-making in animal shelters involves evaluating and categorizing an animal's behavior and temperament. Temperament refers to the animal's innate nature – traits the animal is born with or that have been selectively bred for in purpose-bred animals. Unlike behavior, temperament tends to remain relatively stable over time.

Those decisions ultimately determine the pet's shelter journey, trajectory, resolution, and ultimately its fate. When deciding on a shelter pet's admission to a resolution flow plan, considerations must extend beyond the mutual enjoyment of the adopter and the pet to include the safety of the family and the broader community where the pet will live. It is for this reason that animal shelters have been working on trying to develop reliable, repeatable, feasible, and predictive testing tools for decades.

The idea started with the first formal psychological test signifying an important development in the realm of standardized measurement instruments, published by van der Borg et al. (1991). This work is considered foundational in the field and advanced the use of systematic behavioral assessments in shelter environments. van der Borg et al. (1991) developed a structured shelter behavior test battery designed to "*predict*" later problem behaviors – including aggression, fear, obedience issues, and separation-related problems. This test represented a culmination of work focused on designing an instrument that was theoretically grounded, empirically validated, and statistically robust – a hallmark of the rigorous psychometric practices that were being emphasized in the early 1990s. Their study is cited frequently as one of the earliest and most influential attempts to empirically validate in-shelter assessments for predicting postadoption behavior. The paper added to the growing body of literature around empirical assessments, influencing how constructs were operationalized and measured. Consequently, various animal temperament tests were developed and tested over the years, such as the American Society for Prevention of Cruelty to Animals (ASPCA)'s Safety Assessment for Evaluating Rehoming (SAFER), Canine Behavioral Assessment and Research questionnaire (C-BARQ) (Hsu and Serpell 2003), Matchup II (Marder et al. 2013), Sue Sternberg's Assess-a-Pet, etc., to name a few.

The results of such tests should, in the ideal case, ensure safe placement and humane treatment of the animals. They should also help understand the individual needs based on the pets' behavior and temperament. They aim to reduce stress and improve the success rate and safety of adoptable or rehabilitated animals. With such tests, we wish to help shelter teams, potential adopters, and volunteers gain insights into how a pet might behave in various situations and environments. We hope to see how they interact with various people and other animals and whether they have any behavioral challenges that need addressing before or after adoption. Findings of such testing intend to ensure better matching, a smoother transition into their new homes, and ideally reduce the likelihood of future behavioral issues or returns. While shelter workers and scientists disagree on the approach to such testing, most agree that logical, systematic methods should be followed, based on facts, analysis, and a clear set of criteria.

Authors reviewing the van der Borg data have recalculated sensitivity, positive predictive value (PPV), as well as negative predictive value (NPV) from the published data and concluded that a positive test result had a substantial false-positive rate – i.e. many dogs labeled problematic in the shelter did not show those behaviors in the home (Patronek et al. 2019; Clay et al. 2020a). Subsequent empirical re-evaluations by researchers like Christensen (2007) and others tracked in follow-up field studies adopted dogs and found substantial rates of postadoption aggression even among dogs that "passed" shelter tests and conversely that many failing dogs improved at home – reinforcing limited predictive power (Christensen et al. 2007). Poulsen et al. (2010) and later investigators evaluated variants of shelter test batteries and emphasized methodological issues (standardization, interrater reliability, and test timing) that affect predictive validity (Poulsen et al. 2010).

In more recent years, those existing "standardized" temperament tests have come under further scrutiny. Patronek, in his 2016 paper "*No Better Than Flipping a Coin*," critically examines the reliability of current animal temperament and behavior assessments in shelter animals (Patronek and Bradley 2016). He and his team of researchers argued that many standardized tests are not consistently predictive of future behavior or even suitability for adoption matching. The authors highlight the variability and limitations of these tests, suggesting that reliance on them can lead to misjudgments and unfavorable outcomes for animals.

Things began to change as major shelter organizations revisited long-standing assumptions about in-shelter behavior evaluations. In its *Position Statement on Shelter Dog Behavior Assessments*, the ASPCA (2018) emphasized that shelters should gather as much information as possible about a dog's behavior – but that "behavior assessments have not proven highly accurate or precise when used to predict aggression after adoption" and such decisions *should not be based solely on a dog's behavior during a single assessment* unless the aggression is truly egregious. The statement also urges shelters to balance information gathering with the overarching goal of moving dogs into homes or appropriate placements as quickly as feasible.

Increasingly, animal welfare advocates are demanding a more holistic, individualized approach to assessing animal welfare and behavior, rather than overestimating the predictive power of standardized tests in which animals are placed in artificial situations and subjected to battery tests. Historically, these assessments focused on observing an animal's reactions to staged scenarios such as being approached by strangers, being handled near high-value food items, interacting with other animals, or responding to physical restraint, sudden noises, or fast movements.

In response to concerns about these artificial setups, some shelters have shifted toward gathering behavior information from the person surrendering the pet. While this approach can provide useful context, it also does not always offer a complete or accurate picture. Owner reports may reflect different environments, management styles, or expectations, and they often fail to predict how the animal will behave under shelter conditions – or in a future home.

Research has shown that many traditional shelter behavior questionnaires and assessments may be biased or limited in their ability to characterize dogs' true behavior, particularly when owner reporting and shelter conditions differ. Segurson et al. (2005), for example, evaluated a behavioral intake questionnaire and found significant discrepancies in reported problem behaviors based on context and reporting conditions. Highlighting the challenges of using these tools as reliable predictors of future behavior (Segurson et al. 2005).

The main question remains: Does behavior and temperament testing improve animal welfare, enhance the adoption success, and result in placing pets in homes where they can thrive?

Here is the crux of temperament testing for shelter pets: ***Sensitivity and Specificity***

Science has shown that there is no test to date that accurately predicts a pet's future behavior in an adopter's home environment. The challenge lies in the predictive value or *sensitivity and specificity* of such tests. Sensitivity and specificity are two key metrics used to evaluate diagnostic screening tests. They tell us how *trustworthy* and *effective* a test is at identifying an individual with or without a certain medical or behavioral condition. They inform us of how well a test identifies *true positives* and *true negatives*. Sensitivity and specificity matter because they are essential for making informed case trajectory decisions.

The *sensitivity* of a test measures the proportion of an individual with the *condition correctly identified* by the test. High sensitivity means few false negatives.

Example: A dog displaying food aggression during a temperament test in the shelter remains food aggressive in a home environment.

Advocates of adopting that dog out despite positive test results don't believe that the test performed was sensitive. They are willing to take the risk of making the dog available for adoption despite a positive test result because the test may have been false. After all, the dog that tested aggressively in the shelter may be friendly in the new home. The test would not be sensitive, and the test failed the dog.

The *specificity* of a test measures the proportion of individuals without the condition who are *correctly identified as negative*. High specificity means few false positives.

Example: A dog that does NOT react aggressively during the food test in the shelter temperament test remains friendly in any home environment around food.

Advocates of putting pets through a set of rigorous or repeated testing before adopting don't trust their test is specific. They are not willing to take the risk and are holding pets back for repeated testing before adoption. Their internal dialogue may include, "What if the pet was not correctly identified as negative? What if the test yielded an incorrect result with a kibble diet, but with a chew bone would be positive. How about canned food? How about we test the pet again tomorrow?" The pet that tested negative in the shelter may be aggressive in the new home when given a rawhide bone due to the different context.

What does science say about food aggression testing in the shelter?

A retrospective cohort study at the Animal Rescue League of Boston compared shelter behavior evaluations with owner reports of food aggression after adoption (Marder et al. 2013). Ninety-seven dogs were assessed using the Match-Up II program. Of the 20 dogs labeled food aggressive (FA+) in the shelter, only 55% showed the behavior at home. Among the 77 dogs labeled FA−, 22% were still reported to display food aggression postadoption. Thus, shelter detection of food aggression had limited predictive value, while the absence of aggression in the shelter was a better indicator of its absence in the home.

Perhaps the most striking finding was that most adopters – including those whose dogs showed food aggression in the home – did not consider the behavior a serious problem. Nearly all respondents stated that they would adopt the same dog again, regardless of food-related aggression.

Such findings challenge the overall value of formal food-aggression testing in shelters, particularly given the substantial time, effort, and resources required. This raises a critical question for shelters and behavior programs: If traditional evaluations have limited predictive accuracy and low perceived relevance to adopters, how can we best identify traits such as friendliness, fear, aggression, or adaptability and use them to match pets and adopters in a way that promotes safe, successful placements? What makes this issue even more complicated is that variability in testing conditions – such as differences in environment, handler skills, animal stress levels, and prior experiences – can produce inconsistent results.

Human psychologists recognize that judging personality from a single encounter is often inaccurate. Similarly, a pet's behavior can vary with environment, stress, and social interactions, so multiple observations over time and in various situations are necessary. Individual differences among animals further compound the variability seen in shelter behavior evaluations, leading to significant disagreement about the reliability and predictive value of such tests for ensuring successful adoptions and safe placements.

Structured, consistent behavior observations allow shelters to identify behavioral patterns, inform decisions about housing, training, and adoption and support the pet's wellbeing. Evaluations are not meant to predict the future with certainty, but to minimize risks and ensure each pet is placed in a suitable environment where it can thrive, promoting positive results for both pets and adopters.

5.3 Contemporary Approach on How to Conduct Behavior Assessments in Shelter Pets

5.3.1 Problem-Oriented Veterinary Behavioral Record (POVBR)

Any behavior assessment should be conducted in a timely manner, with objective data collected and findings documented in a clear, efficient, and transparent manner. In the end, the data should improve animal wellbeing, inform case trajectory strategies (CTS), and result in adoptable pets being placed in suitable environments. A structured approach to behavior observations is to record them in the *Problem-Oriented Veterinary Behavioral Record (POVBR)*. This is a document that aims to summarize the behavior and welfare status of pets. It emphasizes the importance of making informed, thoughtful decisions to achieve a positive resolution for both pets and adopters. Analyzing past behaviors and observing patterns based on existing data allow us to make better predictions about pets' coping strategies and adaptability to new situations and environments (Clay et al. 2020b). It is the goal of this type of documentation that anyone trained in the approach can and should collect and document observations.

Problem-oriented approaches are not new. This chapter focuses on applying them to animal shelter behavioral health and wellbeing. Many shelters already use health charts to track appetite, elimination, and emotional status (see Chapter 7). Extending this approach to pets with specific behavioral concerns or conditions allows shelter team members to confidently address issues, design targeted treatment plans, and improve CTS and resolution.

It begins with compiling a comprehensive problem list, which forms the basis for developing management or treatment plans for behavioral issues. Like medical conditions, behaviors must be recorded objectively, transparently, and measurably. While this practice may initially feel unfamiliar, accurate documentation allows timely intervention, informs prognosis, and supports sound, data-driven decision-making in the shelter.

To create a POVBR document, we use four categories – commonly called *SOAP* – to systematically collect information, interpret it, and develop a treatment plan.

5.3.1.1 "S" for Subjective Data

Subjective information includes observations and reports about the pet – its history, behaviors, and interactions as described by owners, team members, or volunteers. This may involve emotional interpretations, anthropomorphism, or lay "diagnoses." While such input should be recorded with care, it provides valuable context for understanding the pet's behavior and needs.

Challenges and Tips: How is information tracked in the shelter and who records it? The most effective approach is nonjudgmental, using open-ended questions or a standardized intake form to ensure accurate, consistent documentation.

5.3.1.2 "O" for Objective Data

Objective information includes measurable, observable data collected by trained personnel and updated consistently throughout a pet's journey. It is especially valuable when pets are transferred, helping evaluate progress, treatment effectiveness, and guide care decisions. Accurate objective data also supports prognostic assessment, reflects wellbeing over time, and promotes clear communication among all team members, veterinarians, and adopters.

Challenges and Tips: Team members must be trained to document objectively. Key questions include: How is information tracked and recorded? Who records it and who is trained to evaluate it? Video surveillance – during playtime, out-of-shelter experiences, or in foster homes – can be very useful. Having multiple trained observers helps ensure consistency and reliability.

5.3.1.3 "A" for Assessment

Along with documenting observed problems, a thorough analysis of the situation is conducted – often the most challenging step in the SOAP process. Collecting objective data is essential and provides a factual, unbiased foundation for evaluating a pet's health and behavior. Comprehensive analysis identifies underlying issues, supports targeted treatment plans, and enables well-informed decisions that improve case resolution. The assessment summarizes the evaluator's impressions, offering an objective description of observed behaviors. Any trained team member or volunteer familiar with behavior documentation can perform these assessments.

The Assessment Should Answer the Following Three Key Questions

1) Triggers: What elicits or does not elicit the wanted or unwanted behavior? Who or what sets it off? Who or what makes the pet calm?
2) Thresholds: When, where, how, and how often does the behavior occur – or not occur?
3) Motivation: Why is the behavior happening? Understanding this requires careful, objective observation and interpretation of body language. In most cases, additional or specialized training is needed to answer this question accurately.

With an accurate history and careful observations, these key questions can be answered, guiding the CTS and creating an individualized care plan for pets with behavioral challenges.

Challenges and Tips: Team members must be trained to read subjective and objective data to reach objective conclusions for an assessment. It is important to clarify who conducts the evaluation, and having multiple trained observers ensures consistency and accuracy.

5.3.1.4 "P" for Plan

A well-structured plan is crucial for ensuring that the pet receives timely and appropriate care and treatment based on the collected data. The plan outlines the necessary steps and interventions required to address any identified issues, providing a clear roadmap for team members and volunteers to follow. This helps to ensure that everyone is aligned in their efforts, leading to more consistent and effective care for the pets in the shelter.

Included in any comprehensive plan should be the following:

- CTS: Resolution options, treatment options, prognosis, expected length of stay (LOS), and end-point discussions.
- Resolution options: Adoption, return to owner, return to field, foster, transfer, and euthanasia.
- Management: Avoiding triggers, keeping below threshold, providing appropriate enrichment, and choice of humane tools.
- Treatment: Behavior modification steps, with or without psychotropic medications or nutraceuticals.
- Education to leadership, DVMs, teams, volunteers, adopters, and all other stakeholders.

Challenges and Tips: Assess plans frequently and adjust as needed. If there is no progress, revise or discontinue the plan. Always set a timeline, monitor outcomes, and maintain transparency throughout the process.

5.3.2 Creating the Problem List

This process involves compiling all available data and problems for a pet. Both behavioral and medical concerns must be included in the problem list compilation. By identifying all the problems, we get a more complete picture of the pet. Based on the problem list, a detailed CTS and care plan can be developed and carried out, and a prognosis may be presented. A problem list needs to be compiled as early as possible in the process of a pet's shelter stay. This allows for the development of an appropriate journey and efficient and sustainable use of an organization's resources.

Accurate history-taking provides the data for the problem list, using all available information. This ensures that relevant details are considered, supporting an effective problem list and a targeted CTS – in some cases helping to identify interventions before a pet even enters the shelter.

5.3.2.1 Where Does the Information Come From?

5.3.2.1.1 Intake Information

This data is often subjective. It is the pet's story. It allows for what untrained people say, including emotional interpretations, anthropomorphism, or lay term "diagnosis." It is appropriate to limit, but not to disregard, such information. It can be collected with a combination of open- and closed-ended questions or an intake questionnaire. Most importantly, people providing this type of information should never feel judged.

Type of History for Shelter Pets

Owner surrender: Pre-surrender interviews or forms can be used to learn as much as possible about the medical and behavioral history of the pet to be surrendered. When we learn more about the pet, providing behavioral or medical resources to the owner can delay or prevent surrender in an ideal setting.

Stray/surrender: In the case of an animal surrendered as a stray, the finder typically has some information about where, how, and when the pet was found, captured, and transported. All of that information should be documented. In order to simplify the process and ensure consistency in documentation, template forms can be helpful.

Return to shelter: No matter how long a pet lived in the home, if they are returned to the shelter, they should be treated as if surrendered by their owner. Any time spent in a home can provide a lot of relevant information.

Custody cases: A shelter often faces the most challenges when it comes to custody cases. By using the data provided here, we can strive to provide the correct form of enrichment and a better environment for the pet and improve its wellbeing during its often long stays.

Other intakes: Regardless of how a pet enters the shelter, any type of information collected can be useful and should not be underestimated or neglected to capture in the POVBR.

5.3.2.1.2 Information from Observations

Objective Documentation and the Importance of Measurable, Descriptive Data Accurate and objective documentation is essential for assessing behavior, guiding treatment planning, and ensuring consistent communication across teams. Behavioral data should be recorded as it is observed, not as it is interpreted. This distinction is critical in shelter settings, where decisions must be based on factual, reproducible information rather than assumptions or subjective impressions.

For example, instead of stating that a dog is "freaked out" or is a "scaredy cat," the record should accurately reflect what the observer saw:

- *"When the handler reached toward the dog, the dog lowered its head, crouched, pulled its ears backwards, tucked its tail, dilated its pupils and growled."*

This type of description provides *specific, observable, measurable data*, removing personal interpretation or bias. Not all team members or volunteers will initially be able to identify multiple behavioral cues, but even reporting one observable detail (e.g. "*ears back*" and "*tail tucked*") is valuable. Over time, as training increases awareness, team members will naturally develop greater skills in noticing and describing behaviors in detail.

Objective documentation also applies to incidents of aggression. Any form of aggression – especially bites – must be recorded using a numerical bite scale rather than subjective terms such as *snapping*, *nipping*, or *mauling*. Such terms vary widely in meaning and may minimize or exaggerate the seriousness of the event.

Using structured rating tools ensures consistency. While the Dunbar and Yin scales are widely used, the authors suggest a Bite Severity Classification (BSC) that focuses on contact and injury severity without requiring detailed anatomical assessment (see Table 5.1). This makes it more practical for shelter team members and volunteers who may not be trained to interpret wound depth or tissue damage.

Whenever possible, photographs of injuries should be included in the record to support documentation and enhance accuracy.

Table 5.1 Bite Severity Classification

Level	Severity Category	Description
1	No Contact	Warning signals only: growling, freezing, hissing, spit-stomping (cats), air snap, lunging without contact
2	Contact, No Injury	Contact with clothing, leash, or skin without visible marks or injury
3	Contact with Minor Injury	Bruising, red marks, torn clothing; skin intact with no puncture or abrasion
4	Broken Skin – Superficial Injury	Scratches or shallow punctures affecting the surface layer of skin only
5	Broken Skin – Deep Injury	Full-thickness puncture or abrasion where the tooth penetrates through the outer skin layer
6	Multiple Deep Injuries	Multiple (>2) deep punctures and/or one significant deep laceration
7	Sustained Attack	Grab-and-shake, failure to release without external intervention and/or fatal injury

The Problem List: A Foundation for Data-Driven Case Planning The problem list is a consolidated summary of all concerns identified at admissions into the shelter and during ongoing shelter observations. It should:

- Use a numerical format.
- Provide clear, objective descriptions for each problem.
- Include both behavioral and medical issues.
- Be updated regularly as new information becomes available.

A detailed, objective problem list helps determine how many challenges an animal presents with, which in turn guides the CTS, including:

- Medical evaluation.
- Treatment planning.
- Safety considerations.
- Need for foster placement.
- Suitability for behavior modification.
- Adoption counseling or risk communication.

An example of a detailed problem list for a two-year-old, 60 lbs, male neutered mix breed dog in shelter X in California, created five hours after admission.

Problem List

1) Diarrhea: Watery, eating and drinking well, no vomiting.
2) Hacking coughing: Nonproductive, Temp 102.3, bright and alert.
3) Growling when restrained for medical treatment – ears back/tail down otherwise loose body language when meeting unfamiliar people or other dogs.
4) Cowering at loud or sudden noises such as doors slamming in shelter – ears back/tail down, not able to accept treats during these events.

Integrating medical and behavioral information into a unified record is essential for comprehensive care and effective decision-making. In many shelters, medical and behavioral issues are documented separately, often in different systems. This separation can obscure a pet's overall welfare, leading to miscommunication, prolonged suffering, caregiver stress, and inefficient use of resources.

Ideally, a diagnosis can be made for each listed problem before making a treatment plan. A diagnosis is the identification of the nature of an illness or other problem by examination of the clinical signs, interpreting test results and naming the medical condition (e.g. "canine parvovirus" or "hip dysplasia" or "separation anxiety" or "fear aggression"). In most countries, including the United States, United Kingdom, Canada, and Australia, diagnosing a disease or condition in animals is a legally restricted act. This is part of the Veterinary Practice Act (or equivalent), which defines what only a licensed veterinarian is allowed to do. Veterinarians receive extensive training and unique ability to recognize complex patterns of clinical signs, rule out differentials, and understand how conditions can interact or present across species.

In reality, in most shelters, it is often impossible to determine the full etiology of a behavior or medical issue. Commonly, clinicians must choose treatments based on a *"working" diagnosis*. Importantly, only veterinarians can legally diagnose medical or behavioral conditions; animal trainers, nonveterinary behaviorists, vet techs, shelter staff, and pet owners cannot. Creating a problem list, however, is not diagnosing. Team members can be trained to observe and report behaviors – e.g. "This dog shows signs of fear – as determined by body language – when approached by strangers" – without labeling it as a medical or behavioral diagnosis. This distinction is critical: misdiagnosis by unqualified individuals can worsen conditions, lead to inappropriate treatment, compromise animal wellbeing, and create legal liability for the organization.

A problem list ideally leads to a diagnosis, guiding treatment of specific medical or behavioral conditions, improving resource use, and providing a prognosis. However, trained team members can accurately document behavior observations and success criteria and measure progress without making a medical or behavioral diagnosis.

5.3.3 Designing the Behavior Treatment Plan

The treatment plan for any behavioral challenge – whether at home or in a shelter – requires a structured, multifaceted approach based on a five-step process. Completion typically takes six to eight weeks, though timelines vary with the individual animal, the severity or chronicity of the condition, and available resources. While shelters may not implement all five steps fully, familiarity with Steps 1–3 is essential, as they form the foundation of any effective behavioral intervention.

The program is flexible: Steps can be applied independently or in combination, depending on the pet, case specifics, shelter resources, and handler expertise. This subchapter outlines a *generic treatment framework* that can be adapted to address a wide range of behavioral problems in shelter pets.

5.3.3.1 Step 1. Management

The first and most critical step in any behavioral treatment plan includes safety measures and avoidance strategies. This step is critical as it focuses on managing the condition rather than treating it. The goal is to prevent the behavior from worsening and to protect both the pet and those interacting with it.

This step is similar to giving a dog with diarrhea a bland diet – while not curing the condition specifically, it will prevent further harm. For aggressive behavior, avoiding triggers that elicit the unwanted behaviors reduces injury risk, lowers stress, and increases the chances of a positive outcome. Safety and avoidance can begin once a problem list and behavioral triggers have been identified and require no specialized tools – just structured management, consistent handling, and clear communication among teams and volunteers.

Strict management forms the foundation of any behavioral plan, enabling safe progress in subsequent steps. However, avoiding triggers in a shelter can be challenging due to unpredictable environments, high noise levels, limited space, and frequent changes in caretakers. If triggers cannot be reliably avoided, it may indicate that the shelter is not suitable for caring for that pet, prompting consideration of alternatives such as foster placement, transfer to a specialized facility, immediate adoption, or even compassionate euthanasia.

Even if early progress seems slow, consistent avoidance is essential. Every rehearsal of unwanted behavior strengthens it, making prevention critical to rehabilitation. All interactions should be documented in the POVBR, noting when behaviors occurred or were successfully avoided, to support objective decision-making and track progress.

Ultimately, avoidance serves both as a safety measure and a treatment strategy, protecting team members, volunteers, and pets while improving the likelihood of successful behavior modification.

5.3.3.2 Step 2. Interactions and Environment

Predictability and structure are the two components lacking for most pets in shelters. However, they are essential for creating a stable and reliable environment. Stress and anxiety can occur in an environment that is unpredictable and where the pet has no control. This stress can manifest itself in medical or behavioral issues, such as excessive barking, destructive behavior, or even aggression. This may further reduce their chances of being interacted with while at the shelter or adopted. Additionally, an unpredictable environment can hinder their ability to form positive relationships with humans, impacting their overall wellbeing. When pets know what to expect, they feel more secure and are more predictable in their own behavior. Predictable routines and structured processes help pets and care teams alike. Behavior modification is more efficient, and it reduces misunderstandings or errors.

Ways to achieve predictability with pets in shelters are by providing time-scheduled interactions, creating pleasant in-kennel experiences, and making every interaction with humans enjoyable and uniform. A good way to achieve this is by using a consistent approach to rewarding positive behaviors every time they are noticed. We have to stress here that a punishment-based approach causes more harm than good. It can lead to increased fear and anxiety in pets, making them more likely to exhibit aggressive, fearful, or avoidant behaviors. Furthermore, punishment can damage trust between the animals and their caregivers. This hinders the development of the strong, positive bond necessary for successful rehabilitation and adoption (see Chapter 9).

5.3.3.3 Step 3. Tools

The goal of step 3 is to gather, acquire, or collect any objects, devices, tools, and humane equipment needed to carry out a specific task and implement a behavior modification plan more efficiently or accurately. Using such tools should enhance the handler's abilities, simplify their tasks, and improve the welfare of shelter animals. The list is endless and can be broken down into categories.

Physical tools: Set up specific training areas, leashes, baby gates, kennels, crates, screen doors, window coverings, tethers, head halters, harnesses, basket muzzles, clickers, target sticks, remote feed or toy dispensers, treats and treat pouches, relaxation mats, treadmills, different kinds of litterboxes and litter, nail caps, scratching posts, anxiety wraps, calming caps, ear muffs, toys, balls, treadmill, noise canceling machines, mobiles, various surfaces, stairs, etc.
Digital tools: Video cameras, radios, TV, computers, laptops, tablets, phones, recording systems software, Microsoft Excel, Adobe, Salesforce, AI, Photoshop, etc.
Cognitive tools: Feed or toy dispensing devices, food puzzle games, relaxation music (Through a dog's ear), various scents, safe herbs, etc.
Scientific tools: Thermometer, decibel meter, etc.
Educational tools: Training material, PowerPoint, books, lectures, YouTube videos, simulations, learning apps, etc.

5.3.3.4 Step 4. Reintroduction and Exposure

The pet must be prepared for exposure and reintroduction to triggers or situations that elicit problem behaviors, while continuing Step 1 avoidance. Reintroduction occurs gradually, once the pet has learned and practiced basic behaviors that are incompatible with unwanted behaviors and help focus attention on the handler (e.g. sitting quietly instead of lunging, looking at the handler instead of fixating on an object) in the absence of the trigger(s).

These behaviors should first be practiced and rewarded in a calm environment or at a distance from the trigger, allowing the pet to remain relaxed and focused. With this technique, over time, the pet learns to associate previously stressful stimuli with calm behavior and positive outcomes, reducing unwanted responses.

Using a cue-response-reward (C-R-R) approach reinforces reliable performance of trained behaviors in different situations. Consistently recognizing and rewarding behaviors incompatible with unwanted actions builds confidence, provides clear expectations, and facilitates a smoother transition into an adopter's home. This approach is simple to apply and transfers easily to a new home, providing additional consistency for the pet.

A series of gradual steps and intensities is used to reintroduce triggers identified during assessment – this is *desensitization with counterconditioning (DS/CC)* (see Chapter 9). Common methods involve altering the intensity or distance of the stimulus, such as location, loudness, speed, movement, duration, type of stimulus, or its response. DS/CC begins at the *lowest intensity* that elicits no signs of unwanted behavior, anxiety, or concern. The stimulus is presented while the pet is rewarded for relaxed, positive behaviors. Short, repeated sessions reinforce these responses, always ending with a reward. Depending on the severity and chronicity of the condition, this process can take weeks, months, or a lifetime.

In shelter settings, pets should not be expected to complete this step before adoption. It is more realistic to provide a trigger-free environment or ensure transparency with adopters, informing them of the need to continue the plan at home as needed.

5.3.3.5 Step 5. Medications and Nutraceuticals

Psychoactive medications and anxiety-reducing nutraceuticals are often included in treatment plans for pets with behavioral problems. They are especially helpful when triggers cannot be fully avoided or when fear and anxiety significantly disrupt daily functioning. Medications may also be indicated for severe, chronic, or treatment-resistant behaviors, as they can lower overall arousal or fear, making the pet more receptive to learning, behavior modification, and improving overall well-being and safety.

These types of medication can improve the pet's anxiety and improve learning. It can decrease the pet's reactivity and increase their responsiveness. Some medication will take effect faster, while others may take longer to reach full effect. The medical team needs to consider any health concerns when prescribing psychoactive drugs. The medical team must work closely with the behavior and adoption teams. It is essential that all team members involved in the pet's care – including veterinarians, behavior team, management, and adoption counselors – are informed about the CTS, the expected LOS, and whether the pet can or should be adopted while on these medications. Clear communication ensures consistency in care and transparency with potential adopters and supports appropriate follow-up and monitoring to maintain the pet's wellbeing and treatment success.

The medical team should be regularly updated on behavioral changes to assess medication efficacy. These medications are rarely a cure and should always be part of a documented management plan. Used judiciously, they can improve animal welfare and they should not be reserved as a last resort, as delaying treatment can allow conditions to worsen.

Most psychoactive medications for shelter pets are used off-label; therefore if the pet is adopted while on such medications, adopters must be informed of potential side effects and interactions with other medications. Anxiety-reducing supplements and pheromones can also provide valuable support, either as stand-alone interventions for milder cases or as adjuncts to medication, promoting emotional stability and overall wellbeing (see Chapter 10).

5.4 Behavioral Health Assessment Staging (BHAS)

5.4.1 BHAS as a Behavioral Triage and Monitoring System – See Appendix C for the Guide

The Behavioral Health Assessment Staging (BHAS) is a structured monitoring system developed by the author (WS) to support objective, consistent decision-making for shelter pets with behavioral concerns. Once a shelter pet has been identified with a behavior condition or problem and an individualized behavior plan has been established, the BHAS is implemented to track progress and guide the CTS.

Conceptually, BHAS aligns with the Asilomar Accords framework by supporting transparent, welfare-based decision-making; however, it differs in function and purpose. While Asilomar categories classify shelter pets by adoptability and outcome status (e.g. healthy, treatable, or unhealthy), BHAS provides a dynamic, longitudinal assessment of behavioral health. Pets may move between BHAS stages over time as their behavioral condition improves or deteriorates, allowing teams to track progress, allocate resources appropriately, and intervene early when wellbeing declines.

The BHAS functions as a behavioral equivalent of a medical triage and treatment monitoring system. Just as patients are reassessed at defined medical checkpoints, BHAS allows team members and volunteers to follow each shelter pet's behavioral trajectory over time, using objective criteria rather than isolated incidents or subjective impressions.

Each BHAS stage represents both the pet's clinical status and its progression over time. Once a treatment plan is initiated, improvement is expected within a defined and predetermined interval (days, weeks, or months), depending on the specific problem being addressed. If improvement is observed, the plan continues. When progress stalls, the case requires reassessment – analogous to a medical patient not responding to initial therapy. At this point, the treatment plan must be adjusted, which may include modifying environmental management, changing training or behavior-modification strategies, or initiating, adjusting, or discontinuing psychoactive medications or nutraceuticals.

If, at the subsequent checkpoint, the shelter pet continues to show no improvement or clinical decline, the pet's behavioral prognosis must be reevaluated. At this stage, alternative CTS – such as transfer to a specialized program, return to owner, placement in a working or sanctuary setting, or advanced intervention – should be explored, similar to referral or escalation of care in medical cases.

Throughout this process, BHAS ensures that all team members and volunteers receive consistent updates, promoting transparency, continuity of care, and shared understanding of the pet's status. When no viable alternatives remain – due to lack of placement options, failure to respond to treatment, or progression to a critical behavioral health state that compromises wellbeing or safety – compassionate euthanasia becomes a medically and ethically indicated outcome, comparable to end-of-life decisions made for pets with severe, nonresponsive medical disease.

By framing behavioral care within a triage-based model, BHAS supports defensible, welfare-centered decisions and reinforces that behavioral illness deserves the same structured, compassionate, and objective approach as physical illness.

BHAS is a *five-stage classification system* used to describe the severity, stability, and treatability of behavioral conditions in dogs and cats housed in shelters. The scale is designed to mirror medical triage systems in both tone and function, using clear terminology, defined criteria, and visual cues to support rapid understanding and alignment across teams.

5.4.2 Purpose

The BHAS provides a shared language for behavior teams, medical teams, animal care teams, and volunteers. It supports:

- Clear communication across departments.
- Objective assessment of behavioral health over time.
- Appropriate treatment planning and resource allocation.
- Consistent timely monitoring of improvement, stagnation, or decline.

By anchoring observations to defined stages, BHAS reduces subjective interpretation and helps ensure that decisions are based on observable trends rather than isolated incidents.

5.4.3 Using BHAS

- Assign a BHAS stage based on the pet's current problematic and dysregulated behavior.
- Reassess at minimum on a weekly basis to track response to treatment and stability over time. Reassessment(s) may occur more frequently based on bite incidents or increase in frequency or intensity of the behavior problem.
- Use the assigned stage to guide handling protocols, enrichment plans, treatment intensity, and communication.
- BHAS stages provide prognostic guidance, not a fixed outcome.
- Shelter pets can move up and down the scale based on their behaviors.

5.4.4 Adoption Guidance

Shelter pets classified in Stages 1–3 are considered appropriate for adoption placement. Pets in Stages 4–5 will require further intervention, stabilization, or welfare-based decision-making before adoption can be ethically or safely considered.

Overall, the BHAS offers a practical, welfare-centered framework. It is meant to serve as a tool that allows shelters to monitor behavioral trajectories with the same rigor and objectivity applied to medical conditions, supporting humane, transparent, and defensible outcomes.

5.5 Challenges and Limitations

5.5.1 Risk Assessment for Shelter Pets with Behavioral Disorders

(With Emphasis on Aggression, Fear, Frustration, and Separation-Related Behaviors)

Risk assessment in shelters must extend beyond the question of *"Is this animal dangerous?"* to include the risk of worsening mental health, prolonged suffering, self-injurious behavior, team member injuries, and ethically indefensible outcomes. Behavioral disorders – particularly aggression – are among the most challenging cases shelters face and require structured, objective evaluation and an intentional CTS.

The BHAS and the Risk Assessment Checklist are most powerful when used together. They are especially useful for pets in BHAS categories 4–5 or for any pet with a bite history, worsening behavior, or declining wellbeing. When a pet is not improving – or is deteriorating despite intervention – these tools help identify escalation and impaired wellbeing across the Five Domains. This applies not only to aggression cases but also to severely fearful, shut-down, or anorexic pets that are suffering and unable to cope in the shelter environment. By integrating both BHAS and the risk assessment, teams gain a clearer understanding of the pet's journey and can make compassionate, timely, and defensible decisions.

This framework is designed to help:

- Systematically assess behavioral risk.
- Identify contributing factors and triggers.
- Evaluate safety and welfare implications.
- Determine appropriate CTS, including management, foster, transfer, or compassionate euthanasia.

It is especially intended for organizations without a formal behavior program, offering a repeatable method for evaluating complex cases.

5.5.2 Core Risk Assessment Domains

5.5.2.1 Trigger(s) That Elicit the Problem Behavior

Identify what consistently precedes the behavior.

- **Trigger type**:
  - Person (adult, child, unfamiliar, or familiar)
  - Dog
  - Other animal
  - Object, situation, sound, and handling
- **Context**:
  - On-property/off-property
  - Owner or handler present/absent

- **Predictability**:
  - Predictable and consistent
  - Unpredictable or escalating

Unpredictable triggers significantly increase risk.

5.5.2.2 Motivation for the Behavior

Understanding motivation is essential for prognosis and management.

- Aggression
  - Defensive (fear-based and distance-increasing)
  - Offensive (approach-oriented and proactive)
- Escape-driven behavior
- Frustration-related behavior
- Separation-related distress
- Fear or anxiety without overt aggression

Defensive and escape-motivated behaviors may respond differently to intervention than offensive aggression.

5.5.2.3 Frequency of the Behavior

Assess how often the behavior occurs.

- Rare/intermittent/frequent/daily
- Has frequency increased over time?
- Can the behavior be interrupted once initiated?

High-frequency behaviors with poor interruptibility carry greater risk.

5.5.2.4 Intensity and Interruptibility of Behavior

Evaluate what actually happens when the behavior occurs and determine whether the pet can be distracted or redirected from the problematic behavior pattern.

Interruptibility

- Can be easily interrupted/redirected
- Can sometimes be interrupted/redirected
- Cannot be interrupted/redirected

Nonbite Behaviors (BSC Level 1/2)

- Growling
- Lunging
- Contact with clothing (no skin)

Bite Behaviors (BSC Level 3–7)

- Severity of bite (use standardized bite scales)
- Number of bites (single vs. multiple)
- Location of bites (hands, face, and extremities)
- Escalation over time

Repeated, escalating, or multiple-bite incidents significantly increase risk.

5.5.2.5 Size and Physical Capability of the Animal

Physical risk is directly influenced by size and strength.

- Small
- Medium
- Large
- Giant

Larger animals with the same behavioral profile carry inherently higher injury risk.

5.5.2.6 Predictability and Recovery

Assess emotional regulation and recovery after an incident.

- Presence of warning signals (growling, freezing, and avoidance)
- Speed of recovery after trigger removal
- Ability to disengage and return to baseline

Poor recovery and absence of warning signals increase risk.

5.5.2.7 Prior History and Pattern

Review all known background information.

- Previous bite or aggression history
- Repeated incidents across contexts
- Prior management strategies and their effectiveness
- Previous behavior modification or medication trials
- Pattern stability vs. deterioration

5.5.2.8 Concomitant Medical Factors

Medical conditions can exacerbate behavior and increase risk. A veterinarian should diagnose or rule out medical conditions.

- Pain (orthopedic, dental, otitis, and GI)
- Neurological disease
- Endocrine disorders
- Sensory deficits
- Medication side effects

Untreated pain or medical disease worsens prognosis and welfare.

5.5.2.9 Management Feasibility in the Current Environment

Assess whether the shelter can safely and humanely manage the animal.

- Staff safety and skill level
- Ability to prevent exposure to triggers
- Adequacy of housing, enrichment, and predictability

- Risk of recurrence under shelter conditions
- Impact on the pet's welfare and mental health

A pet may be "manageable" short-term but deteriorate with prolonged confinement.

5.5.2.10 Risk Is Not Only About Safety

Risk assessment must also include:

- Risk of behavioral deterioration
- Risk of chronic fear, frustration, or shutdown
- Risk of moral distress for staff and caregivers
- Risk of prolonged confinement with poor quality of life

A pet that can be physically managed but is psychologically deteriorating remains at a high risk from a welfare standpoint.

5.5.2.11 Outcome Trajectories to Consider

Following the assessment, shelters should identify a realistic and ethical pathway:

- In-shelter management with intervention
- Foster placement (with appropriate support and safety planning)
- Transfer to a specialized organization
- Compassionate euthanasia, when risk and suffering cannot be ethically mitigated

Compassionate euthanasia for behavioral conditions should be considered a *welfare-based medical decision*, not a failure – particularly when safety, predictability, and quality of life cannot be ensured.

5.5.2.12 Goals of a Risk Assessment Framework

Shelter teams should be able to:

- Objectively formulate a behavioral problem list.
- Identify triggers, motivation, and risk modifiers.
- Evaluate both safety and welfare risks.
- Develop a clear, documented care trajectory plan.
- Support transparent, defensible decision-making.

This Risk Assessment Checklist provides a structured, objective method to evaluate both safety risk and welfare risk in shelter pets exhibiting behavioral concerns. This structured approach helps shelters move away from reactive, emotionally driven decisions toward consistent, ethical, and evidence-informed care – even in the absence of specialized behavior teams. By scoring 10 key domains – including trigger predictability, motivational basis of behavior, frequency and intensity of incidents, bite severity, warning signals, medical contributors, and the feasibility of safe management – the tool generates a total risk score (0–31) that guides CTS decisions. Risk categories (low, moderate, high, and critical) support consistent, transparent, and ethically defensible outcomes ranging from in-shelter behavior plans to foster or transfer or – when necessary – compassionate euthanasia.

The checklist emphasizes that high risk does not mean a *bad* animal, but rather a *mismatch* between the pet's needs and available resources. It promotes team alignment, protects the pet's wellbeing and team safety, and enhances organizational sustainability. This tool is designed to support shelters in making humane, informed, and consistent decisions for pets with dysregulated behaviors.

See Appendix D for Risk Assessment Checklist with Scoring Weights for Shelter Pets with Behavioral Disorders

5.5.3 Compassionate Euthanasia for Pets with Behavioral Conditions

This part of the chapter outlines the criteria for making compassionate euthanasia decisions for shelter pets with severe behavioral conditions. The word euthanasia comes from the Greek *eu* (good) and *thanatos* (death), meaning "*a good death*." In practice, this refers to a death that occurs at the right time, preventing unnecessary pain, fear, or suffering.

Euthanasia decisions are among the most emotionally challenging choices faced by pet owners, shelter professionals, volunteers, and veterinarians. It can be difficult enough when a pet is terminally ill and suffering from physical decline; however, determining the right course of action for an otherwise young and physically healthy pet with serious behavioral concerns is much more complex.

Each case must involve careful evaluation of all alternatives, including adoption, foster, management, treatment, or transfer options. Euthanasia should never be a default decision, but rather a thoughtful and deliberate act made with compassion, guided by the principles of welfare, safety, and quality of life – for both the pet and the surrounding community.

An owner's decision to pursue or decline euthanasia is influenced by a range of factors, including empathy, knowledge of animal health and wellbeing, interpretation of behavioral or medical evidence, moral or cultural beliefs, financial limitations, caregiver burden, and sometimes anthropomorphic reasoning. In a shelter environment, these same factors apply but are often amplified by complexity. Shelter pets typically have multiple advocates – veterinarians, behavior specialists, leadership, team members, volunteers, and sometimes rescue partners and the community at large – each bringing their own perspectives and ethical frameworks. This collective involvement, while valuable, can make the decision-making process both emotionally charged and logistically challenging.

Furthermore, every euthanasia decision in a shelter has broader implications. It not only affects the individual pet but also can impact the wellbeing and resources of the entire population within the facility. Decisions made for one pet may influence the organization's capacity and SoS, affect population flow, and even alter transfer opportunities for healthy animals in other shelters. Thus, euthanasia considerations in shelters must always balance individual welfare with population-level management to ensure that overall animal wellbeing and community safety remain at the forefront.

A shelter must thoughtfully consider its obligations to the organization, the team members, and volunteers and – most importantly – the pets in its care.

Euthanasia decisions for medical conditions often face less scrutiny than for behavioral issues, but pets suffering or posing safety risks should always be considered under the same welfare-based framework. Treating euthanasia for behavioral reasons differently can increase stress and emotional burden for the team responsible for these decisions. A critical aspect of this responsibility is establishing a clear, consistent stance on euthanasia for behavioral cases. Regular, neutral, and structured discussions – held proactively rather than during emotionally charged crises – promote balanced, ethical, and compassionate decision-making.

To support these conversations, shelters should implement a nonjudgmental and transparent process for evaluating cases. The use of a POVBR, the BHAS and the risk assessment framework is invaluable in this regard, as it ensures that behavioral and medical concerns are documented systematically and chronologically from intake onward.

Finally, regular CTS discussions – involving medical, behavioral, and leadership teams – are essential to ensure that decisions remain active, evidence-based, and welfare-centered. This proactive approach fosters team alignment, reduces moral distress, and upholds both the ethical and operational integrity and sustainability of the organization.

The following are two important points to be considered for euthanasia for pets with severe behavioral dysregulation discussions:

1) Safety-based decisions: The pet is aggressive and is considered not safe for humans or other animals. Euthanizing aggressive pets seems easier on paper than it actually is. All the conditions of these pets need to be taken into consideration. A veterinarian or in some cases a behavior specialist may be able to provide a specific diagnosis and prognosis based on the review of a well-kept POVBR, BHAS, or careful assessment of the pet's condition(s). Euthanasia should be an ethical and well-considered decision, made with full awareness of the organization's responsibilities and the potential adopter's liability.
2) Welfare-based decisions: The pet may or may not be aggressive but is suffering from debilitating fears, phobias, or anxieties. A shelter or even a home environment may face limitations in providing an adequate quality of life for such pets. If behavioral or medical conditions significantly impair a pet's ability to function normally or experience comfort and wellbeing, euthanasia should be considered as a humane option. The availability of a shelter or an adopter's resources, time, and expertise needed to safely and effectively manage the pet's condition must also be carefully evaluated as part of the decision-making process.

Questions to Facilitate the Discussions

Is the pet coping with the current situation? Are all five domains addressed appropriately?
Is the pet able to move unassisted, interact with other animals/people, and able to perform normal species-specific behaviors?
Is the pet's condition severe or chronic?
Is the condition challenging to manage for an average pet owner?
Is the condition causing unnecessary suffering?
What is the long-term prognosis for the pet's life in another home?
Will the pet require continuous treatment, medication, or management?
Is the pet a hazard to itself, other animals, or humans?
Is there a reasonable home available?
Where is the line between realism and optimism?

5.5.4 Complicated Medical Cases

Treating complex medical cases in shelter pets presents significant practical and ethical challenges, particularly in high-intake or resource-limited organizations. Teams must balance animal welfare, public health, and limited resources while determining whether a condition is treatable and if the pet will be adoptable afterward. Long-term medical cases can strain shelter capacity – consuming staff time, space, and funding – while also increasing stress and lowering quality of life for the affected pet.

Each case must be carefully evaluated to ensure both the pet's wellbeing and the shelter's SoS. Training and enrichment should be tailored to the abilities of the sick or injured pet, as mental stimulation remains essential to their wellbeing. When possible, such pets should be placed in foster care until recovery or adoption. In select cases, adoption "*as is*" – where the adopter assumes responsibility for ongoing care – can be an appropriate and compassionate option.

5.5.5 Combination of Medical and Behavioral Cases

Pets with multiple behavioral issues, or a combination of medical and behavioral conditions, are among the most challenging cases and often have a poor long-term prognosis. Pets who are in chronic pain, fear, or distress – physically or emotionally – can have a severely impaired quality of life. The complexity of treatment for a pet with concurrent medical and behavioral conditions along with safety concerns and resource limitations may have a combined negative on the pet's overall quality of life. Each issue may compound the others, making resolution, management, and treatment extremely difficult.

These pets are challenging to rehome for several interconnected reasons: practical, clinical, and ethical.

Several conditions can interact and worsen one another – for example, anxiety and aggression. Treating one issue may not necessarily improve the others and, in some cases, may even exacerbate them. Identifying the root cause can be especially difficult when medical and behavioral signs overlap, such as when pain contributes to aggression. Additionally, medications used for behavioral disorders (e.g. selective serotonin reuptake inhibitors [SSRIs]) may conflict with treatments for physical illnesses. Chronic medical conditions like arthritis or neurological disease can also reduce the effectiveness of behavior modification and make a pet more irritable or reactive, further complicating treatment and welfare outcomes.

Generally, complex conditions require long-term behavioral modification, medical management, and specialized environments. Most shelters cannot handle such high-need pets due to a lack of resources (time, money, expertise, and capacity to care). And even with proper treatment, the pet may remain chronically anxious or fearful of handling, may become unsafe to people and other pets, or generally unable to enjoy a normal life.

It is also important to remember that most adopters seek safe, healthy, and low-maintenance companions. As a result, pets with complex medical or behavioral issues often have limited adoption prospects, leading to prolonged shelter stays and, in some cases, euthanasia after extended treatment efforts. This reality underscores the ethical and practical challenges shelters face in balancing the wellbeing of these pets with the expectations and capabilities of potential adopters.

To avoid this dilemma, shelters should have a clear process in place. Early CTS planning is needed, especially when addressing complex cases. All behavior and medical information regarding the pet's conditions, treatment plans, and potential challenges should be transparent and readily available in the POVBR. The BHAS will describe the severity, stability, and treatability of behavioral conditions.

Humane endpoints should be defined early in the process and be part of the CTS. Humane endpoints are predetermined criteria that signal when continued treatment or intervention is no longer in the pet's best interest – typically when suffering cannot be alleviated, wellbeing continues to decline, or risks to the animal or people become unacceptable. Establishing these thresholds in advance promotes welfare by preventing prolonged distress, ensuring timely decision-making, and guiding the team toward compassionate, ethical outcomes. Clearly defining humane endpoints also helps the care team form an accurate picture from the start and implement tailored interventions. Ongoing tracking of progress and regular welfare assessments are essential before continuing any treatment plan.

Ideally, individualized care plans can be developed in collaboration with behaviorists and the veterinary medical teams so that both medical and behavioral needs are addressed simultaneously. Additionally, increasing community outreach and education can help find foster homes or adopters who are uniquely suited to handle the unique challenges of these special needs animals.

In summary, euthanasia decisions are never easy, and they shouldn't be. All reasonable outcome options should be discussed for each individual pet as a team. When the caretakers can make an active decision as a team, taking into account the organization's mission, values, and SoS, the team can ensure that the decision aligns with the best interests of the pet, the organization, and the community it serves. Transparency and collaboration among team members are essential to making compassionate and responsible choices. Furthermore, there must be space for grieving; self-care is essential, and maintaining healthy boundaries is vital. In this challenging field, caring for ourselves allows us to continue caring for the animals – and each other – with compassion and resilience.

References

American Society for the Prevention of Cruelty to Animals (ASPCA) (2018). Position statement on shelter dog behavior assessments [Online]. Available at: https://www.aspca.org/about-us/aspca-policy-and-position-statements/position-statement-shelter-dog-behavior-assessments (accessed 22 January 2026).

van der Borg, J.A.M., Netto, W.J., and Planta, D.J.U. (1991). Behavioural testing of dogs in animal shelters to predict problem behaviour. *Applied Animal Behaviour Science* 32 (2–3): 237–251. https://doi.org/10.1016/S0168-1591(05)80047-4.

Christensen, E., Scarlett, J., Campagna, M., and Houpt, K.A. (2007). Aggressive behavior in adopted dogs that passed a temperament test. *Applied Animal Behaviour Science* 106: 85–95. https://doi.org/10.1016/j.applanim.2006.07.002.

Clay, L., Paterson, M., Bennett, P. et al. (2020a). Do behaviour assessments in a shelter predict the behaviour of dogs post-adoption? *Animals* 10 (7): 1–13. https://doi.org/10.3390/ani10071225.

Clay, L., Paterson, M., Bennett, P. et al. (2020b). In defense of canine behavioral assessments in shelters: outlining their positive applications. *Journal of Veterinary Behavior*. Elsevier Inc. https://doi.org/10.1016/j.jveb.2020.03.005.

Hsu, Y. and Serpell, J.A. (2003). Development and validation of a questionnaire for measuring behavior and temperament traits in pet dogs. *Journal of the American Veterinary Medical Association* 223 (9): 1293–1300. https://doi.org/10.2460/javma.2003.223.1293.

Marder, A.R., Shabelansky, A., Patronek, G.J. et al. (2013). Food-related aggression in shelter dogs: a comparison of behavior identified by a behavior evaluation in the shelter and owner reports after adoption. *Applied Animal Behaviour Science*. Elsevier B.V. 148 (1–2): 150–156. https://doi.org/10.1016/j.applanim.2013.07.007.

Patronek, G.J. and Bradley, J. (2016). No better than flipping a coin: reconsidering canine behavior evaluations in animal shelters. *Journal of Veterinary Behavior: Clinical Applications and Research*. Elsevier Inc. 15: 66–77. https://doi.org/10.1016/j.jveb.2016.08.001.

Patronek, G.J., Bradley, J., and Arps, E. (2019). What is the evidence for reliability and validity of behavior evaluations for shelter dogs? A prequel to "no better than flipping a coin". *Journal of Veterinary Behavior*. Elsevier Inc. 31: 43–58. https://doi.org/10.1016/j.jveb.2019.03.001.

Poulsen, A.H., Lisle, A.T., and Phillips, C.J.C. (2010). An evaluation of a behaviour assessment to determine the suitability of shelter dogs for rehoming. *Veterinary Medicine International* 2010: https://doi.org/10.4061/2010/523781.

Segurson, S.A., Serpell, J.A., and Hart, B.L. (2005). Evaluation of a behavioral assessment questionnaire for use in the characterization of behavioral problems of dogs relinquished to animal shelters. *Journal of the American Veterinary Medical Association* 227 (11): 1755–1761.

6

Animal Care Trajectory Strategies: Planning Care and Outcome

6.1 Defining Animal Care Trajectory Strategies (CTS) and Its Benefits

Traditionally, many animal shelters use a practice known as pathway planning, which can also be described as an animal care trajectory strategy (CTS). A trajectory strategy is a proactive, structured approach to guiding pets through the shelter system toward an appropriate outcome and is a hallmark of progressive, humane animal welfare organizations.

This approach focuses on determining the optimal care plan and pathway for each individual animal or defined group of animals. It encompasses designing strategies with a series of coordinated steps that begin prior to admission and continue throughout the animal's stay, adapting as needed based on medical, behavioral, and welfare assessments. By intentionally managing each pet's journey – rather than reacting to crises – CTS supports timely decision-making, efficient use of resources, and improved welfare outcomes. Having a clear, proactive plan for each pet's journey through the shelter system is essential to delivering humane, effective care. A CTS provides a shared roadmap that considers all species and all conditions – healthy, medical, and behavioral – rather than addressing needs in isolation or reacting to critical events as they arise.

When trajectory planning is proactive, shelters can anticipate care needs, align medical and behavioral interventions early, and reduce unnecessary length of stay (LOS). This allows pets to move through the system with fewer disruptions, lower stress, and better welfare outcomes. In contrast, a reactive approach to population management often results in bottlenecks, escalating stress within the pet population, and frequent emergencies that demand immediate attention but divert resources away from long-term solutions.

This dynamic closely mirrors the four-quadrant framework of *urgent vs. important* decision-making. Reactive sheltering is dominated by tasks that are *urgent but not always important*: crisis behavior escalations, disease outbreaks, overcrowding, and professional burnout. While these situations require immediate action, they consume time and resources that could otherwise be invested in *important but not urgent* work – such as preventive medical care, early behavioral intervention, community support programs, and team training.

A well-defined CTS shifts organizational focus toward the *important and proactive* quadrant. By planning animal flow in advance, shelters can allocate resources more effectively, reduce crisis-driven decision-making, and maintain steadier operations. Medical, behavioral, and operational teams are better able to coordinate care, preventing problems rather than continually responding to them.

Importantly, a CTS strengthens an organization's ability to fulfill its mission. When expectations, pathways, and decision points are clearly defined, teams can communicate consistently across departments and with the community they serve. This shared understanding improves transparency, builds trust, and allows the organization to have a broader and more sustainable impact – helping more animals, more effectively, with the resources available.

Ultimately, shelters that adopt and adhere to a clearly articulated animal CTS experience better population flow, reduced stress, fewer emergencies, and stronger outcomes. By focusing on planning rather than reacting, organizations can create systems that support both animal wellbeing and organizational sustainability.

This approach is especially critical for organizations caring for pets with medical and/or behavioral conditions. These populations typically require more time, expertise, and resources than healthy pets.

Without a clear CTS in place, the naturally quicker placement of easy-to-adopt pets can inadvertently leave pets with greater needs unintentionally left behind. Over time, this imbalance contributes to prolonged LOS, increased stress, declining wellbeing and difficult ethical dilemmas for both pets and teams.

An effective CTS intentionally accounts for the entire shelter population, not just those with the shortest or simplest journey to adoption. The goal is not to move some pets through the system as quickly as possible, while others remain stalled for weeks, months, or even years, but rather to establish a reasonable and humane flow-through rate for all pets, adjusted for individual needs and conditions based on the scope of sustainability (SoS) (see Chapter 1) of the organization.

When pets with complex medical or behavioral needs are not incorporated into population-level planning, they consume disproportionate resources in a reactive manner, often during crises. In contrast, a proactive trajectory strategy anticipates these needs early, allocates appropriate resources, and sets realistic timelines for assessment, treatment, and outcome decisions. This prevents bottlenecks, reduces cumulative stress on animals and teams, and supports more equitable care across populations.

By designing a system that balances speed with support – rather than prioritizing ease over need – organizations can maintain steady population flow, protect welfare, and uphold their mission. A clearly defined, communicated, and consistently applied trajectory strategy allows shelters to serve all pets responsibly, ensuring that no subset is inadvertently left behind due to lack of planning or capacity.

By establishing a clear, equitable CTS, organizations become more operationally sustainable. They are better able to define and maintain their scope of care. The organizations can retain the capacity to respond to extraordinary community needs, such as hoarding situations, natural disasters (fires, floods, etc.), disease outbreaks, and other emergency events without compromising ongoing welfare standards.

6.2 Shelter Metrics – The Role of Data in Successful Care Trajectory Strategy

For any strategy to be effective and sustainable, an organization must be able to measure what is happening and use that information to guide decisions. Data-driven decision-making is not a new concept in animal sheltering; shelters have long collected metrics to document operations, demonstrate accountability, and report outcomes. What has changed over the past 10–20 years is how data is used – shifting from retrospective reporting to real-time, decision-support tools that directly influence animal welfare and lifesaving capacity.

Historically, shelter data focused primarily on output metrics, such as total intake, adoptions, transfers, euthanasia numbers, and reclaim rates. These metrics were essential for transparency, but offered limited insight into *why* pets are entering shelters, *how long* they stay, or *what interventions* improved outcomes.

Over time, shelters began tracking more process-oriented metrics, including:

- LOS by species and condition
- Live release rate (LRR)
- Return-to-owner (RTO) rates
- Transfer and foster utilization
- Spay/neuter compliance.

More recently, data systems designed specifically for shelters have enabled organizations to monitor population flow and welfare indicators, such as:

- LOS stratified by health, age, and behavioral status
- LOS by stage: time spent in each step of the shelter pathway (intake, evaluation, treatment, and adoption-ready) used to identify delays and improve flow
- Foster LOS and conversion to adoption
- Kennel capacity and housing utilization
- Disease incidence and outbreak tracking
- Outcomes for pets with medical and/or behavioral treatment plans
- Behavioral progression metrics linked to assessment tools (e.g. Behavioral Health Assessment Staging [BHAS] stages)

These advances allow shelters to move beyond asking "*How many pets did we save?*" to asking "*Are pets moving through the system in a timely, humane, and sustainable way?*" When integrated into an animal CTS, data help organizations identify bottlenecks, allocate resources equitably across populations, and intervene early when wellbeing or capacity thresholds are at risk.

Ultimately, data-informed trajectory planning strengthens an organization's ability to fulfill its mission. By grounding decisions in objective metrics rather than crisis response alone, shelters can improve consistency, increase lifesaving impact, and protect teams and animal wellbeing, while maintaining operational flexibility to respond to community-wide needs.

6.2.1 Past

In the 1990s, the "*no-kill*" movement gained prominence, emphasizing that pets should not be euthanized solely due to lack of space. Shelters achieving an LRR of 90% or higher were commonly labeled "no-kill," with euthanasia reserved for pets with poor medical or behavioral prognoses.

Over time, the term has become increasingly polarizing, particularly between municipal shelters and private organizations. Private nonprofits often have greater control over intake, while municipal shelters must accept all animals from their jurisdictions, placing them under different operational and ethical pressures. This disparity has at times contributed to public misunderstanding and criticism, which can hinder effective shelter operations and reduce community trust.

Municipal shelters have evolved significantly and now serve as both pet and community advocates. When pets in their care experience severe, unrelenting physical or behavioral decline with poor quality of life, shelters must make compassionate, welfare-based decisions. Prolonged confinement under these conditions is neither humane nor beneficial for the pet or the population as a whole.

A sustainable sheltering system requires balancing the needs of individual pets with the capacity to serve the broader community. Moving beyond outcome labels and toward a shared, humane sheltering framework – where shelters and rescues collaborate rather than compete – supports transparency, trust, and better outcomes for pets and people alike.

6.2.2 Present

Modern animal sheltering relies on data-informed decision-making to guide population management and support animal welfare. One of the most critical metrics is LOS, defined as the time from admission (intake) to outcome. Prolonged LOS is associated with decreased shelter capacity, increased disease risk, higher operational costs, and reduced welfare for pets, teams, and volunteers. Monitoring and actively managing LOS is therefore essential to maintaining both humane care and organizational sustainability. Another key metric is LRR, which represents the proportion of pets that leave the shelter through adoption or transfer. While LRR provides an important population-level snapshot, it is most effective when interpreted alongside LOS and other capacity metrics.

A data-driven approach allows shelters to optimize admissions and animal flow. Systems that identify animals suitable for early placement or fast-tracking can reduce bottlenecks, shorten LOS, and lower disease transmission risk (Cho et al. 2015). Effective population management requires aligning operational capacity with intake and care demands.

To support timely outcomes, shelters must understand their functional capacity, including:

- Adoption and transfer rates
- Admissions (intake) volume
- Foster availability
- Vaccination and deworming capacity
- Veterinary examination and surgical capacity
- Medical and surgical treatment needs
- Behavior intervention and environmental enrichment requirements.

Tracking these metrics allows organizations to assess whether current practices are sustainable and aligned with their mission (Srinivasa et al. 2022).

Housing data are equally important. Overfilling kennels or permanently closing kennel partitions to increase capacity can elevate stress, injury risk, and disease transmission. Maintaining available space for cleaning, isolation, and quarantine is critical to infection control and team safety. Full occupancy limits flexibility and increases the likelihood of operational disruptions during disease outbreaks.

Finally, data support collaborative partnerships. By understanding which pets are likely to move quickly through their system and which may benefit from transfer, shelters can work effectively with trusted rescue partners and other organizations to reduce LOS and improve outcomes across the community.

6.2.3 Future

The future of animal sheltering lies in predictive, integrated, and individualized data use. Rather than relying solely on retrospective reporting, shelters will increasingly use data to forecast LOS, resource needs, and outcomes for pets based on medical, behavioral, and social variables.

In this model, organizations maintain dynamic benchmarks for average LOS by condition – for example, uncomplicated kennel cough vs. pneumonia, dermatophytosis in kittens, or dental disease requiring surgical intervention. Understanding these timelines allows shelters to make informed admission decisions, anticipate foster or medical capacity needs, and prevent throughput constraints before they occur.

Foster care programs will become fully integrated into population management systems. Future data platforms will track foster caregiver availability, preferences, skill sets, and historical outcomes, allowing shelters to match pets to foster homes with the same intentionality used in adoption matching (Hawes et al. 2018). Real-time dashboards may support rapid placement through targeted outreach – via social media, text alerts, or internal messaging – maximizing foster utilization and reducing shelter overcrowding.

Behavioral data will also play a central role. Shelters will increasingly categorize behavior concerns by severity, context, and treatability, distinguishing between developmentally normal behaviors, stress-induced shelter behaviors, and clinically significant maladaptive behaviors. In the near future, the use of data – combined with tools such as BHAS and risk-assessment checklists – will allow organizations to track and forecast behavior-related LOS, allocate training and enrichment resources more effectively, and identify when escalation or alternative care trajectories are warranted.

Looking ahead, shelters will also incorporate community capacity data into decision-making. Information from relinquishment trends, adoption returns, housing patterns, socioeconomic indicators, and availability of positive reinforcement trainers, behavior, and veterinary professionals – both local and virtual – will help determine which medical and/or behavioral cases a community can realistically support. This approach acknowledges that adoptability is not solely an animal factor, but a match between animal needs and community resources.

Ultimately, the future of shelter data use is not about collecting more data but about using the right numbers at the right time to guide humane, transparent, and sustainable decisions. By integrating medical, behavioral, foster, and community data into cohesive CTS, shelters can move from reactive crisis management to predictive, welfare-centered population care – expanding their impact while protecting both pets and the people who care for them.

Future shelter data systems should also integrate animal population metrics with workforce and team development data to support sustainable operations and prevent professional burnout.

Key People Indicators That Can Be Tracked Include

- Team turnover and retention rates, stratified by role and tenure
- Vacancy duration and time-to-hire, which affect workload and morale
- Overtime hours and schedule variability, including consecutive long shifts
- Sick leave and unplanned absences, as early indicators of fatigue or stress
- Workers' compensation claims and injury rates, particularly bite or handling injuries
- Caseload distribution, including time spent assigned to high-intensity populations (e.g. isolation, severe behavior, and critical care)
- Training hours and competency coverage, ensuring team members are supported rather than overextended
- Employee assistance program (EAP) utilization or wellness check-in participation, when available and appropriate
- Exit interview themes, identifying systemic stressors rather than individual failures.

When analyzed alongside animal data – such as LOS, disease outbreaks, or high-risk medical and or behavioral cases – these metrics allow leadership to anticipate strain points and adjust staffing, intake, and trajectory decisions proactively. Incorporating team development data into population planning supports team wellbeing, operational resilience, and consistent animal care, reinforcing that sustainable lifesaving depends on caring for both pets and the people who serve them.

In addition to animal and people and culture metrics, future shelter data systems should capture cost, time, volunteer, and resource-utilization data to fully understand operational impact and sustainability. Relevant metrics include:

- Cost per animal per day and cost per outcome, stratified by health and behavioral status
- Staff time allocation by function (husbandry, medical care, behavior work, enrichment, and adoption support)
- Dietary needs and costs, including prescription diets, supplements, and feeding frequency adjustments
- Enrichment resources, tracking type, frequency, team/volunteer time required, and impact on behavior or LOS
- Medical resource utilization, including diagnostics, medications, surgical time, isolation housing, and recheck frequency
- Behavioral resource utilization, such as trainer hours, behavior consults, safety equipment, and medication management
- Volunteer hours, roles, and retention, including time spent in high-impact areas such as enrichment, socialization, and foster support.

When combined with LOS, BHAS stage, and outcome data, these metrics allow shelters to identify which interventions are most effective, which populations require disproportionate resources and where efficiencies can be gained without compromising welfare. Volunteer and enrichment data, in particular, highlight often underrecognized contributions that significantly reduce stress, improve behavior, and support faster, healthier outcomes.

Integrating cost, time, and resource-use data enables organizations to plan realistically, allocate equitably, and advocate transparently for funding and community support – strengthening both SoS and animal wellbeing.

Shelter metrics have only begun to scratch the surface of what is possible. As data systems continue to evolve, shelters are moving beyond basic reporting toward integrated, real-time tools that inform welfare-centered decision-making. Improved surrender and preadmission data – capturing the true drivers of relinquishment – can help organizations identify where prevention efforts should be focused and which community support systems are most likely to keep pets with their families.

When shelters truly understand why pets are entering in the first place, they can shift resources upstream, designing targeted interventions such as housing support, medical assistance, behavior education, or temporary foster options. Combined with emerging technologies, including artificial intelligence and predictive analytics, these insights have the potential to move sheltering from reactive intake management to proactive prevention systems.

The future of sheltering lies in using data, not only to improve outcomes for animals already in care but also to reduce the need for sheltering altogether – ultimately improving wellbeing for animals, people, and the communities they share. Looking ahead, these tools have the potential to transform animal sheltering from a reactive system into a proactive, predictive care model, enhancing the wellbeing of the animals entrusted to shelters while supporting the people who care for them. The new era of animal sheltering is not just data-informed – it is pet-centered, humane, and deeply hopeful.

6.3 Admissions Strategy: Intake Planning as the Foundation of Sustainable Care

A successful animal CTS begins before an animal ever enters the shelter. Sustainable sheltering requires intentional planning that asks not only *what outcomes are possible* but also *what the organization can realistically and humanely handle*. This includes consideration of species, medical complexity, behavioral needs, staffing, housing, foster capacity, financial resources, and community support systems. Defining the SoS allows organizations to serve animals effectively without compromising welfare, team wellbeing or long-term organizational stability.

Traditionally, shelters have been viewed by the public as the default solution for any unwanted or at-risk animal. While shelters can and do provide lifesaving care, they are also inherently stressful environments and placement is never guaranteed. A modern CTS recognizes this reality and shifts the focus from reactive intake toward active population management and prevention, while maintaining compassion for people and pets in need.

A well-designed animal CTS depends on a thoughtful, adoption-driven admissions strategy. Regardless of whether an organization operates a brick-and-mortar facility or is foster-based, all shelters are constrained by space, time, staffing, and financial resources. Even foster-based organizations are limited by the number of available foster homes, the skills of those caregivers, and the level of medical and behavioral support the organization can provide.

Most shelters rely on successful adoptions to create capacity for new admissions. Increasing the speed and volume of appropriate, successful adoptions directly expands an organization's ability to help additional animals. In this sense, capacity is not static – it is dynamic and driven by outcomes. For municipal shelters with open-intake obligations, this planning is even more critical, as they must preserve ongoing capacity for community relinquishments, stray animals, emergency walk-ins, pets displaced by incarceration, neglect or hoarding cases, natural disasters, and disease outbreaks.

6.3.1 Adoption-Driven Capacity and Flow

While the public may assume that every empty kennel represents a failure to help, the opposite is true. Shelters must maintain a buffer of open space to protect animal welfare, prevent disease spread, preserve behavioral health, and keep operations functional. By operating proactively, preserving flexible space, and managing intake based on true capacity for care (C4C), shelters keep animals healthier, move them through the system faster, and ensure that more pets – and the right pets – find homes. This approach also supports a stable *SoS* and reduces professional burnout.

6.3.1.1 Where the "Shelter Math" Becomes Magical

A persistent misconception is that reducing intake or leaving kennels open means helping fewer animals. In reality, running below capacity allows shelters to save *more*, not fewer. With a smaller population, stress decreases, disease risk drops, and staff have enough time for proper care and adoption counseling, resulting in a lower LOS. And when LOS shortens, each kennel can house more pets per year.

For Example

- 50 kennels + 30-day LOS = ~600 animals/year
- 50 kennels + 15-day LOS = ~1,200 animals/year

Cutting LOS in half doubles the number of animals cared for annually – without adding a single kennel. In other words: Avoiding overcrowding doesn't limit lifesaving – it *multiplies* it.

6.3.1.2 Side Note: Cohousing Should Never Be Used Simply to "Save Space"

Cohousing should not be implemented as a *space-saving* tactic. While cohousing can offer valuable social enrichment when done strategically, it must *only* occur under the right conditions. Each decision should be based on careful evaluation of species, size, age, health status, behavior, and true social compatibility, with ongoing monitoring for stress, resource guarding, or conflict.

When cohousing is appropriate, shelters should adhere strictly to the Association of Shelter Veterinarians' Guidelines for Standards of Care (DeTar et al. 2022). Poorly planned cohousing often leads to increased stress, disease transmission, injury risk, and ultimately higher resource use, undermining both wellbeing and C4C. In short, cohousing can be an enrichment tool and should not be used as a space-management strategy.

Even when the goal is not to increase adoption numbers, reducing LOS has profound organizational benefits. Cutting care days in half directly reduces the cost of housing each animal, freeing resources that can be reinvested into mission-critical areas. With fewer daily care demands, shelters expand their SoS – allowing them to accept more behaviorally or medically complex cases, stabilize high-risk pets, or redirect funds toward essential community programs such as spay/neuter, vaccine clinics, or pet retention support. In short, shorter LOS doesn't just help more pets move through the system faster and healthier – it increases the shelter's capacity to serve the community and to care for pets with greater needs.

Intentionally preserving open kennels is a strategic, humane, and mathematically sound approach to saving the most lives. Sadly, organizations that operate continuously at or near 100% capacity face more disease outbreaks, increased staff turnover, and greater operational instability. Tools, such as the C4C framework developed by the UC Davis Koret Shelter Medicine Program, provide evidence-based guidance for determining appropriate housing capacity and should be integrated into admissions planning. Maintaining intentional open space is a form of risk management and welfare protection. In addition to assessing the needs of each individual animal, shelters must consider the broader impact of every admission or housing decision on the entire population in their care – what we refer to as the organization's SoS.

6.3.2 Scheduled Admissions and Intake Control

Whenever feasible, a scheduled admissions strategy benefits both shelters and the communities it serves. Encouraging the public to contact the organization in advance allows shelters to plan admissions volume deliberately, align staffing and housing, and preserve space for urgent needs. Ideally, shelters maintain a guaranteed buffer of empty kennels reserved for emergencies such as found animals or urgent owner relinquishments. Without this buffer, shelters are forced into undesirable alternatives – turning people away, group housing incompatible animals, emergency transfers, or making difficult population-level decisions under pressure. Proactive scheduling reduces these risks by aligning admissions with available resources and preserving welfare-based decision-making.

6.3.3 Admissions Assessment and Early Decision-Making

The initial assessment at admissions is critical in determining each pet's trajectory. Detailed observations should be documented to establish the pet's handleability and care needs, ensuring that the teams and volunteers interact safely and appropriately. These assessments do not necessarily determine adoptability, but they can protect both people and pets by setting handling expectations.

If a pet retreats, freezes, or appears shut down during intake, this should be documented. When capacity allows, a decompression period of 24–72 hours may be provided before reassessment. Shelters operating near capacity may need to shorten this window, balancing welfare with operational realities.

Pets displaying overt aggression during admissions require immediate trajectory decisions. Safety risks to team members, volunteers, and the community must be carefully weighed alongside welfare considerations, with outcomes ranging from transfer or specialized placement to euthanasia when risk and prognosis are unacceptable.

6.3.4 Behavior Capacity and Adoption Sustainability

A shelter behavior program should be modeled on adoption-driven sustainability. Understanding which pets the local community can realistically support is essential. Distinguishing between normal species-specific behaviors (neurotypical), behaviors that are normal, but considered nuisance behaviors, and true behavioral disorders that reflect dysregulation or clinical concern is essential for determining appropriate behavioral pathways (see Chapter 4).

- Nuisance behaviors (e.g. jumping, barking, biting [bite severity classification, BSC 1–2] [see Chapter 5], or scratching) are often developmentally normal or environmentally influenced and many respond well to training and management. Whether these behaviors continue to be problematic in a new home depends greatly on the adopter's expectations, tolerance, and the specific environment. What one person sees as a nuisance, another may view as completely acceptable. Conversely, behaviors that were not problematic in the shelter may become undesirable in the adopter's home. These pets benefit from take-home behavior plans, postadoption follow-up, access to training, educational support, and the appropriate tools to help families guide and reinforce desired behaviors (see Chapter 13).
- Behavior problems involve maladaptive or dysregulated behavior challenges, such as fear, anxiety, repetitive behaviors, or aggression. In addition to standard supports, these pets may require psychoactive medication, ongoing behavior counseling, and timely postadoption follow-up to support long-term success.

This tiered approach allows shelters to allocate behavior resources strategically while maximizing placement success.

6.3.5 Surrenders, Diversion, and Community Support

Economic pressures – housing instability, rising costs of living, and limited access to veterinary care – are major drivers of pet relinquishment. A sustainable admissions strategy prioritizes diversion with dignity, offering support, guidance, or referrals whenever possible rather than defaulting to shelter intake.

Effective diversion and prevention programs include:

- Pet food pantries
- Low- or no-cost vaccination and preventative care
- Accessible spay/neuter services

- Community veterinary clinics for minor medical issues
- Targeted community services (e.g. fence repair, training support, and in-home assistance for seniors)
- Community cat programs utilizing trap–neuter–return
- Community rehoming boards and facilitated rehoming events.

These programs reduce unnecessary shelter entry, preserve human–animal bonds, and allow shelters to focus resources where they are most needed.

6.3.6 Admissions Strategy as a Sustainability Tool

An intentional admissions strategy is not about limiting help – it is about maximizing impact. By planning intake proactively, aligning it with adoption-driven capacity, supporting diversion, and integrating medical and behavioral realities, shelters can maintain steady population flow, protect wellbeing and remain resilient in the face of emergencies.

When shelters actively manage admissions, they help not only the pets within their walls but also the broader community – recognizing that while shelters can be a refuge, they are also stressful environments and placement is never guaranteed. A sustainable CTS ensures that shelter care is used when it is truly the best option and that when pets do enter, they receive thoughtful, humane, and goal-directed care.

6.4 Outcome Options and Measuring Success Beyond Live Release Rate

Historically, LRR has been one of the most visible and widely referenced shelter metrics. For many years, it served as a proxy for organizational success and lifesaving efforts, and it remains an important population-level indicator. However, as sheltering practices, data systems, and community expectations have evolved, it has become increasingly clear that LRR alone tells only part of the story. LRR does not capture the complexity of admissions obligations, differences in community demographics, availability of resources, or the quality of care provided to pets during their stay. Nor does it reflect the ethical, medical, and behavioral decision-making required for pets with severe illness, declining welfare, or significant safety risks. Holding shelters solely accountable to a single outcome metric oversimplifies the work and can unintentionally incentivize practices that compromise welfare, transparency, or sustainability.

Modern, progressive sheltering requires a shift toward both quantitative and qualitative outcome measures, evaluated within the context of an organization's mission, capacity, and community role. These measures include LOS, medical and behavioral improvement, successful placement matching, postadoption retention, team and volunteer sustainability, and the pet's quality of life throughout their trajectory – not just the final outcome.

6.4.1 Outcome Options Within a Trajectory Strategy

A well-designed CTS recognizes that adoption is not the only humane or appropriate outcome. Ethical population management requires a range of outcome options that reflect individual pet's needs and community resources.

Outcome strategies may include:

- Adoption
- Transfer to other shelters or rescue organizations
- Working cat programs (barns, bodegas, warehouses, businesses, facilities, emotional support, and mascots)
- Working dog programs (prison programs, therapy, emotional support, service, facility, search, and rescue)
- Sanctuary placement, when appropriate and available
- Compassionate euthanasia, when welfare, safety, or prognosis warrant

Each option should be considered within the framework of welfare, safety, sustainability, and realistic long-term outcomes.

6.4.2 Cooperation Between Shelters and Rescue Organizations

Collaboration between shelter and rescue organizations is not optional – it is essential. When animal welfare organizations work toward a shared goal rather than competing, they create a network that allows pets to be placed where they are most likely to thrive.

Transfer decisions should be based on fit, not volume. A pet that struggles in one environment may do well in another with different housing design, population density, or community exposure. For example, a shy or noise-sensitive dog may decline behaviorally in an urban shelter with narrow walkways and constant exposure to barking dogs, yet improve significantly in a quieter facility with calmer surroundings. Successful partnerships are mutually beneficial and often flexible. Transfers may occur at a one-to-one ratio or, depending on capacity and adoptability, one pet in exchange for several others. Community preferences matter: some regions adopt small dogs quickly, while others favor larger breeds or specific types. Understanding these dynamics allows organizations to reduce LOS and improve welfare without overwhelming any single system.

6.4.3 Working Cat Programs

Working cat programs provide meaningful outcomes for cats who are not suited for traditional homes but can live safely and humanely in environments where rodent control is desired. Equestrian facilities, warehouses, farms, and industrial sites are often willing to provide food, water, and shelter with minimal human interaction required.

Community-based placements – including business mascots, bookstores, bodegas, and cat cafés – can also increase exposure and adoption opportunities while benefiting both cats and organizations. In all cases, placement decisions must prioritize safety, health, and realistic expectations for care.

6.4.4 Working Dog Programs

Shelter dogs may be excellent candidates for working roles when temperament, motivation, and health align. These programs not only provide outcomes for dogs with longer lengths of stay but also deliver meaningful benefits to the community.

Examples include:

- Prison dog programs, which benefit both dogs and incarcerated individuals by improving adoptability and vocational skills
- Therapy, facility, and psychiatric service dog programs
- Search and rescue and detection programs, which often seek high-drive, active dogs
- Specialized working roles, matched carefully to behavioral suitability.

These programs require thoughtful screening and strong partnerships but can significantly expand outcome options beyond adoption alone.

6.4.5 The Role of Sanctuary

Sanctuary placement is often viewed as an ideal alternative to euthanasia; however, true sanctuaries with adequate funding, staffing, space, and enrichment are rare. Ethical sanctuaries must meet high welfare standards, provide lifelong care, and have clear protocols for medical and behavioral decline.

Organizations considering sanctuary placement must perform due diligence to ensure compliance with Association of Shelter Veterinarians (ASV) guidelines and the Five Domains of Welfare. Sanctuary should never be used as a default solution to avoid difficult decisions, nor should it place animals into conditions worse than shelter care.

6.4.6 Measuring What Matters

As sheltering evolves, success must be measured by how pets are cared for, not just how they exit.

A modern outcome framework considers:

- Animal welfare throughout the stay
- Transparency and ethical decision-making
- Timeliness and appropriateness of placement
- Sustainability for staff, volunteers, and resources
- Community impact and prevention of future intake

While LRR remains a meaningful data point, it must be interpreted in context and alongside a broader set of indicators. When shelters are evaluated holistically, organizations are empowered to make humane, defensible decisions that reflect both compassion and responsibility.

In summary, an effective animal CTS integrates admissions planning, population flow, outcome diversity, community partnerships, and data-informed evaluation. By moving beyond single-metric definitions of success and embracing a systems-based approach, shelters can reduce crowding, improve welfare, support teams' wellbeing and better serve both pets and communities. Sustainable sheltering is not defined by speed alone, nor by labels – but by thoughtful planning, collaboration, and a commitment to doing what is best for each pet within the realities of capacity and care.

References

Cho, Y., Lee, Y., Hwang, B. et al. (2015). Data analysis for improving population management in animal shelters in Seoul. *Korean Journal of Veterinary Research* 55 (2): 125–131. https://doi.org/10.14405/kjvr.2015.55.2.125.

DeTar, L., Doyle, E., O'Quin, J. et al. (2022). The Association of Shelter Veterinarians' guidelines for standards of care in animal shelters. *Journal of Shelter Medicine and Community Animal Health*. Available at: http://journal.um-surabaya.ac.id/index.php/JKM/article/view/2203.

Hawes, S., Kerrigan, J., and Morris, K. (2018). Factors informing outcomes for older cats and dogs in animal shelters. *Animals* 8 (36): https://doi.org/10.3390/ani8030036.

Srinivasa, D., Mondal, R., Rentzell, K., and Protopopova, A. (2022). Interviews with Indian animal shelter staff: similarities and differences in challenges and resiliency factors compared to western counterparts. *Animals* 12 (19): 2562. https://doi.org/10.3390/ani12192562.

7

Stress Management for Shelter Pets

7.1 Recognizing and Understanding Stress in Shelter Pets

This chapter was designed to inspire and empower organizations with practical, achievable solutions – from small, incremental changes to larger programmatic shifts – that can be tailored to any shelter, regardless of size or resources. The goal is to encourage each organization to evaluate stress levels within their population and select strategies that best support the wellbeing and create a calmer, more humane shelter experience for every pet in their care.

Stress is a normal part of life and occurs when the body is pushed out of balance by internal or external stimuli. Not all stress is harmful; in fact, a moderate level of stress can support learning, adaptation, and resilience. However, when a pet experiences high-intensity stress or prolonged exposure without relief, stress becomes chronic and can negatively affect both mental and physical health, in particular when the animal has little ability to escape, control, or reduce the stressor.

These conditions are often present in the shelter environment. Pets are abruptly removed from their previous living situations – whether owned homes or free-roaming environments – and placed into unfamiliar surroundings. They are exposed to new animals, people, foods, lighting, sounds, odors, and unpredictable schedules. They do not understand where they are, why they are confined, or how long they will remain there. In addition, they may be restrained for examinations, vaccinations, and medical procedures, which can further increase stress.

Every animal copes with stress differently. Some adapt quickly, while others show fear, frustration, heightened reactions, or disengagement. Individual differences in genetics, prior experiences, health status, and emotional resilience influence how each pet responds. Recognizing these differences is essential for providing appropriate handling, enrichment, decompression time, and individualized care that supports welfare and improves outcomes. Refer to Chapter 4 for a more in-depth reading on how stress affects shelter pet's behavior.

It is important that team members and volunteers are trained to recognize stress body language and how to respond appropriately with each species and each individual. The use of standardized guidelines helps the team members and volunteers determine the level of wellbeing the shelter pet is experiencing. The authors have created a *Wellbeing Scale*, in which higher scores indicate better overall wellbeing experienced by the pet. Think of the scale as a 5-out-of-5 star rating, with 5* representing optimal physical and mental wellbeing and 1* indicating severe distress and high risk. The Canine and Feline Wellbeing Scales provide a structured framework for evaluating emotional and physiological states in shelter and clinical environments.

Each level on the scale is defined by observable behaviors and physical indicators, allowing team members and volunteers to assess wellbeing objectively. The scale also serves as a decision-making tool, guiding safe handling, appropriate interventions, and tailored enrichment and supports a welfare-centered care trajectory strategy (CTS).

We find that using this Wellbeing scale daily helps assess and safeguard the physical and emotional state of every pet in shelter care. It requires minimal time, yet provides tremendous benefits, allowing team members and volunteers to identify stress early, reduce risk, improve welfare outcomes, and create a more positive, humane shelter experience for every pet.

The consistent implementation of the Wellbeing Scale enhances (see Table 7.1):

Table 7.1 Canine and Feline Wellbeing Scale (Descending Scores-Reduced Wellbeing)

Star Rating	Wellbeing State	Canine Indicators	Feline Indicators
5*	Relaxed and Social	Consistent appetite; voluntarily seeks interaction; friendly demeanor; relaxed posture and facial expression; normal grooming, rest, sleep and play; occasional panting with soft lip commissures; eager, consistent engagement with reinforcers	Consistent appetite; voluntarily seeks interaction; relaxed posture; friendly demeanor; normal grooming, rest, sleep and play; readily engages with reinforcers
4*	Mild Stress/ Generally Coping *(1–2 signs may be present)*	Paw lift; occasional lip licking; tail occasionally lowered; ears slightly back/side; mild fidgeting but settles; accepts treats/toys/attention; may initially avoid then solicit interaction; occasional panting with slightly tight mouth	Occasional vocalizations; may initially avoid then approach; accepts treats/toys/attention; mild restlessness that resolves
3*	Mild to Moderate Stress	Partially dilated pupils; initial gaze avoidance; takes treats with hard mouth; panting with tight mouth; occasional barking, jumping or hiding; furrowed brow; slow/cautious movement; head turning without retreat; inconsistent engagement with reinforcers; hesitant but not avoidant of staff	Occasional hiding; partially dilated pupils; gaze avoidance; increased respiratory rate; slight decrease in appetite or grooming; head turning without withdrawal; inconsistent interest in reinforcers; occasional meowing or pawing; hesitant but not avoidant
2*	Significant Distress/ Shutdown or Defensive (Not Aggressive)	Escape attempts; hiding or immobility; trembling or fidgeting; tucked tail; ears back; dilated pupils; increased respiratory rate; excessive panting; tense or closed mouth; poor appetite; reduced exploration; resistant or avoidant of interaction; fight/flight/freeze responses; inconsistent or absent response to reinforcers	Trembling; poor appetite; dilated pupils; feigned sleep; persistent hiding; decreased grooming; occasional piloerection; increased respiratory rate; fight/flight/freeze responses; refusal of reinforcers; avoidant or resistant; tucked tail; lowered head; ears to side; occasional swatting, hissing or growling; decreased play
1*	Severe Distress/ High Risk (Aggressive)	Growling, snarling, snapping; lunging or charging; frantic escape attempts; excessive panting with tight mouth; repetitive barking, pacing, spinning, mouthing or jumping; destructive behavior; refusal of reinforcers; intolerance of handling or routine procedures	Spitting, hissing, screaming; lunging, swatting, stomping; attempts to scratch, bite or grab; piloerection; tail lashing; fleeing on approach; open-mouth breathing; rapid respiration; intolerance of handling; refusal of reinforcers; overturned kennel items; offensive approach toward staff; repetitive pacing, vocalizing, or pawing at enclosure

- Standardized behavioral assessment across team members and departments.
- Safe and appropriate handling decisions.
- Targeted intervention and enrichment planning.
- Early identification of stress-related welfare concerns or escalating distress.
- Clear documentation and communication across all teams managing animal care.

7.2 The Physiological Cost of Fear and Chronic Stress in Shelter Environments

Not all stress is harmful. Short-term (acute) stress can be adaptive and play an important role in learning and survival. Acute stress triggers a rapid physiological and behavioral response, including increases in cortisol, blood glucose, heart rate, respiratory rate, and blood pressure. These responses serve an important purpose, and in healthy individuals, these changes are temporary and the body typically returns to baseline once the stressor has passed.

For example, a dog that jumps onto a kitchen counter and accidentally knocks over a metal baking sheet and is startled by the loud noise. He immediately flees the room. Following this incident, the dog may temporarily avoid the kitchen or the counter. However, within hours, the healthy dog will return to the kitchen to drink water or eat without any residual effect. In this case, the stress response did not cause lasting harm.

7.2.1 Effects of Prolonged Stress Exposure

In contrast to acute stress, *chronic or prolonged stress* can have significant negative effects on both behavior and health. Pets exposed to ongoing stress may develop fear, anxiety, frustration, impulsivity, reactivity, repetitive behaviors, self-injury, or aggression. In the shelter environment, these pets often struggle to present well to potential adopters; they may appear frozen and withdrawn, vocalize excessively, pace, or repeatedly jump at kennel doors or toward people. Chronic stress also weakens immune function, making pets more susceptible to illness and further compromising their ability to cope.

Whenever a pet appears unwell or exhibits new or worsening changes in behavior, a medical evaluation is essential to rule out underlying disease, pain, or discomfort that may reduce physical capacity, affect coping ability, or exacerbate stress-related behaviors. Addressing medical conditions is a critical component of improving overall welfare and supporting behavioral resilience.

Stress-related behaviors frequently lead to reduced adopter interest and longer shelter stays. Importantly, many pets do not show meaningful behavioral improvement while remaining in the shelter environment, further decreasing their chances of adoption. As a result, shelter pets experiencing high or prolonged stress are often overlooked despite having the potential to thrive in a more suitable setting.

7.2.2 Physiological Stress Pathways

High stress levels activate two primary biological systems: the sympathetic nervous system (SNS) and the *hypothalamic–pituitary–adrenal (HPA) axis*. Together, these systems help the body respond to perceived threats by releasing stress-related hormones, including dopamine, epinephrine, norepinephrine, and cortisol (Lupien et al. 2009).

Some pets are highly resilient and adapt within hours or days. Others may require weeks or months to adjust. A subset of pets can cope temporarily, but eventually experience coping exhaustion, leading to declining mental health, negative emotional states, and reduced overall wellbeing.

Activation of the SNS is associated with heightened arousal, vigilance, and emergency responses. Physiological effects include decreased gastrointestinal motility, pupil dilation, vasoconstriction, bronchodilation, and the release of adrenaline from the adrenal glands – commonly referred to as the *"fight-or-flight"* response.

The HPA axis plays a central role in regulating longer-term stress responses. Stress triggers the hypothalamus to release corticotropin-releasing hormone (CRH), which stimulates the pituitary gland to release adrenocorticotropic hormone (ACTH). ACTH then acts on the adrenal glands to release glucocorticoids, primarily cortisol.

In contrast, the parasympathetic nervous system (PNS) supports rest and recovery. It regulates functions such as digestion, growth, heart rate reduction, respiration, salivation, elimination, and reproductive processes. The PNS is most active during sleep and after eating.

7.2.3 Cognitive, Emotional, and Health Consequences of Chronic Stress

Stress negatively affects working memory and memory retrieval, with the amygdala playing a key role in how emotional stress influences memory processing. The release of norepinephrine during stressful events affects memory consolidation within the amygdala, reinforcing fear-based learning.

Chronic stress can lead to structural and functional changes in the amygdala, hippocampus, and prefrontal cortex (McEwen and Morrison 2013). These changes are associated with impaired cognition, increased anxiety, altered mood regulation, and reduced behavioral flexibility (Roozendaal et al. 2009).

Beyond behavioral effects, chronic stress exacerbates underlying medical conditions and contributes to disease across species, including humans, dogs, and cats. Stress impacts nearly all body systems, including the gastrointestinal, urinary, dermatological, respiratory, cardiovascular, immune, reproductive, and growth systems (Mills et al. 2014). Over time, this physiological burden significantly compromises welfare and overall health.

7.2.4 Effects of Stress on Laboratory Results

Animals experiencing moderate to high levels of stress commonly exhibit stress-induced alterations in laboratory values, which can complicate the interpretation of diagnostic results (Puurunen et al. 2018). These changes may reflect physiological responses to stress rather than underlying pathology and should be interpreted within the context of the animal's emotional state and handling experience.

Common stress-related laboratory findings include:

- Blood glucose: Transient hyperglycemia due to catecholamine and cortisol release
- Creatine kinase (CK): Increased levels associated with physical struggling, restraint, or muscle exertion during blood collection
- Lactate: Elevated concentrations, particularly in stressed cats, reflecting anaerobic metabolism and sympathetic activation
- White blood cell count: A classic *stress leukogram* characterized by neutrophilia and monocytosis with concurrent lymphopenia and eosinopenia
- Platelets: Platelet clumping, which may falsely suggest thrombocytopenia, especially in cats.

Additional findings have been described in fearful dogs, including increased plasma concentrations of glutamine and γ-glutamyl glutamine (γ-Glu Gln) (Puurunen et al. 2018).

Stress-induced hypertension, which may occur in shelter environments, has the potential to influence symmetric dimethylarginine (SDMA) values (Puurunen et al. 2018). Elevated SDMA is commonly associated with acute kidney injury and chronic kidney disease. Research suggests that a heightened and prolonged state of fear can lead to sustained psychological stress, which in turn may adversely affect renal function. These findings highlight the importance of considering emotional stress as a contributing factor when interpreting blood work in shelter pets.

7.2.5 Medical Conditions That May Mask or Cause Behavior Problems

Distinguishing primary behavior concerns from medically driven behavior changes can be challenging. Many medical conditions cause pain, discomfort, or physiological dysregulation that may present as fear, aggression, withdrawal, reactivity, or decreased tolerance to handling.

Conditions Commonly Associated with Pain

- Dermatitis/Otitis externa
- Orthopedic pain/Osteoarthritis/Intervertebral Disc Disease
- Gastrointestinal pain or discomfort
- Periodontal Disease

7.2.6 Medical Conditions That Can Cause Behavioral Changes

Hypersensitivities (Atopic Dermatitis, Flea Allergy Dermatitis, Adverse Food Reactions)

- Pruritus (itching)
- Cutaneous inflammation
- Secondary skin infections

Endocrinopathies

- Hypothyroidism: Lethargy, weight gain, reduced engagement, and "tragic" facial expression
- Hyperadrenocorticism: Polyuria, polydipsia, muscle weakness, and wasting
- Hypoadrenocorticism: Lethargy, vomiting, diarrhea, increased thirst and urination, and unintentional weight loss

Gastrointestinal Disease

- Food allergies or intolerances
- Inflammatory bowel disease
- Pancreatitis
- Hepatic lipidosis

Neurological Disease

- Seizure disorders (including idiopathic epilepsy)
- Cognitive dysfunction
- Intracranial disease (e.g. neoplasia, inflammation, infection, trauma)
- Neuropathic pain
- Vestibular disease

7.2.7 Organ System Responses to Stress

7.2.7.1 Gastrointestinal Response to Stress

Stress decreases parasympathetic tone, resulting in reduced salivation and decreased blood flow to the gastrointestinal tract, while increased sympathetic activation suppresses gastrointestina motility. In animals with preexisting gastrointestinal disease (e.g. inflammatory bowel disease), stress amplifies monocyte-mediated inflammation and further impairs motility (Schneider et al. 2023). Clinical signs include hyporexia or anorexia, diarrhea, colitis, pica, and psychogenic polydipsia. Chronic glucocorticoid exposure promotes intestinal inflammation, reduces smooth muscle contractility, and delays gastrointestinal transit. Similar associations between stress, abdominal pain, diarrhea, and fatigue have been documented in humans (Mawdsley and Rampton 2005; Schneider et al. 2023).

7.2.7.2 Urogenital Response to Stress

Stress commonly alters elimination behaviors in shelter pets. Dogs and cats may exhibit inappropriate urination or defecation, increased urinary frequency, straining, or hematuria. In cats, stress is a well-established trigger for feline idiopathic cystitis (FIC), mediated by neuroendocrine dysregulation and altered bladder permeability. Stress-related catecholamine release and altered autonomic balance contribute to lower urinary tract inflammation and pain (Buffington 2011; Stella et al. 2011).

7.2.7.3 Dermatological Response to Stress

Stress increases epidermal permeability, leading to increased shedding and impaired skin barrier function. Displacement behaviors such as scratching and licking cause microtrauma, further compromising the skin barrier and altering the skin microbiome, which increases susceptibility to secondary bacterial infections (pyoderma). Dogs with chronic pruritic disease and concurrent fear or anxiety are often more irritable and less tolerant of stressors, with an increased risk of aggressive behavior. In cats, stress reduces grooming behavior; when combined with stress-induced immunosuppression, this contributes to the high prevalence of dermatophytosis in shelters. Bidirectional interactions between stress, pruritus, and anxiety have been documented across species, including humans and animal models (Griffin and DeBoer 2001; Paus et al. 2006).

7.2.7.4 Metabolic Response to Stress

Prolonged stress shifts metabolism toward gluconeogenesis through the breakdown of fat and protein stores, particularly when food intake is reduced. This contributes to muscle wasting, weakness, fatigue, and increased morbidity in vulnerable populations such as neonates, geriatric animals, and those in poor body condition. Overweight adult cats experiencing stress-related anorexia are at high risk for hepatic lipidosis, a life-threatening condition that frequently results in euthanasia if untreated (Center 2005).

7.2.7.5 Cardiovascular Response to Stress

Stress activates the sympathetic nervous system, leading to tachycardia, hypertension, and transient cardiac murmurs. Sustained sympathetic activation increases cardiovascular workload and may exacerbate underlying heart disease. In humans, chronic stress is associated with myocardial infarction, arrhythmias, stress cardiomyopathy, stroke, and sudden cardiac death, highlighting the systemic cardiovascular consequences of prolonged stress exposure (Steptoe and Kivimäki 2012).

7.2.7.6 Growth and Reproductive Effects of Stress

Stress suppresses reproductive function and growth through inhibition of gonadotropin release and diversion of metabolic resources away from development. Outcomes include smaller litters, low birth weight, poor growth, and increased neonatal mortality. Exposure to elevated cortisol levels in utero or early life can alter brain development, resulting in increased anxiety, impulsivity, and reduced stress tolerance later in life (Lupien et al. 2009).

7.2.7.7 Immune System Response to Stress

Chronic stress causes immunosuppression through sustained glucocorticoid release. This inhibits cytokine production, delays lymphocyte maturation, induces lymphopenia, and promotes lymphocyte apoptosis. Stress also reduces vaccine responsiveness, increases susceptibility to infection and sepsis, and delays wound healing (Dhabhar 2014; Hekman et al. 2014)

7.3 Minimizing Stressors in the Shelter Environment

Understanding the profound negative impact that prolonged stress can have on shelter pets underscores the importance of minimizing time spent in the shelter environment. The best outcome for pets exhibiting signs of stress is adoption and timely exit from shelter care.

For pets who remain in the shelter, environmental optimization is essential to support both physiological and psychological wellbeing. Meaningful improvements can be made regardless of a facility's age, size, or design. When shelters are evaluated through the pets' sensory experience – what they see, hear, smell, and feel – targeted modifications can be implemented to reduce stress and enhance welfare.

The recommendations that follow are not intended as an all-or-nothing standard. Rather, the authors aim to raise awareness and provide practical, scalable solutions that can be adapted to organizations of all sizes and resource levels. Even small changes, implemented at the right time, in the right space, for the right pet, can significantly improve welfare outcomes.

7.3.1 Environmental Modifications

7.3.1.1 Visual Sensitivity and Stress in Shelter Pets

Both dogs and cats have receptors in their eyes that are sensitive to movement. They both have greater peripheral vision. The tapetum lucidum, the reflective layer at the back of the eye that causes the familiar "eye shine," enhances vision in low-light conditions by reflecting light back. This allows dogs and cats to make better use of limited available light (Beaver 2003; Byosiere et al. 2018). Humans are often unaware that dogs have a visual acuity of approximately 20–40% of human vision, meaning dogs see less fine detail and rely more on movement, contrast, and other senses to interpret their environment. While they can see a person or an object that is 20 m away, the image is fuzzy (Byosiere et al. 2018). It is only when the person or object is in closer proximity that they can see the details and features. This may explain why some dogs bark at familiar people until the person is closer and then the dog stops barking because they recognize them.

Cats have good visual acuity for objects approximately 25 cm to 2 m away. For objects closer than about 25 cm, their ability to focus decreases and they rely more heavily on their whiskers (vibrissae) to gather spatial and tactile information, effectively helping them "see" what is too close for clear vision (Beaver 2003; Bradshaw et al. 2012).

Bright, fluorescent lighting can be harsh and overstimulating for shelter animals, contributing to stress and discomfort.

7.3.1.1.1 Reducing Visual Stress: Simple, Effective Strategies

- Use LED instead of fluorescent lights.
- Avoid lights shining directly into kennels or cages.
- Use softer, warm-spectrum lighting where possible.
- Reduce overall light intensity, especially in resting areas.
- Use spot lighting for rooms where extra brightness is needed.
- Create consistent lighting schedules to reduce unpredictability.
- Install a dimmer switch so the intensity of light can be regulated.
- Use 60 W lighting. Use small headlamps for spot lights when needed.
- Use natural light when available, while preventing glare and overheating.
- Turn off or dim lights during overnight hours to support normal circadian rhythms.
- Provide darkened retreat spaces (hide boxes, covered kennels, partially draped enclosures).

Dogs and cats also differ from humans in how they perceive color. Dogs primarily see blue, green, and yellow wavelengths, with reduced sensitivity to reds (Byosiere et al. 2018). Cats can perceive some colors as well, but they are more responsive to brightness, contrast, and object size than to color alone. Research suggests cats can distinguish between certain color combinations, including red vs. green, blue vs. green, and blue vs. yellow (Clayton and Kamback 1966; Loop and Bruce 1978). Using colors that shelter pets can actually perceive – especially high-contrast blues and yellows – can help reduce stress and improve environmental clarity. Without these cues, animals may experience their surroundings largely as gradations of black, gray, and white, which can make spaces feel more confusing and overstimulating. Thoughtful color choices can therefore support orientation, comfort, and overall wellbeing.

Limiting visual overstimulation can significantly reduce stress in shelter pets. Closing doors to block views of busy hallways or applying opaque window films helps reduce exposure to constant motion that can trigger anxiety (see Figure 7.1). Simple solutions such as opaque cloth or plastic

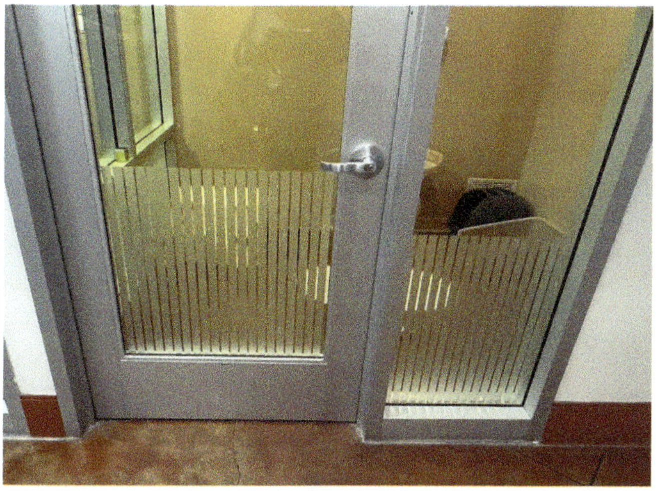

Figure 7.1 Opaque Strips on Door

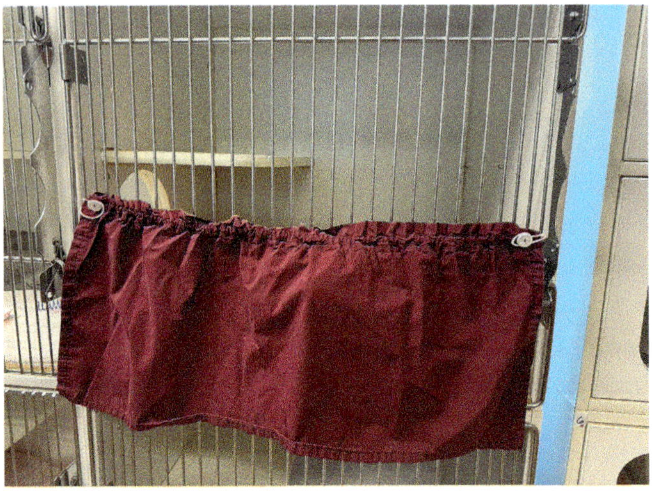

Figure 7.2 Cloth Curtain Hide

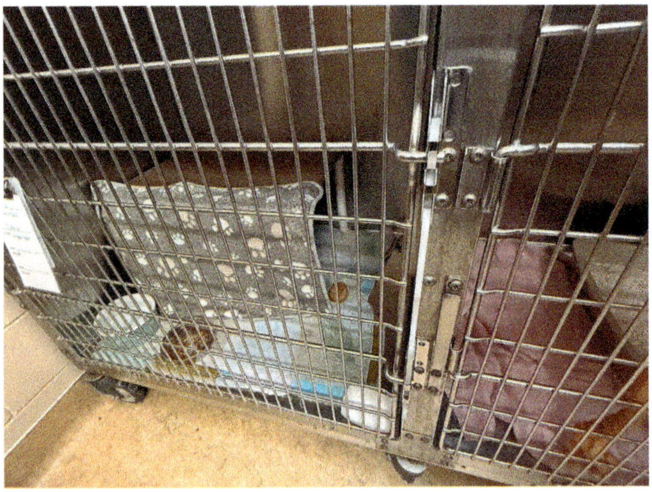

Figure 7.3 Blanket Hide

curtains are often effective and inexpensive (see Figures 7.2 and 7.3). Providing hide or retreat spaces – for example boxes or crates placed inside cages or kennels – can immediately lower stress by giving animals control over their environment (see Figure 7.4). Several research studies have shown that cats prefer access to a hide rather than perches in the shelter setting (Vinke et al. 2014; Ellis et al. 2017). Draping a towel or sheet over the front of a cat's enclosure is another easy way to reduce visual exposure and supports a sense of safety.

7.3.2 Olfactory Sensitivity and Stress in Shelter Pets

Dogs and cats experience the world primarily through scent, and their olfactory sensitivity far exceeds that of humans. A cat's sense of smell is estimated to be about 14 times stronger than a human's with roughly twice as many olfactory receptors (Padodara and Jacob 2014; Chung et al. 2018).

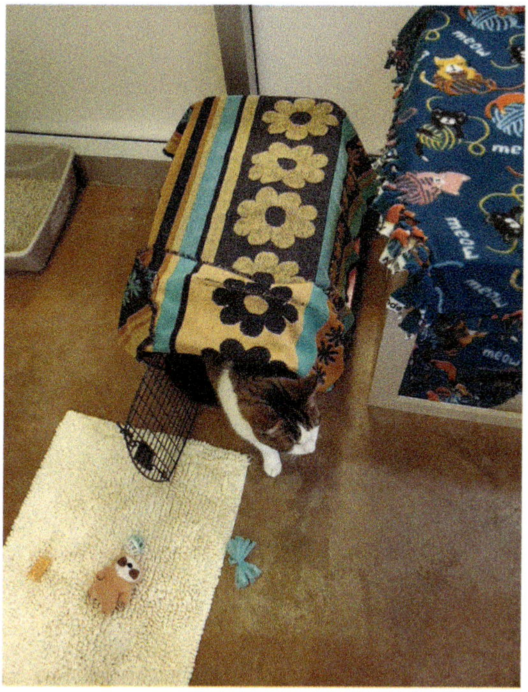

Figure 7.4 Cat with Carrier Hide

Dogs are even more sensitive, with a sense of smell estimated to be 10,000–100,000 times greater than humans and approximately 300 million olfactory receptors (Padodara and Jacob 2014).

Because of this heightened ability, shelter pets are far more affected by odors – both pleasant and unpleasant – than people realize. Strong or unfamiliar smells can quickly increase stress, trigger avoidance behaviors, disrupt feeding, and rest and interfere with emotional regulation.

7.3.2.1 Reducing Olfactory Stress: Simple, Effective Strategies

- Avoid harsh chemical odors: Strong-smelling cleaners such as bleach and ammonia can provoke negative emotional responses. Their fumes may cause nasal irritation or a stinging sensation, similar to what humans experience, but intensified by animals' sensitive noses.
- Ensure kennels are fully dry and odor-free: Animals should only be returned to kennels or cages once surfaces are completely dry and free of residual chemical odor, as lingering smells can prolong stress.
- Use low-odor disinfectants when possible: Accelerated hydrogen peroxide-based cleaners effectively disinfect surfaces with minimal odor, shorter contact times, and reduced need for personal protective equipment. This is beneficial for both animals and staff.
- Reduce scent disruption during cleaning: For dogs, instead of moving them into holding kennels during cleaning, shelters should consider potty walks or playgroups when appropriate. These activities reduce stress, allow normal behavior, and limit exposure to strong cleaning odors.
- Spot clean for fearful animals – especially cats. For fearful dogs and cats that are difficult to remove from enclosures, spot cleaning is recommended whenever possible. This is especially important for cats, as removing all items from a kennel eliminates familiar scent cues. Leaving bedding, hides or objects carrying the cat's own scent helps preserve a sense of safety and stability.

- Use calming scents cautiously: Certain mild scents, such as lavender or chamomile, may reduce anxiety in some animals. However, essential oils should never be applied directly to pets or to surfaces they may lick. Lavender oil can be toxic to cats if ingested or absorbed through the skin. If used, it should be placed on cotton pads or balls to lightly scent the room, never in direct contact with the animal.

7.3.3 Pheromones

Pheromones are chemical messages that are detected by the animal's vomeronasal organ. Pheromones are species specific, meaning cats only respond to cat pheromones and dogs only respond to dog pheromones. These chemical messages can influence the social behavior of dogs and cats (Frank et al. 2010). Cats have several facial pheromones, F1–5, produced by their cheek glands. The F2 pheromone is used in sexual display by male tomcats. The F3 pheromone is involved in facial marking. Its use was shown to reduce urine marking, scratching, excessive grooming and anxiety. Additional studies noted improvement in the cats' feeding and play behavior as well as level of activity (Pageat and Gaultier 2003). The pheromone may also function by facilitating stress reduction. The F4 pheromone is known as the allomarking pheromone and assists a resident cat accept the introduction of a new cat into the household. The F4 pheromone can also reduce the cat's aggression from human handling (Pageat and Gaultier 2003).

Canine and feline mammary glands have specialized glands that release pheromones that are released by lactating mothers while their litters are nursing. The pheromone functions to provide a message of safety and security. See Chapter 10 for more on Pheromone therapy.

7.3.4 Auditory Sensitivity and Stress in Shelter Pets

Dogs and cats experience the shelter environment very differently from humans, particularly when it comes to sound. Both species have large, mobile aural pinnae that rotate to pinpoint the direction of sound, making them highly sensitive to auditory stimuli. Adult cats hear frequencies ranging from 48 Hz to 85 kHz, and adult dogs from 67 Hz to 45 kHz, far exceeding the human hearing range of 64 Hz to 23 kHz (Strain 2017). Sounds above 20 kHz are considered ultrasonic, meaning many noises inaudible to humans may still be clearly perceived by shelter pets (Kruger et al. 2021).

This heightened hearing makes dogs and cats particularly vulnerable to loud, sudden, repetitive, or unpredictable sounds, all of which are common in shelters. Chronic exposure to noise can increase stress, disrupt rest, heighten reactivity and impair emotional regulation.

7.3.5 Reducing Auditory Stress: Small Changes, Big Impact

- Voice modulation matters: Team members and volunteers should use calm, controlled tones when speaking around shelter pets. Raised or excitable voices can increase stress or over-arousal, especially in fearful or excitable animals. Individual responses vary: some shy pets respond to gentle, higher-pitched voices, while others do better with soft, low tones. So observation is key.
- Minimize startling noises: Avoid slamming doors, drawers, windows, or kennel doors. Handle equipment carefully to prevent sudden loud sounds that may startle animals.
- Manage noise exposure for sensitive animals: For pets sensitive to sound, closing doors or windows during periods of heavy foot traffic or machinery use can significantly reduce overstimulation. Other animals may tolerate or even enjoy activity, reinforcing the need for individualized housing decisions.

- Reduce metal noise in housing: Stainless steel cages and kennels can amplify sound. When possible, choose alternative materials or install plastic or coated door slides. Regularly oil hinges and latches to prevent squeaking or clanging, which can be highly stressful.
- Use sound buffering intentionally: White noise machines can help mask unpredictable shelter sounds. Portable or Bluetooth speakers may be used to play species-appropriate music, classical music at ~60 BPM, reggae, or audiobooks, all of which research has shown can reduce stress and promote relaxation.
- Designate quiet spaces: Whenever possible, shelters should create quiet wards for shy, fearful, or highly stressed animals. House dogs and cats separately to reduce cross-species noise stress.
- Address barking proactively: In dog housing areas where barking escalates as people walk past kennels, team members or volunteers can toss treats while walking by, helping dogs associate foot traffic with positive outcomes. After several days, treats can be delivered only during pauses between barks, reinforcing quieter behavior. Many shelters observe a noticeable reduction in barking volume within a week with consistency. (Protopopova and Wynne 2015; Baldan et al. 2023)

7.3.6 Tactile (Touch) Sensitivity and Stress in Shelter Pets

Touch is a critical but often overlooked aspect of how dogs and cats experience the shelter environment. Both species rely on tactile input to interpret pressure, texture, temperature, and surface stability. When these needs are unmet, animals may experience discomfort, insecurity, and increased stress.

Shelter environments often rely on hard, durable surfaces that provide little physical comfort. Whenever possible, animals should be given choice in resting surfaces, allowing them to self-regulate comfort and reduce physical strain. Tactile comfort is closely linked to emotional regulation, particularly for cats, who benefit from environments that support both rest and retreat.

Tactile exploration also plays an important role in enrichment. Dogs use their mouths to gather sensory information and regulate stress, while cats may bite, mouth or carry objects during play. Providing safe, varied tactile enrichment supports both mental and physical wellbeing.

By addressing tactile needs through thoughtful housing design and enrichment, shelters can reduce stress and significantly improve comfort and emotional wellbeing using simple, low-cost strategies.

7.3.7 Reducing Tactile Stress: Simple, Effective Strategies

- Provide elevated resting options to reduce pressure on joints and avoid cold floors.
- Offer cats both hide and perch options, such as a cardboard box placed on its side.
- Provide cats with at least two scratching options (cardboard, sisal, carpeted surfaces).
- Create scratching posts for cats using carpet remnants attached to 2×4 boards or posts.
- Supply dogs with chew toys made from various safe materials to meet oral sensory needs.
- Closely monitor dogs that shred toys or attempt to ingest bedding, stuffing, or squeakers.
- Provide cats with toys of different textures to support biting, carrying, and play behaviors.
- Use box walls as visual barriers to help separate food, resting, and litter areas in tight spaces.
- Provide choice in resting surfaces, offering both hard flooring and soft or cushioned options (beds, mats, hammock-style beds).
- Place area rugs or rubber mats in slippery or high-traffic areas for dogs hesitant on smooth surfaces.

- Use low-cost, replaceable materials such as yoga mats or plastic shelf liners that are easy to sanitize.
- Position hide boxes with openings facing the back of the enclosure to allow full retreat and a sense of safety.

These small, intentional adjustments can significantly reduce tactile stress while improving comfort, engagement, and overall wellbeing for shelter pets.

7.3.8 Gustatory (Taste) Sensitivity and Stress in Shelter Pets

Taste plays a smaller, but still meaningful role in how shelter pets experience stress and enrichment. Most shelters rely on strict, consistent diets to reduce the risk of gastrointestinal upset and diarrhea, which can be difficult to manage in a group setting and may complicate medical decision-making when infectious diseases are a concern. Consistency is therefore essential for health monitoring and disease control.

However, a completely monotonous diet can contribute to reduced appetite, frustration, and disengagement, particularly in stressed animals. Carefully managed gustatory enrichment can stimulate appetite, increase motivation and support emotional wellbeing without compromising medical safety.

Offering very small amounts of bland, familiar ingredients (when medically appropriate) can engage taste and scent while minimizing risk. Likewise, using the animal's own diet in creative ways helps preserve dietary consistency while adding novelty and enrichment. When paired with mental engagement – such as food puzzles – gustatory enrichment can reduce boredom, support coping, and promote more positive shelter experiences.

7.3.9 Reducing Gustatory Stress: Simple, Effective Strategies

- Maintain a consistent base diet to support gastrointestinal health and disease monitoring.
- Break up dietary monotony with tiny portions of treats, used strategically and sparingly.
- Repurpose the pet's regular canned diet into baked, dried treats to maintain consistency.
- Crumble approved food items over kibble to encourage eating without changing the diet.
- Closely monitor animals using puzzle toys to ensure they do not damage or ingest pieces.
- Use small amounts of bland, low-risk foods (when approved) to stimulate appetite and interest.
- Use puzzle feeders or food-dispensing toys to add mental and physical stimulation during meals.

When applied thoughtfully, gustatory enrichment can enhance engagement, reduce stress, and improve overall welfare, while still respecting the medical and operational realities of shelter care.

For more details on sensory enrichment, see Chapter 8.

7.4 Implementing Stress-Reduction Techniques

As mentioned in earlier chapters, the best way to reduce fear, anxiety, and stress when interacting or handling shelter pets is recognition through reading their body language. An organization should implement stress reducing techniques in the team member and volunteer training, such as body held at a sideways angle, minimize direct eye contact, and avoid reaching over the pets' heads. Then they can maximize the care provided to the shelter pets through their daily interactions and management.

Any shelter should periodically re-examine how they are managing and treating the animals in their care – there is almost always room for improvement. The *Canine & Feline Wellbeing Scale* provides a structured way to guide handling, medical care, and behavioral support. Pets rated as relaxed or *5-star* are generally comfortable with handling and can tolerate gentle restraint. These animals typically accept treats, can be easily redirected with food or toys, and often can be positioned for procedures with minimal prompting.

In contrast, shelter pets with *1–2 star ratings* are highly stressed and may display fear-based aggression. These animals require a careful, experienced approach to handling and restraint. While no animal should ever be handled heavy-handedly, pets in this category often tolerate only *very light restraint* and teams must be prepared to use safety tools and advanced handling skills to reduce risk.

Traditionally, many veterinary professionals were taught to use strong manual restraint – pinning or holding pets firmly for procedures. However, in many cases, *minimal restraint and a light, supportive touch* accomplish the task more effectively and without inducing additional fear or emotional trauma. When animals are frightened, their first instinct is to struggle or escape; forceful handling tends to escalate distress and risk of injury for both the pet and the handler.

For pets requiring minimal restraint, *towels, blankets, or soft wraps* are often safer and less stressful than direct physical restraint. A towel gently wrapped around the body or neck is far less threatening than placing an arm over a dog's shoulders or scruffing or stretching a cat. Gentle, supportive restraint reduces fear while maintaining safety for the animal and the team.

Regardless of the pet's wellbeing rating, *planning ahead* is essential. Preparing the environment, gathering necessary equipment in advance and coordinating with the team help ensure procedures are efficient, handling time is minimized and stress is reduced for animals, staff and volunteers alike.

7.4.1 Step 1: Preparation

- Gathering all necessary supplies
- Determining what procedures are needed
- Determining the location where the procedure will be performed.

The medical team and animal care team should work collaboratively to determine whether a shelter pet would benefit from pre-procedure pharmaceuticals. Animal care staff interact with pets daily and can provide valuable insights into how an individual animal responds to handling, stress, and unfamiliar interactions. This information helps the medical team select the most appropriate approach and anticipate challenges.

Input from the animal care team also supports decisions about medication selection and route of administration (oral vs. intramuscular), balancing effectiveness with the pet's tolerance and safety. Prior to any procedure, teams should create a clear list of essential vs. optional tasks, completing the most critical procedures first. Any additional procedures completed beyond those priorities should be considered a bonus, helping reduce overall stress while ensuring necessary care is delivered.

7.4.2 Step 2: The Team

- Which team members will be participating in the handling and treatment?
- The roles of each participant need to be clarified.
  - Who will deliver the oral medication?
  - Who and how will the intramuscular injection be administered?

- How much time will be spent trying to perform a task and when is it time to stop and try again if needed?
- How many attempts will be used for restraining before choosing another approach (e.g. sedation)?

The more stressed a shelter pet is, the more experienced the handler should be, in order to complete procedures efficiently and minimize stress and risk for the animal, team members, or volunteers.

7.4.3 Step 3: Transport

Transporting pets within a shelter is stressful for animals and staff and is often inefficient, so movement should be minimized whenever possible. When transport is necessary, plan routes to limit exposure to people and other animals. Use radios or clear communication so hallways are temporarily clear. Small dogs and cats should be transported in carriers supported from the bottom or sides, not carried by the handle, to prevent swaying and motion sickness.

Dogs reluctant to walk should not be dragged on leash or routinely picked up. Lifting dogs – especially those over 30 lbs – increases stress and risk of injury to both people and animals. Instead, use food or toy lures, carriers, carts, familiar handlers, or calm canine companions. Spatial pressure with tools like an exercise pen can help guide movement when needed.

Whenever possible, perform procedures in the animal's current housing by bringing supplies to them. This reduces transport stress, saves time, and lowers the risk of animals developing negative associations with new locations or approaches.

7.4.4 Step 4: Procedure and Handling

The fourth step includes medication administration (if needed), handling and completion of the required procedure(s). Handling should always begin with no or minimal restraint, paired with high-value treats or toys to reduce stress (see Figures 7.5–7.7). Most dogs and cats can tolerate brief handling (approximately three to five seconds) before stress escalates, though individual tolerance varies.

Each pet should have a customized handling plan documented in their shelter record. If the initial approach is unsuccessful, pause, regroup and reassess before escalating. Consider whether

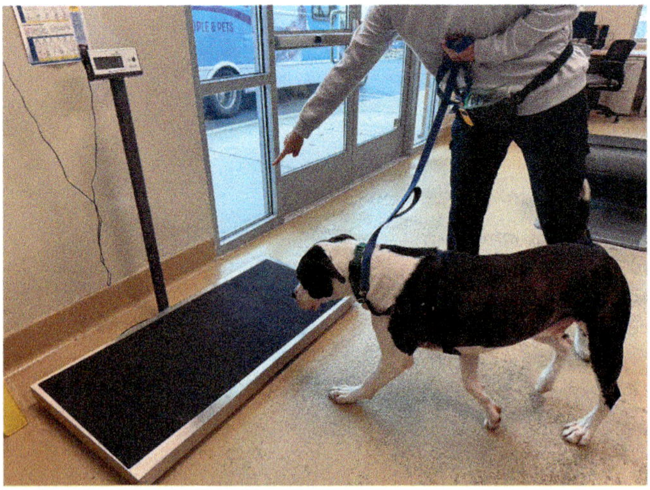

Figure 7.5 Placing Dog on Scale

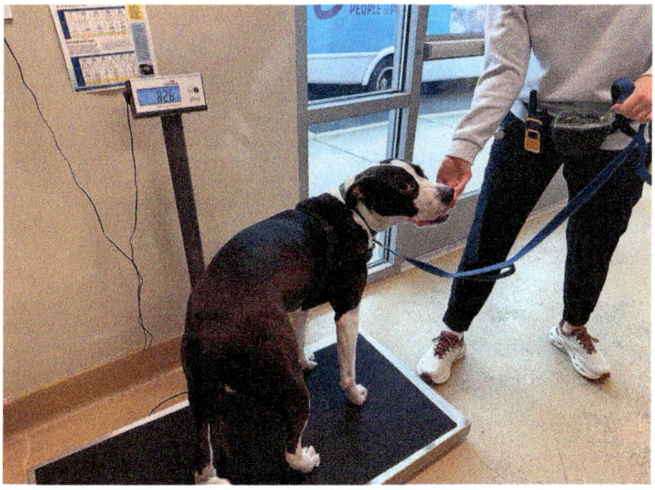

Figure 7.6 Positioning on Scale

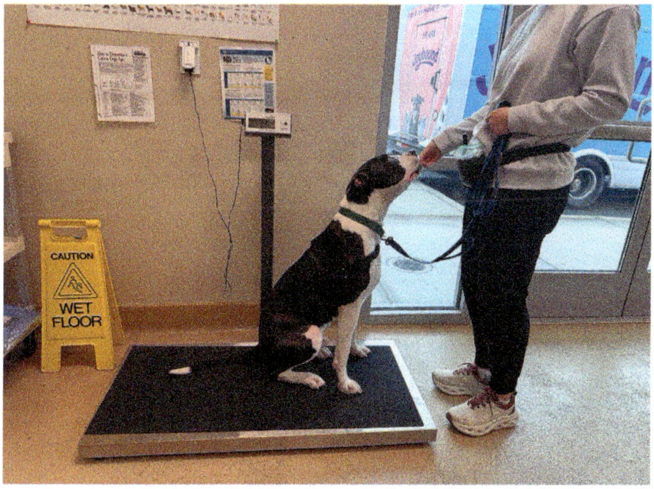

Figure 7.7 Rewarding on Scale

additional tools or a different technique are warranted. If a second attempt is not successful, it may be best to reschedule the procedure for later in the day or after oral anti-anxiety medication, rather than continuing and increasing stress.

Keep in mind, some shelter pets will remain highly stressed despite best efforts to reduce environmental and handling stressors. When interaction, movement, handling or restraint is necessary, it is essential to use appropriate tools and thoughtful planning to complete tasks safely, efficiently and with the least amount of stress possible for both the animal and the people involved.

7.4.5 Tool Use and Handling Skills

Training must emphasize that tools are not always the first or best option. Improper or premature use can increase stress and injury risk. For example, a cat that escapes a cage does not automatically require capture with a net. Many cats can be safely guided into a carrier using treats, toys, exercise pens, or gentle spatial pressure. When lifting small pets is unavoidable, towels or blankets should be used to wrap and support the animal, reducing fear and risk of injury. All team members should be trained not only in the safe use of handling and restraint tools but also in the decision-making needed to determine *when* those tools are appropriate. Effective shelter handling relies on using a thoughtful humane approach first and escalating to using more restraint only when necessary. This protects safety, preserves animal wellbeing, and ensures that team members and volunteers feel confident and supported in their work.

Leash-handling skills for example are essential for anyone walking dogs. Team members and volunteers must learn how to redirect dogs safely when they pull or lunge, using proper body positioning and leash leverage rather than pulling straight back – a technique that often increases arousal and instability.

However, it is important to recognize that handling skill is not a single dimension. Instead of dividing people into "experienced" and "inexperienced," shelters should acknowledge that different pets require *different kinds* of experience, and that everyone can contribute meaningfully at some level.

For example:

- *High-arousal, strong, or adolescent dogs* benefit from handlers who are physically skilled, confident, and practiced in leash management and redirection.
- *Shy, fearful, or behaviorally sensitive dogs and cats* benefit from calm, emotionally attuned handlers who excel at reading subtle body language and maintaining a gentle, low-pressure approach.

Both roles require experience – just *different* forms of experience. By recognizing this diversity of strengths and matching pets with handlers whose skills align with their needs, shelters can expand the pool of capable caregivers, improve safety and welfare, and create a more inclusive and empowered team environment.

Dog-to-dog altercations – whether occurring during playgroups, in shared housing or in high-arousal areas – require specialized training and should only be managed by team members or volunteers who have been specifically trained in safe intervention techniques. The risk of injury to both people and dogs is significant, making preparation and skill essential. To ensure safety, tools for interrupting aggressive behavior or separating fighting dogs must be readily accessible throughout the shelter and clinic.

Dog-fight response training is critical. Team members should:

- Call for immediate assistance and avoid intervening alone.
- Never place hands between fighting dogs or attempt to grab collars directly.
- Use leashes, loud noises, visual barriers, or physical dividers (e.g. exercise pens and pig boards) to create space and stop the fight.
- Reserve advanced techniques – such as hind-leg lifts or break stick use – for highly trained staff only, as these methods carry a high risk of redirected bites.
- Once separated, immediately place physical barriers between the dogs and remove each dog from the area to prevent re-engagement.

7.4.6 Shelter Handling and Safety Tools

7.4.6.1 For Dogs

General Handling and Safety Management

- Crates
- Large towels and/or blankets

- Basket muzzles
- Elizabethan collars (E-collars)
- Slip leashes

For Dogs Who Are Potentially Aggressive

- Rabies pole
- Noise makers (e.g. two metal bowls clanged together, air horn)
- Exercise pen for barrier creation
- Pig board/animal separator
- Break stick
- Water hose
- Citronella spray

7.4.6.2 For Cats

General Handling and Management

- Carriers
- Exercise pen (as a temporary barrier or room divider)
- Towels and blankets

For Cats Who Are Potentially Aggressive

- Catch net
- Small plastic laundry basket (for safe containment or exam assistance)

7.5 More Options for Decreasing Stress in Shelter Pets

Many dogs in the shelter are stressed by confinement. Some dogs are more resilient than others. Researchers found that cortisol levels of dogs dropped when they were fostered overnight (Gunter et al. 2019) and increased when dogs returned to the shelter. However, the dogs were able to sleep for longer periods of time while in foster and upon their return to the shelter. Deep sleep has a restorative effect on mental health. While it may be more difficult to have the public foster dogs for a long period of time, incorporating a one-night sleep over, helps alleviate stress in the shelter dogs and may help to build more resiliency.

Some organizations incorporate a daytime outing program for dogs. This program provides the dogs a break from the shelter and an opportunity for increased exercise. Gunter et al. (2021) found that short excursions of 2–2.5 hours away from the shelter did not reduce cortisol levels of dogs. Instead, the stress levels were elevated and the dogs spent more time in higher activity. The benefit of this program was providing more exposure of adoptable dogs to the eyes of the public and offering additional information handlers can provide about the dog's behavior out in public. Potential adopters do want to know how the dog behaves around other dogs, strangers, children, bicycles, scooters, cars, etc. Another study indicated that dogs that participated in a day time outing program or short-term foster stays had an increased likelihood of being adopted compared to the other dogs that did not participate in those programs (Gunter et al. 2023). Programs involving community members were more successful when compared to programs where only team members or volunteers were involved. Again, this highlights the importance of community engagement and a community approach to reducing the shelter population.

There is only one study that evaluated how temporary fostering affected the stress levels of cats. Vitale et al. (2022) found that neither an overnight nor one week foster increased the cats' stress levels or social interactions with people (Vitale et al. 2022). However, it was also noted that the cats did not have increased cortisol levels nor exhibited increased fear or aggression while in the foster home. Based on the authors' personal experience in two shelters, fearful cats who were not eating or coming out of their hides in the shelter were able to eat consistently and did come out of hiding more often in foster care. After one week of foster care, the cats were brought back to the shelter and the majority of the cats had gained in resiliency. They may still hide during the day and may need to be lured out with toys or treats. The majority of the cats were able to consistently eat after being fostered. Organizations that allow the public to adopt the cats while in foster may see more success. According to the Shelter Animals Count (2025), foster based organizations had a higher adoption rate of 75% in 2025 compared to the national shelter average of 56%.

Play group for dogs is another popular program that allows dogs to continue to interact with their peers and build social relationships. It is important that organizations continue to use positive reinforcement when allowing dogs to play. The use of any punitive techniques on dogs while interacting with other dogs will only inhibit behaviors and not teach them how to behave appropriately with other dogs. Team members and volunteers should receive sufficient training to ensure that they can read body language and know when to intervene before altercations erupt between dogs. Ideally, there should be at least one person per dog and at minimum one person per two dogs for maximum safety. For dogs under 20 lbs, one person may be able to supervise as many as three small dogs. A safety kit needs to be available in case play escalates into an altercation. Organizations should consider having two play groups, one for large dogs and one for smaller dogs. Having a specific shy dog play group can do wonders for increasing sociability, confidence and adoptability of the smaller behaviorally challenged dogs.

Another program is neighborhood wellbeing walks. The volunteers are guided on a group walk with 4–10 dogs around the neighborhood. Each handler has a dog. This experience allows the dogs to be exercised, interact with people and other dogs, and be exposed to the outside world. This is also a good way to train volunteers and improve upon their handling skills. An experienced team member should be going up and down the line assisting with each volunteer or dog to ensure every person and dog has a good experience.

Cat social visit programs should be incorporated in all shelters. Different protocols may be needed depending upon how the cats are housed. In some organizations, the adoptable cats are kept in rooms where the volunteers can enter and interact with cats. In other organizations where all the cats are kept in cages, a different method must be utilized in which volunteers can interact with cats through the bars. In most of these facilities, it would be unsafe for the volunteers to open the cage doors to interact due to the higher risk of the cats escaping the cage. However, fishing pole type toys can be used between the kennel bars to stimulate their senses and engage the cats in a good play session.

In summary, while no shelter can remove every source of stress, every shelter can make meaningful change. Thoughtful programs, compassionate handling, and intentional environmental modifications can significantly reduce stress and help shelter pets build resilience, confidence, and trust.

References

Baldan, A. L., Ferreira, B. L., Warisaia, V., Feuerbacher, E. N., Monticelli, P. F., and Gunter, L. M.(2023) Reducing barking in a Brazilian animal shelter: A practical intervention. *Applied Animal Behaviour Science*, 265, 105992. https://doi.org/10.1016/j.applanim.2023.105992.

Beaver, B.V. (2003). *Feline Behavior: A Guide for Veterinarians*, 2e. Philadelphia: Saunders.

Bradshaw, J.W.S., Casey, R.A., and Brown, S.L. (2012). *The Behaviour of the Domestic Cat*, 2e. Wallingford: CABI Publishing.

Buffington, C.A.T. (2011). Idiopathic cystitis in domestic cats — beyond the lower urinary tract. *Journal of Veterinary Internal Medicine* 25: 784–796.

Byosiere, S.E., Chouinard, P.A., Howell, T.J., and Bennett, P.C. (2018). What do dogs (*Canis familiaris*) see? A review of vision in dogs and implications for cognition research. *Psychonomic Bulletin and Review* 25 (5): 1798–1813. https://doi.org/10.3758/s13423-017-1404-7.

Center, S.A. (2005). Feline hepatic lipidosis. *Veterinary Clinics of North America: Small Animal Practice* 35(1 SPEC. ISS.): 225–269. https://doi.org/10.1016/j.cvsm.2004.10.002.

Chung, B.S., Chung, M.S., Lee, S.-B. et al. (2018). Sectioned images of a cat head to contribute to learning of its sectional anatomy. *International Journal of Morphology* 36 (2): 537–543. https://doi.org/10.4067/S0717-95022018000200537.

Clayton, K.N. and Kamback, M. (1966). Successful performance by cats on several colour discrimination problems. *Canadian Journal of Psychology* 20 (2): 173–182. https://doi.org/10.1037/h0082940.

Dhabhar, F.S. (2014). Effects of stress on immune function: the good, the bad, and the beautiful. *Immunologic Research* 58 (2–3): 193–210. https://doi.org/10.1007/s12026-014-8517-0.

Ellis, J.J., Stryhn, H., Spears, J., and Cockram, M.S. (2017). Environmental enrichment choices of shelter cats. *Behavioural Processes* 141: 291–296. https://doi.org/10.1016/j.beproc.2017.03.023.

Frank, D., Beauchamp, G., and Palestrini, C. (2010). Systematic review of the use of pheromones for treatment of undesirable behavior in cats and dogs. *Journal of the American Veterinary Medical Association* 236 (12): 1308–1316. https://doi.org/10.2460/javma.236.12.1308.

Griffin, C.E. and DeBoer, D.J. (2001). *The ACVD task force on canine atopic dermatitis (XIV): psychological stress and canine atopic dermatitis. Veterinary Immunology and Immunopathology* 81: 153–159.

Gunter, L.M., Feuerbacher, E.N., Gilchrist, R.J., and Wynne, C.D.L. (2019). Evaluating the effects of a temporary fostering program on shelter dog welfare. *PeerJ* 7: e6620. https://doi.org/10.7717/peerj.6620.

Gunter, L.M., Gilchrist, R.J., Blade, E.M. et al. (2021). Investigating the impact of brief outings on the welfare of dogs living in US shelters. *Animals* 11 (2): 548.

Gunter, L.M., Blade, E.M., Gilchrist, R.J. et al. (2023). The influence of brief outing and temporary fostering programs on shelter dog welfare. *Animals* 13: 3528. https://doi.org/10.3390/ani13223528.

Hekman, J.P., Karas, A.Z., and Sharp, C.R. (2014). Psychogenic stress in hospitalized dogs: cross species comparisons, implications for health care, and the challenges of evaluation. *Animals* 4 (2): 331–347. https://doi.org/10.3390/ani4020331.

Kruger, M.C., Sabourin, C.J., Levine, A.T., and Lomber, S.G. (2021). Ultrasonic hearing in cats and other terrestrial mammals. *Acoustics Today* 17 (1): 18–25. https://doi.org/10.1121/at.2021.17.1.18.

Loop, M.S. and Bruce, L.L. (1978). Cat color vision: the effect of stimulus size. *Science* 199 (4334): 1221–1222.

Lupien, S.J., McEwen, B.S., Gunnar, M.R., and Heim, C. (2009). Effects of stress throughout the lifespan on the brain, behaviour and cognition. *Nature Reviews Neuroscience* 10 (6): 434–445. https://doi.org/10.1038/nrn2639.

Mawdsley, J.E. and Rampton, D.S. (2005). Psychological stress in IBD: new insights into pathogenic and therapeutic implications. *Gut* 54 (10): 1481–1491. https://doi.org/10.1136/gut.2005.064261.

McEwen, B.S. and Morrison, J.H. (2013). The brain on stress: vulnerability and plasticity of the prefrontal cortex over the life course. *Neuron*. Elsevier Inc. 79: 16–29. https://doi.org/10.1016/j.neuron.2013.06.028.

Mills, D., Karagiannis, C., and Zulch, H. (2014). Stress-its effects on health and behavior: a guide for practitioners. *Veterinary Clinics of North America: Small Animal Practice* 44 (3): 525–541. https://doi.org/10.1016/j.cvsm.2014.01.005.

Padodara, R.J. and Jacob, N. (2014). Olfactory sense in different animals. *Indian Journal of Veterinary Medicine* 2 (1): 1–14. Available at: https://www.researchgate.net/publication/262932824.

Pageat, P. and Gaultier, E. (2003). Current research in canine and feline pheromones. *Veterinary Clinics of North America: Small Animal Practice* 33 (2): 187–211. https://doi.org/10.1016/S0195-5616(02)00128-6.

Paus, R., Theoharides, T.C., and Arck, P.C. (2006). Neuroimmunoendocrine circuitry of the "brain-skin connection". *Trends in Immunology* 27 (1): 32–39. https://doi.org/10.1016/j.it.2005.10.002.

Protopopova, A., and Wynne, C. D. L. (2015) Improving in-kennel presentation of shelter dogs through response-dependent and response-independent treat delivery. *Journal of Applied Behavior Analysis*, 48(3), 590–601. https://doi.org/ 10.1002/jaba.217.

Puurunen, J., Tiira, K., Vapalahti, K. et al. (2018). Fearful dogs have increased plasma glutamine and γ-glutamyl glutamine. *Scientific Reports*. Springer US 8 (1): 15976. https://doi.org/10.1038/s41598-018-34321-x.

Roozendaal, B., McEwen, B.S., and Chattarji, S. (2009). Stress, memory and the amygdala. *Nature Reviews Neuroscience* 10 (6): 423–433. https://doi.org/10.1038/nrn2651.

Schneider, K.M., Blank, N., Alvarez, Y. et al. (2023). The enteric nervous system relays psychological stress to intestinal inflammation. *Cell* 186: 2823–2838.e20. https://doi.org/10.1016/j.cell.2023.05.001.

Shelter Animals Count (2025). *2025 mid-year analysis: national shelter data report*. New York: Shelter Animals Count/ASPCA. Available at: https://www.shelteranimalscount.org/ (accessed 19 January 2026).

Stella, J.L., Lord, L.K., and Buffington, C.A.T. (2011). Sickness behaviors in response to unusual external events in healthy cats and cats with feline interstitial cystitis. *Journal of the American Veterinary Medical Association* 238 (1): 1–7. https://doi.org/10.2460/javma.238.1.67.Sickness.

Steptoe, A. and Kivimäki, M. (2012). *Stress and cardiovascular disease. Nature Reviews Cardiology* 9: 360–370.

Strain, G.M. (2017). Hearing disorders in cats: classification, pathology and diagnosis. *Journal of Feline Medicine and Surgery* 19 (3): 276–287. https://doi.org/10.1177/1098612X17695062.

Vinke, C.M., Godijn, L.M., and van der Leij, W.J.R. (2014). Will a hiding box provide stress reduction for shelter cats? *Applied Animal Behaviour Science* 160: 86–93. https://doi.org/10.1016/j.applanim.2014.09.002.

Vitale, K.R., Frank, D.H., Conroy, J., and Udell, M.A.R. (2022). Cat foster program outcomes: behavior, stress, and cat–human interaction. *Animals* 12: 2166.

8

Enrichment Programs for Shelter Animals

8.1 Importance of Enrichment for Behavioral Wellness

In this chapter, we provide definitions of enrichment, behavioral wellbeing, and how to quantify stress. We offer solutions to minimize discomfort for dogs and cats while under the care of a non-permanent home – a shelter.

Over the years, our understanding of the human–animal bond has evolved. It is clear that behavior problems in pets can create stress and frustration for owners, weakening the human–animal bond. Pets exhibiting challenging behaviors – such as excessive barking, hissing, scratching, hiding, or other extreme fears – can make daily interactions difficult, reducing the enjoyment of pet ownership. In severe cases, these issues may even lead to relinquishment.

Shelters must recognize that unaddressed behavioral issues can affect both the pet's wellbeing and organizational outcomes. Many pets enter shelters because their behavioral needs were not met in previous homes. Additionally, the shelter environment itself – characterized by stress, confinement, and inconsistent enrichment – can exacerbate existing issues or contribute to new ones. If these problems are not identified and managed early, they can lower adoption rates, increase returns, and negatively impact a pet's long-term success in a new home. Therefore, promoting the mental health and wellbeing of dogs and cats through environmental enrichment is critical, especially during unavoidable periods of shelter confinement.

The goal of any shelter organization, whether it is a small volunteer group or a large nonprofit, remains the same: providing homeless pets with a better life by placing them with loving families and maximizing available resources.

The *Five Freedoms* define the minimal standards for animal welfare, and all pets in shelters should be entitled to them. Chapter 1 introduces the more modern and comprehensive *Five Domains* framework. This approach not only addresses the animal's basic needs but also evaluates the quality of the environment, providing a more complete assessment of welfare. While most shelters adequately address the first three freedoms (freedom from hunger and thirst, freedom from discomfort, and freedom from pain, injury, and disease), the remaining two related to behavioral and psychological needs are frequently overlooked. This is primarily due to limitations in resources, staffing, expertise, and time constraints. Medical needs are often more pressing, which can result in behavioral needs being deprioritized.

Multiple studies in various species have demonstrated the benefits of enriched environment conditions (Mason et al. 2007; Vinke et al. 2014; Amaya et al. 2020). Enrichment includes not only a nutritionally well-balanced diet but also a controlled climate and good hygienic conditions, so the pets' physical needs are well taken care of. Most natural behaviors are severely restricted under standard shelter housing conditions, and the pet's potential for controlling their physical and social environment is markedly reduced. Most animals are motivated to perform a number of behavior patterns, and restriction of those behaviors acts as a stressor. This leads not only to behavioral deterioration but may also result in impaired medical health due to a compromised immune system.

The reasoning behind not providing adequate enrichment for shelter pets is often that these animals generally "only" spend a short time in a restricted environment when compared to zoo and laboratory animals. Of course, this is a poor argument which triggers a moral discussion about whether animals have the foresight for their future. It has been widely demonstrated that the initial few days in a shelter are the most stressful. Exposure to daily stress and fear should not be acceptable even for a short time period. Hence, it is extremely important to start behavioral support during those initial days. Every step during admissions should be guided with the intent of making the pet's experience as low stress as possible and reduce fear and discomfort while getting them ready for adoption.

Both Broom and Johnson (1993) and Leach et al. (2000) suggested an operational definition of "*environmental enrichment*" as any change to the housing system that increases the frequency and diversity of positive natural behaviors, decreases the occurrence of abnormal behavior, maximizes the utilization of the environment, and increases the animal's ability to cope with the challenges of captivity. The quality of any given structure was considered more important than the quantity of space (or size of the enclosure).

8.2 Designing Enrichment Programs for Dogs

The enrichment strategies for dogs in shelters should provide them with interventions that keep them not only physically, but also mentally healthy and engaged. Ideally, their physical environment will allow them to use all their senses, olfactory, auditory, gustatory, and visual, through the introduction of novel smells, foods, sounds, visual displays, and novel objects and experiences. Providing shelter dogs with foraging toys tends to increase their cognitive activity and learning capacity by encouraging them to use their nose, teeth, and paws to work for food (see Figure 8.1). Furthermore, providing dogs with social contact and increased complexity in their housing environment can be beneficial for the pet. However, social enrichment has to be tailored to the pet's needs and must be safe and meaningful (Hubrecht 1993).

When designing and applying an enrichment program for shelter dogs, the following areas should be considered and addressed to promote optimal animal welfare *(Adapted from Bloomsmith et al. 1991)*.

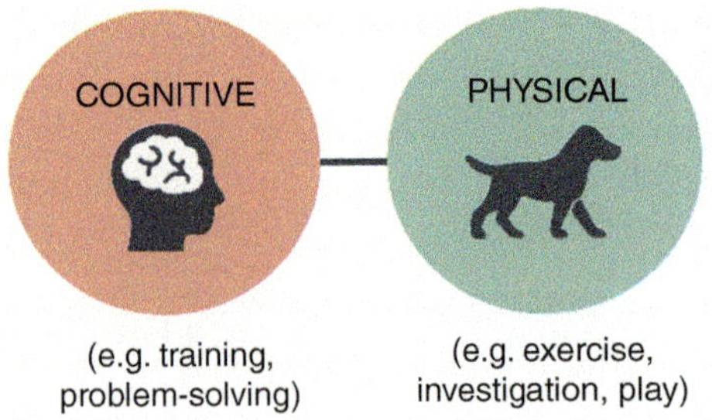

Figure 8.1 Enrichment for Pets Should Fulfill Two Broad Categories: Cognitive and Physical

Engage all the senses: Provide sensory stimulation by including sights, sounds, smells, tastes, and tactile experiences.
Provide for social needs: Allow individuals to interact safely and appropriately with humans and/or other dogs based on individual temperament.
Encourage social or object play: Use safe toys, games, and positive interactions to promote mental stimulation that provides enjoyment for the dog.
Increase physical activity and exercise: Facilitate movement through walks, play opportunities, training sessions, and space exploration based on age, medical needs, and restrictions based on individual temperament.
Encourage problem-solving: Introduce puzzle toys, training exercises, and enrichment challenges that engage cognitive skills.
Provide different feeding opportunities: Rarely should dogs be fed from a food bowl, more beneficial is the use of varied feeding strategies such as scatter feeding, food puzzles, frozen items, or slow feeders to promote natural foraging behavior.

Through taste, smell, and texture, gustatory and olfactory enrichment offers variety and novelty. There are simple ways to provide stimulation to the canine shelter population. Small amounts of treats can be offered, provided that the new foods do not cause gastrointestinal (GI) upset. Novel food items can differ in flavor from the regular diet and may include rabbit, venison, fish, certain safe fruits and vegetables, or small amounts of dairy products (such as plain yogurt or nonfat cottage cheese). Offering the same foods with different textures – for example, hard kibble, soft paste, frozen, or liquids – can also enhance engagement and encourage exploration without jeopardizing GI health. It is important to remember that shelter dogs often come from diverse dietary backgrounds, and their GI health may be sensitive to abrupt changes. To avoid GI upset, monitor individual tolerance and avoid excessive variety. The primary goal is to provide safe, enjoyable, sensory stimulation while maintaining digestive health and consistency in the dog's GI functions.

8.2.1 How to Incorporate Canine Field Trips

To meet dogs' social needs, allow them to interact safely with humans and other dogs according to their individual temperaments. Off-campus enrichment, such as walks, canine field trips, and overnight stays in foster homes, can provide meaningful opportunities for mental and social stimulation.

Benefits for Dogs

- Spending time outside the shelter reduces stress, promotes positive human interactions, and can improve overall wellbeing.
- Field trips and overnight stays allow teams and volunteers to gain insight into a dog's behavior in real-world settings.
- These experiences enhance socialization, expose dogs to new environments, and help them practice appropriate behaviors.

Community Engagement

- Canine field trips and overnight programs foster volunteer engagement, build public awareness, and generate goodwill toward the shelter.
- Community members benefit by engaging in active lifestyles while contributing to animal wellbeing.

Adoption Advantages

- Showcasing dogs in homes, parks, walking trails, or pet-friendly businesses can highlight their personalities beyond the kennel.
- Exposure to different environments and social experiences can make dogs more relaxed, confident, and more adoptable.

Safety First

- All dogs must remain on-leash at all times during outings.
- Use properly fitted, secure equipment such as harnesses, collars, and sturdy leashes to prevent escape.
- Avoid situations that could overwhelm or startle the dog.
- Read body language of all dogs in any group setting closely and carefully.
- Volunteers should always check that equipment fits before leaving the shelter.
- Some dogs may benefit from outings in a stroller (puppies, older or disabled dogs, injured dogs).

Feedback Matters

- After each outing, volunteers should provide detailed feedback about the dog's behavior that should be recorded in the dog's **Problem-Oriented Veterinary Behavioral Record (POVBR)**.
  - Examples:
    - *Pulls on leash*
    - *Jumps up when greeting new people*
    - *Salivated during car ride to the beach*
  - This information helps the behavior team and potential adopters understand the dog's needs and adjust training or adoption counseling accordingly.
  - A template can help get the information needed in a consistent format.

8.2.2 Walks and Outdoor Enrichment

Walks, runs, and hikes are valuable for exercise. To be truly enriching, they must allow for species-typical behaviors and some autonomy.

Teach Volunteers to Make Walks More Engaging

- Allow dogs to sniff, explore, and urine mark safely.
- Encourage natural behaviors like digging, investigating scents, and observing wildlife (from a safe distance).
- Avoid over-controlling the walk; allow the dog to make some decisions about where to go or what to investigate.
- Use clear cues to communicate boundaries and transitions:
  - "Free" or "Sniff": Signals the dog may explore and choose their path.
  - "With me now": Signals the end of free time and a return to structured walking.

Benefits

- Increases mental stimulation and reduces frustration.
- Builds trust and confidence between the dog and handler.
- Helps dogs learn flexibility and self-control in a positive way.

8.2.3 On-Site Enrichment for Dogs That Remain on Campus

Not all dogs are suitable to leave the shelter grounds due to medical, behavioral, or logistical reasons. For these dogs, on-site enrichment opportunities are essential to provide variety, reduce stress, and support emotional wellbeing.

When appropriate, dogs may benefit from having a compatible canine roommate. Social housing – when carefully assessed for safety and compatibility – can provide companionship, encourage play, and reduce anxiety and environmental monotony. Pairings should be made based on individual temperament, play style, and tolerance for sharing space and resources.

Research has shown that pair-housed dogs often exhibit reduced stress-related behaviors and have decreased physiological stress markers (e.g. urinary cortisol:creatinine) compared to singly housed dogs (Hecker et al. 2024). Additional studies also found that some dogs housed together exhibited decreased signs of stress (Hetts et al. 1992; Grigg et al. 2017). Social interactions – particularly friendly play – were associated with lower cortisol levels and improved overall welfare. The scientific findings indicated that there are welfare benefits to social housing arrangements for the mitigation of the stress of kennel environments.

Another valuable option is office time, playroom, enrichment room, or quiet room rotations. Allowing a dog to spend part of the day in an office, staff area, or meeting room provides a change of scenery and exposure to normal daily activities, people, and sounds. Encouraging participation from members of different departments in the organization is often beneficial. A quiet environment can be especially beneficial for shy or stressed dogs, offering a break from the busy kennel environment.

These short breaks or social pairings can:

- Increase relaxation and social confidence.
- Decrease stress-related behaviors (e.g. barking and pacing).
- Help staff and volunteers gather valuable behavior observations in calmer settings.

Thoughtful rotation of dogs through different environments within the shelter – whether it is a shared run, playroom, or office space – greatly enhances overall welfare and provides meaningful enrichment even for dogs who cannot participate in off-site activities.

8.2.4 Benefits and Risks of Play Groups

8.2.4.1 Social Play Can Fulfill Innate Social Needs

Dogs are a social species that evolved from group-living ancestors. Many dogs retain an intrinsic motivation to greet, interact, and even play with other dogs. Especially for younger, energetic dogs, selecting a playmate of similar size and activity level helps ensure balanced, safe interactions. Large size or strength differences can increase the risk of unintentional injury, even during friendly play. When pairing dogs for social play or shared housing, it is essential to confirm compatibility and safety. Dogs should be matched based on temperament, play style, and energy level rather than just availability or space.

8.2.4.2 Promotes Emotional and Behavioral Health

Social play is a form of enrichment and provides mental stimulation, stress relief, and positive emotional experiences. Dogs often exhibit lower stress behaviors (less pacing, barking, or self-directed behaviors) after play sessions. Play associated release of endorphins and dopamine promotes positive affective states. Flower (2016) and Shiverdecker et al. (2013) both found that play and social interaction reduce stress indicators in shelter dogs.

8.2.4.3 Improves Social Skills and Communication

Play can teach young dogs to read and respond to social cues, enhancing their ability to communicate effectively with other dogs and humans throughout life. Puppies can learn to moderate bite inhibition, adjust arousal levels, and respect adult dogs' boundaries. Furthermore, repeated exposure to varied play styles builds resilience and tolerance if done so in a safe setting. Horowitz (2009) showed that during play, dogs use ritualized signals to prevent escalation, suggesting that play has a regulatory function in social behavior (Horowitz 2009).

Shelter playgroup studies report that structured playgroups are generally safe and widely used, and many organizations perceive them as beneficial for dogs' wellbeing. A national survey of US shelters found that most respondents believed playgroups improve knowledge of a dog's behavior, enhance quality of life and welfare, and reduce stress, with relatively low rates of serious fights or injuries in playgroup settings (Shabelansky and Segurson 2018).

8.2.4.4 Reduces Kennel Stress and Improves Shelter Welfare

For shelter dogs, social play can offset the stressors of isolation and confinement. Play provides physical exercise, mental stimulation, and emotional release, which reduce anxiety-related behaviors such as spinning, barking, or barrier frustration. Dogs that appear more relaxed and sociable are more likely to be adopted. Hunt et al. (2022) reviewed enrichment strategies and found that dog–dog play was one of the most effective welfare-improving activities in shelter environments. Some programs have documented decreased kennel stress and improved adoption rates following daily play sessions (Hunt et al. 2022).

8.2.4.5 Encourages Physical Fitness and Cognitive Development

Play contributes significantly to both physical fitness and cognitive development in dogs. It supports motor coordination, cardiovascular health, and learning through problem-solving. Interactive play – such as chasing, wrestling, or tug-of-war – provides valuable aerobic exercise when conducted safely. Rooney and Bradshaw (2003) demonstrated that play strengthens social bonds and facilitates learning, while moderate physical activity supports healthy joint and muscle development. Social experiences beyond play also influence wellbeing: shelter dogs often exhibit elevated stress when housed alone, and the presence of a compatible social companion can buffer these physiological stress responses. Research across species shows that the presence of conspecifics can reduce glucocorticoid levels – a phenomenon known as social buffering – suggesting that well-matched social housing may help mitigate stress and support immune function in dogs (Kikusui et al. 2006).

It is essential to recognize that individual differences strongly influence how dogs interact socially, and not every dog is an appropriate candidate for playgroups. When dogs are thoughtfully selected and paired and when supervision, hygiene, and handling protocols are followed, playgroups can improve short-term wellbeing, reduce stress, and support behavioral health for many shelter dogs. Structured play also builds important social competencies. Bekoff (1995) described play as a critical component of canine social communication in which dogs learn self-control, negotiate social rules, and practice behavioral inhibition. Well-socialized dogs demonstrate more flexible body language and recover more quickly after mild conflicts, reflecting greater emotional resilience and adaptability (Ward et al. 2008). However, these benefits are not universal. Dogs with significant social fear, limited early socialization, past trauma, or medical constraints may find playgroups stressful or unsafe. For these individuals, careful assessment and alternative enrichment strategies are essential to preserve welfare and minimize risk.

Every dog should have a choice and opportunities to engage or retreat. Dogs should never be forced into interactions or punished for showing distance-increasing signals. Every dog should be behaviorally evaluated before play group exposure by an experienced team member. All introductions must be monitored closely, allow for frequent breaks, and monitored for signs of overarousal, fatigue, or tension to avoid injuries. Using metrics to track play group participation and measure outcomes assists in evaluating benefit vs. risks.

8.2.4.6 Risk, Limitations, and Caveats

While many shelter programs anecdotally report positive outcomes associated with canine playgroups – including improved sociability, reduced kennel stress, and enhanced adoptability – controlled, randomized trials remain limited. The existing body of evidence is therefore uneven, and interpretation is complicated by substantial implementation heterogeneity across shelters. Differences in group composition, facilitator training, dog selection criteria, session frequency, and facility design make effect sizes variable and limit the broad generalizability of outcomes.

Given these limitations, it is essential that each shelter systematically evaluates its own playgroup program rather than relying solely on external reports or generalized recommendations. Program effectiveness should be assessed using a combination of operational, behavioral, safety, and welfare-based metrics, allowing organizations to refine protocols within their specific scope of sustainability (SoS).

Key outcome measures to track include:

- Operational outcomes, such as length of stay (LOS), adoption rates, return rates, and the incidence of bites using bite severity classification (BSC) (see Chapter 5) or medical visits associated with playgroup participation. These metrics help determine whether playgroups are meaningfully improving flow-through while maintaining safety.
- Behavioral indicators include changes in kennel behavior – such as barking, pacing, withdrawal, social engagement, or relaxed resting – along with postplay or postinteraction body language and trends documented through validated welfare or behavior-scoring tools. Studies in both dogs and cats suggest that careful, consistent interpretation of these observable changes can provide meaningful insight into overall welfare (Berger et al. 2017a, 2017b).
- Program safety metrics, such as the number of infectious disease cases temporally associated with playgroup participation, the frequency and severity of injuries, and the number of sessions paused or discontinued due to health or safety concerns. These data are critical for balancing enrichment benefits with population-level risk management.
- Physiological measures, when available, including academic studies using biomarkers such as salivary cortisol to assess changes in stress before and after playgroup sessions. While not feasible for most shelters to collect routinely, these measures contribute to the broader scientific understanding of how playgroups may influence stress and wellbeing.

Taken together, these metrics underscore the importance of data-driven program evaluation. Playgroups are not inherently beneficial or harmful; their impact depends on thoughtful implementation, ongoing monitoring, and willingness to adapt based on outcomes. Shelters that track results carefully and adjust protocols accordingly are best positioned to maximize welfare benefits while minimizing unintended consequences.

Quick Operational Checklist (One-Page)

1) Follow veterinary protocols for disease tracking ✓
2) Regular vaccination and health check ✓

3) Behavioral screening and grouping ✓
4) Small group sizes and matched play styles ✓
5) Trained handlers, safety protocols, and tools ✓
6) Incident reports ✓
7) Session logging and regular program review ✓

8.3 Designing Enrichment Programs for Cats

The enrichment strategies used for shelter cats are similar to those for dogs and should focus on keeping them physically active and mentally stimulated. Offering a variety of enrichment options helps reduce stress, prevent undesirable behaviors, and support natural feline behaviors such as climbing, grooming, scratching, hunting, and exploring.

Effective enrichment should include vertical space – such as shelves, cat trees, or window perches – whenever possible (Foreman-Worsley and Farnworth 2019). Boxes are excellent alternatives in small areas and encourage climbing, hiding, and observing. Creating double-compartment cat condos by cutting portals between adjacent cages, a practice pioneered by the UC Davis Koret Shelter Medicine Program, increases available space and allows cats to move between compartments. This approach has been shown to reduce stress, improve welfare, and decrease the incidence of upper respiratory infections. Providing hiding spots, beds, and soft blankets supports comfort and rest, while rotating interactive toys and puzzle feeders encourages play, problem-solving giving cats opportunities for choice and control.

Ideally, a cat's physical environment should allow them to engage all their senses – olfactory, auditory, gustatory, and visual – through the introduction of novel smells, foods, sounds, visual displays, and objects. Food puzzles and interactive feeders provide mental stimulation and encourage problem-solving. Scent enrichment can be offered through prepared scent tubes, towels, rugs, or toys infused with animal scents. Cat-safe herbs, such as catnip, silvervine, or valerian, as well as gentle music, can further diversify a cat's sensory experience throughout the day.

Human interaction also plays an important role. Gentle petting, grooming, and even training sessions address both mental and physical needs. Although often overlooked, cats can benefit significantly from training, including clicker training. This provides structured interactions, strengthens the human–animal bond, supports cognitive development, and offers meaningful enrichment for both cats and visitors.

Interactive toys, including items that flutter, move, light up, or make noise, offer additional enrichment by stimulating stalking and hunting behaviors. These toys can provide a combination of visual, auditory, and tactile engagement, supporting a cat's natural curiosity and drive.

Time spent in secure outdoor enclosures allows cats to engage in species-specific activities and natural exploration. Access to the outdoors, while remaining safe, supports both physical and mental wellbeing.

Providing a variety of hiding and climbing options is essential. Cats naturally seek high vantage points where they can observe their surroundings and feel secure. Likewise, hiding spots offer comfort and safety, especially in multicat housing or during stressful situations (Vinke et al. 2014).

By incorporating some of these strategies, shelters can reduce stress-related behaviors and health issues, reduce anxiety, support natural behaviors, improve overall wellbeing, and enhance adoptability.

8.3.1 Fostering Out Cats with Behavior Conditions

Some cats may benefit from time in a home or foster setting, where stressors such as noise, foot traffic, and confinement are typically reduced. A *Cat Foster Program* study, designed to grant stays of either one night or one week, concluded that short-term fostering may be no more or less stressful for cats than remaining in the shelter environment (Vitale et al. 2022). The study documented that short-term fostering did not produce statistically significant improvements in human-directed social behavior or stress levels nor did cats show increased aggression, fear, or decreased social behavior or elevated urinary cortisol creatinine ratios (UCCR) upon returning to the shelter. However, fostering still provides substantial life-saving benefits, particularly by opening shelter space when capacity is limited.

For cats with behavioral concerns, foster care can offer a valuable real-world assessment by documenting how they transition and adapt to a new home environment. This information can improve care plans, refine adoption counseling, and help reduce returns. However, it is important to recognize that not all foster homes are equally suited for behaviorally challenged cats. Factors such as space, household consistency, distractions, other animals, and caregiver experience can impact outcomes.

There is also a risk of behavior worsening or new issues developing if the foster placement is not well matched to the cat's needs. Cats with behavioral challenges often require more time, structure, supervision, and specific support. These demands can contribute to caregiver stress or burnout and, in some cases, may lead foster families to withdraw from the program altogether. The authors observed that pets with behavioral issues are more likely to be returned from foster care compared with medically managed adult cats or kittens when attempting to develop a behavior-focused foster program. The resources required for training, supervision, and oversight often exceeded the benefits of placing this population in foster care. Effective behavioral intervention demands consistent monitoring, clear protocols, trained teams or volunteers, and frequent input from medical and behavior professionals. When this support is not provided promptly, the result can be repeated foster returns, caregiver frustration, and the loss of valuable foster homes. The authors also reported significant data gaps, including delayed or inconsistent behavioral updates from foster caregivers. These gaps made it difficult to adjust treatment plans in a timely manner and frequently contributed to longer overall shelter stays for behaviorally challenged cats.

While fostering can greatly improve wellbeing for many cats and free up critical shelter space, the authors concluded that cats with behavioral concerns may be better served by remaining in the shelter, provided there is an adequate behavior team and volunteers on-site to offer timely support, consistent structure, and the level of professional oversight required to address complex behavioral needs effectively.

When implementing a foster program, it is essential to establish clear criteria for handling medical emergencies, expectations for return or transition, and guidelines for postfoster adoption decisions. Foster caregivers should understand that fostering does not guarantee the resolution of behavioral issues; rather, it provides valuable information and opportunities to observe the cat's behavior in a home environment.

8.3.2 On Campus – Office Mates

Some cats may benefit from placement in an office setting, either in a larger enclosure or loose in the room when it can be done safely and securely (i.e. without risk of escape). In the author's experience, many team members also enjoyed having a feline office companion, which can enhance both the cat's wellbeing and team engagement.

Enrichment Considerations for Overweight or Senior Cats Include

- Bring items in from outside for the cat to sniff.
- Provide cat grass for the cat to smell and/or eat.
- Allow visual opportunities to observe the world around.
- Provide areas to lie comfortably without the need to jump or climb.
- Provide a snuffle mat or a rolled-up towel that contains hidden treats or enticing smells placed within it.
- Play sounds that contain species-specific noises within their hearing frequency, which may sound soothing, such as the sounds of cats purring.
- Provide scented bubbles that can be blown in their direction. The scents can be food-related or contain natural herbs such as lavender or chamomile.
- Catnip: Not all cats respond to catnip. About 30–40% of domestic cats do *not* show the typical catnip response. The sensitivity is genetically determined. Among those that *do* respond, behaviors vary widely in intensity and type (some playful, some more passive). A recent study found large individual differences and suggested genetic variation in olfactory receptors (Bol et al. 2022). Possible overstimulation or undesirable behaviors are anecdotally reported as well.

8.3.3 A Word of Caution on Laser Use for Cats and Dogs

Laser pointers should be used with great care and never directed toward an animal's or a human's eyes, as this may cause injury.

For cats, lasers activate the appetitive phase of the predatory sequence but do not allow for a consummatory phase, leaving no opportunity to physically "catch" the target. This can create frustration, overstimulation, and lingering arousal. Even when redirected to a toy or treat at the end of play, many cats remain fixated on the moving light and do not fully disengage, making laser play potentially frustrating unless paired with tangible rewards.

For dogs, the risks are even more significant. Laser pointers can trigger compulsive light- or shadow-chasing behaviors, which may persist long after play ends. Many dogs develop obsessive patterns, anxiety, or fixation with reflected light sources, making laser play a poor choice for enrichment and potentially harmful for their mental health.

Due to these concerns, laser devices should be used sparingly and thoughtfully with cats and avoided entirely with dogs to prevent stress, frustration, or the development of compulsive behaviors.

8.4 Creative and Affordable Enrichment Strategies for Shelter Use

As long as safety remains the first priority, creativity in enrichment has virtually no boundaries (see Table 8.1).

- Start safe: Ensure materials are free of hazards, which include no small ingestible parts and no toxic materials.
- Monitor response: Some animals may find certain items stressful or overstimulating, watch for signs of distress.
- Rotate frequently: Change the item or hide-spot every day/other day to maintain novelty.

Table 8.1 Canine and Feline Enrichment Strategies and Descriptions

Strategy	Description
Snuffle Mats and Scent Games	Hide safe scents (herbs, hides, or safe scented spray) Kibble or treats in a mat or rag strips so the animal uses its nose Good for dogs *and* cats
Cardboard, Toilet Paper Rolls, and Safe Household Item Puzzles	Use cardboard tubes, boxes, and plastic bottles with holes for treats Use muffin tins, place treats in the hole, and place a tennis ball on top of the treats Stimulates problem-solving Good for dogs *and* cats
Indoor/Office Environment Changes	For pets that cannot go off-site, rotate them into new areas (office, different room) Change surfaces and textures and hide treats around the room Good for dogs *and* cats
Do-It-Yourself (DIY) Tug or Chew Toys from Old Textiles	Braided T-shirts, old ropes, and fabric scraps Cost effective and engaging especially for dogs
Frozen Treat Blocks or Busy Boxes	Place toys or treats in boxes Freeze treats or toys into large buckets; pets must work to access Freeze wet food in ice cube trays Especially great for hot weather and outdoor spaces Good for cats and dogs
Rotate Toys and Reuse Safe Household Items	Changing the environment and switching "old" toys back in after a break renews interest Use paper bags, boxes, and tubes for cats especially

- Label or track enrichment: In the kennel or cat area, note which items each animal engages with.
- Involve volunteers/fosters/staff from other departments: Many of these do-it-yourself ideas are volunteer-friendly and can build engagement.
- Budget smart: Use donated or recycled materials (old T-shirts, cardboard, plastic bottles, and toilet paper roles) rather than always buying new toys.
- Adapt across species: Many ideas work for both dogs and cats (e.g. scent mats and foraging puzzles), but need to be tailored to size, energy, and species differences.

In summary, environmental enrichment for shelter pets is not a one-size-fits-all approach. It requires daily dedication and effort, but the benefits far outweigh the challenges. Effective enrichment can improve behavioral wellbeing, reduce kennel deterioration, provide clearer behavioral insights for placement decisions, enhance team and volunteer skills and morale, and potentially shorten LOS while improving adoption outcomes. Critically, robust enrichment programs can also greatly expand an organization's SoS by reducing stress-related decline and supporting more stable population flow. Enrichment preferences – and equally important, enrichment aversions – should always be documented in the pet's POVBR to ensure continuity of care and individualized behavioral planning.

References

Amaya, V., Paterson, M.B.A., and Phillips, C.J.C. (2020). Effects of olfactory and auditory enrichment on the behaviour of shelter dogs. *Animals* 10 (4): 1–20. https://doi.org/10.3390/ani10040581.

Bekoff, M. (1995). Play signals as punctuation: the structure of social play in canids. *Behaviour* 132 (5–6): 419–429. https://doi.org/10.1163/156853995X00649.

Berger, J., Ho, F., and Cummings, Z. (2017a). Preliminary report: assessment of stress-and relaxation-related behaviors of kennel-housed dogs (*Canis familiaris*) in a no-kill rescue shelter. Poster presented at WSAVA, Copenhagen (2017).

Berger, J., Ho, F., and Cummings, Z. (2017b). Preliminary report: assessment of stress-, relaxation-, and curiosity-related behaviors of kennel-housed cats (*Felis catus*) in a no-kill rescue shelter. Poster presentation WSAVA Copenhagen.

Bloomsmith, M.A., Brent, L.Y., and Schapiro, S.J. (1991). Guidelines for developing and managing an environmental enrichment program for nonhuman primates. *Laboratory Animal Science* 41 (4): 372–377.

Bol, S., Scaffidi, A., Bunnik, E.M., and Flematti, G.R. (2022). Behavioral differences among domestic cats in the response to cat-attracting plants and their volatile compounds reveal a potential distinct mechanism of action for actinidine. *BMC Biology*. BioMed Central 20 (1): 1–38. https://doi.org/10.1186/s12915-022-01369-1.

Broom, D.M. and Johnson, K.G. (1993). *Stress and Animal Welfare*. London, UK: Chapman & Hall.

Flower, S.M. (2016). The effect of play group on the behavior of shelter dogs. Master's thesis. City University of New York. https://academicworks.cuny.edu.

Foreman-Worsley, R. and Farnworth, M.J. (2019). A systematic review of social and environmental factors and their implications for indoor cat welfare. *Applied Animal Behaviour Science*. Elsevier 220 (July): 104841. https://doi.org/10.1016/j.applanim.2019.104841.

Grigg, E.K., Nibblett, B.M., Robinson, J.Q., and Smits, J.E. (2017). Evaluating pair versus solitary housing in kennelled domestic dogs (*Canis familiaris*) using behaviour and hair cortisol: a pilot study. *Veterinary Record Open* 4 (1): 1–14. https://doi.org/10.1136/vetreco-2016-000193.

Hecker, G., Martineau, K., Scheskie, M. et al. (2024). Effects of single- or pair-housing on the welfare of shelter dogs: behavioral and physiological indicators. *PLoS One* 19 (6 June): 1–22. https://doi.org/10.1371/journal.pone.0301137.

Hetts, S., Derrell Clark, J., Calpin, J.P. et al. (1992). Influence of housing conditions on beagle behaviour. *Applied Animal Behaviour Science* 34: 137–155.

Horowitz, A. (2009). Attention to attention in domestic dog (*Canis familiaris*) dyadic play. *Animal Cognition* 12 (1): 107–118. https://doi.org/10.1007/s10071-008-0175-y.

Hubrecht, R.C. (1993). A comparison of social and environmental enrichment methods for laboratory housed dogs. *Applied Animal Behaviour Science* 37 (4): 345–361.

Hunt, R.L., Whiteside, H., and Prankel, S. (2022). Effects of environmental enrichment on dog behaviour: pilot study. *Animals* 12 (2): 141. https://doi.org/10.3390/ani12020141.

Kikusui, T., Winslow, J.T., and Mori, Y. (2006). Social buffering: relief from stress and anxiety. *Philosophical Transactions of the Royal Society of London, Series B: Biological Sciences* 361 (1476): 2215–2228. https://doi.org/10.1098/rstb.2006.1941.

Leach, M.C., Ambrose, N., Bowell, V.J., and Morton, D.B. (2000). The development of a novel form of mouse cage enrichment. *Journal of Applied Animal Welfare Science* 3: 81–91.

Mason, G., Clubb, R., Latham, N., and Vickery, S. (2007). Why and how should we use environmental enrichment to tackle stereotypic behaviour? *Applied Animal Behaviour Science* 102 (3–4): 163–188. https://doi.org/10.1016/j.applanim.2006.05.041.

Rooney, N.J. and Bradshaw, J.W.S. (2003). Links between play and dominance and attachment dimensions of dog-human relationships. *Journal of Applied Animal Welfare Science* 6 (2): 67–94. https://doi.org/10.1207/S15327604JAWS0602_01.

Shabelansky, A. and Segurson, S. (2018). The use, safety and perception of dog playgroups in animal shelters. Maddie's Fund. Available at: https://www.maddiesfund.org/dog-playgroups-in-animal-shelters.htm (accessed 25 January 2026).

Shiverdecker, M.D., Schiml, P.A., and Hennessy, M.B. (2013). Human interaction moderates plasma cortisol and behavioral responses of dogs to shelter housing. *Physiology & Behavior* 110: 110–117. Key studies & reports (short summaries).

Vinke, C.M., Godijn, L.M., and van der Leij, W.J.R. (2014). Will a hiding box provide stress reduction for shelter cats? *Applied Animal Behaviour Science*. Elsevier B.V. 160: 86–93. https://doi.org/10.1016/j.applanim.2014.09.002.

Vitale, K.R., Frank, D.H., Conroy, J., and Udell, M.A.R. (2022). Cat foster program outcomes: behavior, stress, and cat–human interaction. *Animals* 12 (17): 2166.

Ward, C., Bauer, E.B., and Smuts, B.B. (2008). Partner preferences and asymmetries in social play among domestic dog, *Canis lupus familiaris*, littermates. *Animal Behaviour* 76 (4): 1187–1199. https://doi.org/10.1016/j.anbehav.2008.06.004.

9

Principles of Learning as the Foundation for Behavior Modification in Shelter Pets

9.1 Stress, Learning, and Memory: Why Shelter Environments Matter

Learning is highly dependent on emotional state. Both humans and animals learn most effectively in environments that feel safe, predictable, and low in threat. A useful analogy is human learning: people typically choose calm, quiet environments – such as a library – to study and absorb new information. In contrast, learning is impaired in loud, chaotic, or emotionally charged settings. The same principles apply to shelter pets.

9.1.1 Learning Under Stress vs. Safety

When shelter pets are exposed to prolonged stress, learning and positive behavior change become significantly more difficult. As described in Chapter 7, chronic stress activates two major physiological systems: the sympathetic nervous system (SNS) and the hypothalamic–pituitary–adrenal (HPA) axis. While SNS activation produces the rapid "fight-or-flight" response through the release of catecholamines (e.g. adrenaline), HPA activation leads to sustained cortisol release (Joëls et al. 2006). These responses are adaptive in true emergencies, but their prolonged activation interferes with learning. Elevated cortisol and noradrenaline impair working memory, reduce attention flexibility, and disrupt memory retrieval, making it harder for animals to process new information or apply previously learned behaviors (Lupien et al. 2009).

9.1.2 Stress, Fear, and Memory Storage

Several brain structures are involved in how stress affects learning, most notably the amygdala, hippocampus, and prefrontal cortex (McEwen and Morrison 2013). The amygdala plays a central role in processing fear and emotional salience and acts as a threat detector (Roozendaal et al. 2009). Cortisol and noradrenaline enhance the consolidation of emotionally charged memories in the amygdala, making them stronger, more persistent, and more easily reactivated (Joëls et al. 2006).

This explains why fear-based experiences are remembered differently than positive or neutral ones. In humans, a painful or frightening dental visit is often vividly remembered and easily triggered. Similarly, shelter pets may strongly encode frightening handling, loud noises, or aversive training attempts, while struggling to retain newly taught, low-salience behaviors.

Chronic stress also negatively affects the hippocampus and prefrontal cortex – regions essential for contextual learning, impulse control, and behavioral flexibility – further reducing an animal's ability to learn, generalize, and adapt (Arnsten 2009; Lupien et al. 2009).

9.1.3 Implications for Shelter Training and Behavior Modification

Effective learning requires that the pet's stress level be low enough to allow cognitive engagement. When shelter pets remain in a heightened state of fear or arousal, training progresses slowly, inconsistently, or not at all. Repeated attempts to train under these conditions risk creating frustration for both the pet and the trainer. Resulting in the potential that training sessions themselves become aversive.

For learning-based behavior modification to be successful in shelters, stress reduction must precede or occur alongside training efforts. Creating conditions that promote emotional safety increases the likelihood that new behaviors are learned, retained, and generalized, ultimately improving wellbeing and adoptability.

When animals are experiencing stress levels that are too high to allow effective learning or voluntary engagement, environmental enrichment should be the first intervention. Enrichment strategies that encourage exploration, choice, and problem-solving help activate the brain's natural curiosity while reducing emotional arousal. By shifting the animal from a state of fear or hypervigilance to one of investigation and agency, enrichment creates the foundation necessary for learning to occur. As outlined in Chapter 8, addressing the environment and providing appropriate cognitive and sensory enrichment often precedes and significantly enhances the success of formal training and behavior modification efforts.

9.1.4 Dopamine, Food Motivation, and Learning Under Stress

Learning and memory formation are strongly influenced by emotional state and motivation, with dopamine playing a central role. Dopamine is a key neurotransmitter involved in reward processing, attention, motivation, and the consolidation of learning (Berridge and Robinson 1998). When an animal is emotionally regulated and engaged, dopamine release supports the formation of salient and positive memories (Schultz 2016). This increases the likelihood of new behaviors being learned and retained.

9.1.5 Food, Dopamine, and Memory Formation

Highly palatable food rewards – particularly small, salient morsels – activate dopaminergic reward pathways, reinforcing behavior and enhancing memory consolidation. Gustatory experiences are especially powerful because they engage multiple sensory systems simultaneously (taste, smell, and texture), increasing emotional salience and supporting learning (Fahmie et al. 2015). This is why small, high-value treats are often more effective than large portions: they maximize reward signaling without inducing satiety or disengagement.

Positive, reward-based learning contrasts sharply with fear-based learning. Fear can also produce strong memories, which encode primarily through the amygdala and are associated with avoidance, vigilance, and reduced behavioral flexibility. In contrast, dopamine-mediated learning promotes approach behavior, curiosity, and adaptability, which are essential for successful behavior modification and resiliency.

9.1.6 Treat Acceptance as a Stress Indicator

An animal's response to food provides valuable, real-time information about its emotional state. Refusal of treats, delayed intake or taking food, and then spitting it out are strong indicators that the animal may be experiencing stress levels too high to support effective learning. The animal's nervous system remains in a defensive or survival state where dopaminergic reward pathways are suppressed by stress hormones such as cortisol.

Treat acceptance can therefore be used as a practical welfare and readiness-to-learn indicator during behavior modification, both in shelter environments and in home settings. If an animal is unable or unwilling to eat, the focus should shift away from formal training and toward stress reduction, environmental modification, and enrichment until emotional regulation improves.

9.1.7 Implications for Shelter Behavior Programs

Successful learning-based behavior modification depends largely on the pet's emotional capability to engage. Using food strategically – as a reinforcer *AND* as a diagnostic and therapeutic tool – helps trainers and caregivers assess stress levels, supports dopamine-mediated learning, and builds positive associations. When pets can comfortably eat, explore, and seek rewards, they are more likely to form durable, positive memories that support long-term behavior change.

9.2 Learning in the Shelter Environment: Foundations and Implications

Learning occurs continuously and often outside of conscious awareness. Experiences are encoded as positive, negative, or neutral. Pets are constantly learning from interactions with people, other animals, and their environment. As a result, every shelter experience offers learning value, whether intentional or not.

For this reason, all shelter pets benefit from training while in shelter care. While not every pet requires specialized behavior modification, all team members and volunteers can apply basic learning principles to manage behavior, reduce stress, and improve wellbeing. Even routine interactions – feeding, cleaning, handling, and enrichment – shape how pets perceive and respond to their environment.

9.2.1 What Is Learning?

Learning is the process by which animals and humans form associations about their environment, interactions, or outcomes, resulting in a change in behavior. At the neurobiological level, learning produces synaptic changes in the brain, altering how an animal interprets and responds to future experiences. Because shelter environments are highly stimulating and often stressful, it is essential that handling and training practices are humane, predictable, and science-based. Learning processes are generally categorized into nonassociative and associative learning.

9.2.2 Nonassociative Learning

Nonassociative learning occurs when an animal's response to a stimulus changes without forming an association between multiple stimuli (Forkman 2002). This type of learning includes:

- Habituation: *Decreased* response to repeated, nonthreatening stimuli
- Sensitization: *Increased* response following repeated or intense exposure

Nonassociative learning occurs continuously in shelter environments, often without any deliberate training. Animals may habituate to repeated, nonthreatening stimuli, or they may become sensitized to unpredictable or aversive events. Importantly, the outcome depends on the individual animal's coping capacity, prior experiences, and current stress load.

For example, a dog may habituate to loud noise in the hallway within days – eventually resting or sleeping comfortably in the kennel – while a neighboring dog exposed to the identical stimulus becomes increasingly vocal and reactive, indicating sensitization. The latter dog may sleep less, show reduced appetite, and exhibit escalating fear or anxiety rather than habituation. Over time, chronic stress and impaired coping can contribute to immune suppression, increasing vulnerability to infectious diseases such as kennel cough. This contrast highlights that repeated exposure alone does not guarantee habituation; instead, it may amplify distress and negative learning for some animals (see Chapter 4).

9.2.3 Associative Learning and Conditioning

Associative learning involves forming relationships between events or between actions and consequences. This includes *classical* (Pavlovian) conditioning and *operant* conditioning.

Classical conditioning, first described by Ivan Pavlov (Forkman 2002; Mazur 2013), involves learning through the association of stimuli and applies to involuntary or reflexive responses – *Does that ring a bell?* In Pavlov's classic example, a neutral stimulus (the sound of a bell) was repeatedly paired with an unconditioned stimulus (food), which naturally elicited an unconditioned response (salivation). Through repeated pairings, the neutral stimulus became a conditioned stimulus, capable of eliciting salivation (the conditioned response) even in the absence of food. Classical conditioning is limited to reflexive, involuntary responses and does not involve conscious choice or voluntary behavior (Mazur 2013). For example, salivation (drooling) in response to food is a reflexive response that can be classically conditioned, whereas jumping up, sitting, or moving toward a person are voluntary behaviors and are not governed by classical conditioning.

In shelter settings, classical and operant learning processes occur simultaneously, even though they are described separately in learning theory books. Classical conditioning governs involuntary, reflexive responses, while voluntary behaviors are shaped through consequences. In practice, however, animals experience both at the same time during everyday interactions. Pets learn to associate with people, equipment, locations, and routines with emotional outcomes. These associations can either support or undermine wellbeing, depending on how experiences are structured.

For example, when a kennel is hosed down, a dog may begin trembling, an involuntary fear response that becomes classically conditioned to the sound, sight, smell, or the physical presence of the hose. If a caregiver then enters the kennel and the dog jumps up to seek contact, that behavior is voluntary. Alternatively, the same dog may retreat to the back of the kennel, a voluntary behavior driven by fear, while the trembling itself remains involuntary. In this way, the emotional response (fear or safety) and the behavioral response (approach or avoidance) are learned together.

Over time, dogs may learn that a caregiver predicts a positive experience, eliciting a reflexive, positive emotional response along with voluntary affiliative behaviors such as approaching or jumping. Alternatively, they may learn that certain people, tools, or routines predict threat, eliciting fear responses and avoidance behaviors. The emotional association formed through classical conditioning often determines which voluntary behaviors are expressed. These repeated experiences shape distinct neural pathways in the brain, strengthening circuits associated with safety and reward or, alternatively, fear and avoidance. The emotional associations formed through classical conditioning influence which voluntary behaviors are expressed, reinforcing patterns of response that become more automatic and enduring over time.

This is why every interaction matters. Shelter pets are navigating a novel and often stressful environment and learning is occurring continuously, whether intended or not. Compassion in this context means recognizing the pet's emotional state and adapting handling, transportation, training, and expectations to the individual's capacity to cope. Effective learning and behavior modification must be guided by ongoing welfare and behavioral assessments, not rigid, one-size-fits-all training protocols. By meeting pets where they are emotionally and physically, shelters can reduce fear, support learning, and improve overall welfare.

9.2.4 The Four Quadrants of Operant Conditioning and Their Relevance in Shelters

Operant (instrumental) conditioning governs voluntary behavior and describes how behavior is shaped by its consequences. Early work by Thorndike and later expanded by Skinner demonstrated that behaviors followed by favorable outcomes are more likely to be repeated, a principle known as the Law of Effect (Mazur 2013). In shelter environments, where animals are already experiencing elevated stress and unfamiliar handlers, the choice of learning quadrant has profound welfare and training implications.

9.2.5 The Four Quadrants Explained

The four quadrants of operant conditioning are defined by whether a stimulus is added (+) or removed (−) and whether the goal is to increase (*reinforcement*) or decrease (*punishment*) a behavior (Forkman 2002; Mazur 2013).

- Positive reinforcement (+R): Adding something the animal values (e.g. food, praise, and access) to increase a behavior.
- Negative reinforcement (−R): Removing an aversive stimulus to increase a behavior.
- Positive punishment (+P): Adding an aversive stimulus to decrease a behavior.
- Negative punishment (−P): Removing something the animal wants to decrease a behavior.

Reinforcement strengthens behavior, while punishment suppresses it.

9.2.6 Why Positive Reinforcement Is Crucial for Shelter Pets

Positive reinforcement is especially important for shelter pets because learning requires emotional safety. Shelter animals are already under stress simply due to confinement, novelty, noise, and unfamiliar people. Elevated stress suppresses dopamine release and impairs learning and memory. In contrast, reward-based training activates dopaminergic pathways, increasing motivation, attention, and memory consolidation. Positive reinforcement is effective in changing behavior (Schapiro et al. 2003).

Using positive reinforcement allows pets to learn what to do, not just what to avoid. For example, when a dog learns that sitting calmly during greetings consistently results in a reward that behavior increases over time. The dog also gains predictability and control, both of which are critical for reducing stress and supporting wellbeing.

In shelter settings, the primary goal is usually to *increase desirable behaviors* (e.g. calm leash walking and appropriate greetings), not to suppress unwanted ones. Punishment-based strategies are therefore unnecessary in most cases and carry significant risks.

9.2.7 Shaping (Successive Approximations) Using Positive Reinforcement

Shaping, also known as *successive approximation*, is a core positive-reinforcement technique for teaching new behaviors. Because shelters often lack reliable information about a pet's training history, it is safest to approach each pet as if it is starting on the first day of school. Beginning with simple, achievable behaviors – such as making eye contact or touching a target – allows trainers to gradually build toward more complex, desirable behaviors.

Shaping is particularly well suited to shelter environments where pets are handled by multiple caregivers. Clear criteria and incremental progress allow each handler to build upon the previous handler's work, creating consistency despite staff or volunteer turnover.

9.2.8 Behavioral Variability and Learning

Variability in behavior is a normal and necessary part of learning. During early training sessions, an animal may offer different responses as it explores which behaviors produce reinforcement. This variability supports the emergence of new behaviors. When the desired behavior occurs – even briefly – it can be captured by immediately delivering a reinforcer.

Timely reinforcement is essential. Because primary reinforcers (such as food) may be delivered with a slight delay, conditioned reinforcers (also called markers) are used to bridge the gap between behavior and reward. A conditioned reinforcer is a previously neutral stimulus that gains meaning through repeated pairing with a primary reinforcer. Verbal praise, a clicker, or a marker word becomes reinforcing only after consistent pairing with food (Williams 1991). Over time, the marker itself communicates to the animal that the correct behavior has occurred and that a reward is forthcoming.

9.2.8.1 Example: Teaching a Touch Cue Through Shaping

To teach a dog to touch a hand, the trainer may begin by reinforcing the smallest step toward the goal. If the dog does not initially approach the hand, the first criterion may be simply looking at the hand. Subsequent criteria may include moving the head toward the hand, taking a step forward, and eventually making contact. Each approximation is reinforced until the full behavior is achieved. Once the behavior is reliably offered, a cue can be added to elicit it in the future.

Through shaping, complex behaviors are built gradually, humanely, and with minimal frustration. This approach is particularly effective for shelter pets learning in a new and often stressful environment.

9.2.9 Risks of Punishment in Shelter Environments

Although positive punishment can reduce behavior, it does so by decreasing the motivation to perform the behavior by using fear, pain, or intimidation. For example, stepping on a dog's toes to stop jumping may suppress the behavior, but it also risks creating pain and negative associations with the handler, people in general, or the training environment. Fear-based learning is strongly encoded in the amygdala and can generalize rapidly, leading to increased anxiety, avoidance, or aggression.

From a welfare perspective, the risk–benefit ratio of punishment in shelters is unfavorable, similar to prescribing a medication with serious side effects when safer, effective alternatives exist. Research has consistently shown that aversive training methods are associated with increased fear, anxiety, aggressive behavior, and reduced overall wellbeing (Hiby et al. 2004; Herron et al. 2009) and weaken the human–animal bond (Kwan and Bain 2013).

9.2.10 Negative Punishment in Shelter Training: Limitations and Risks

When behavior reduction is necessary, negative punishment – such as briefly removing attention when a dog jumps – can be effective, *if* the animal is motivated by social interaction. When combined with consistent reinforcement of alternative behaviors, it may reduce unwanted behavior without introducing pain or fear.

However, the effectiveness of negative punishment depends entirely on the pet's underlying emotional state. If a dog jumps out of fear or anxiety, removing oneself may actually function as a reward rather than a punishment, reinforcing the very behavior one is trying to reduce. This illustrates how complex and context-dependent punishment-based strategies can be.

In contrast, reinforcing desired behaviors carries far less risk. While positive reinforcement requires awareness and appropriate timing from the human, errors in timing typically result in slower learning rather than harm. Mis-timed punishment, even once, can have significant negative consequences, including increased fear, avoidance of people or environments, behavioral suppression, emergence of alternative unwanted behaviors, or complete disengagement consistent with learned helplessness.

Given the diversity of handlers, experience levels, and interaction styles in shelter environments, punishment-based approaches – positive or negative – carry a disproportionately high risk compared to their potential benefit. Therefore, focusing on rewarding desired behaviors remains the safest, most effective, and most humane strategy for shelter animals. Small inconsistencies in reinforcement are far less damaging than errors in punishment, the latter having far-reaching and long-lasting negative effects on wellbeing and behavior.

9.2.10.1 Key Takeaway for Shelters

In shelter environments, rewarding desired behaviors is far safer than using punishment. While all four quadrants can influence behavior, positive reinforcement is the most effective, humane, and welfare-supportive approach for shelter pets. It promotes learning through dopamine-mediated reward pathways, builds positive associations with people and environments, and gives animals control and predictability, which are critical factors for stressed pets. Punishment suppresses behavior without teaching alternatives and carries unacceptable risks in an already vulnerable population. Errors in timing with positive reinforcement may slow down the learning process, but errors in punishment – even just once – can increase fear, avoidance, aggression, or behavioral shutdown, causing lasting harm. Most shelter pets experience stress and are handled by multiple people with varying skill levels, who often are unfamiliar with the pet. Prioritizing positive reinforcement is therefore crucial to best protect wellbeing while still supporting learning and positive behavior change.

9.3 Counterconditioning and Desensitization

Counterconditioning and desensitization are learning techniques used to change an animal's emotional response, most often from negative (fear, anxiety, and distress) to neutral or positive. Counterconditioning relies on classical conditioning, in which a previously negative stimulus is paired with something the pet finds positive. It is critical that pairing must involve a stimulus that is genuinely rewarding to the individual pet (e.g. food, play, social interaction, or touch). If the animal is too stressed to experience the pairing as positive, no positive association is formed.

9.3.1 Counterconditioning

Counterconditioning changes a shelter pet's emotional response by pairing the trigger with a reward (Keller et al. 2020). For example, a dog who is fearful of men may receive a highly valued treat every time a man is visible at a safe distance. With repeated pairings, the dog's emotional response shifts from fear to neutrality or positive anticipation. Over time, the previously aversive stimulus begins to predict good outcomes.

9.3.2 Desensitization

Desensitization involves gradual exposure to a trigger at an intensity and pace that does not elicit fear or reactivity. The goal is to increase tolerance without overwhelming the animal. Progress is typically slow and incremental, requiring repeated exposures over time. While the process may appear uneventful, maintaining the animal below threshold is essential for success.

Below-threshold rule: *If the animal is showing fear, avoidance, freezing, reactivity, or refusing to accept the reward, the exposure is too intense and learning is no longer occurring.*

9.3.3 Clinical Relevance in Shelters

Counterconditioning and desensitization are foundational techniques for treating fear, anxiety, and stress-related behaviors in shelter pets, including arousal and aggression. While each technique can be used independently, their combined use produces the most reliable and humane outcomes. Together, they help pets build tolerance to triggers while simultaneously improving their ability to cope emotionally, supporting welfare, learning, and adoptability.

These techniques require intentional planning, skilled implementation, and regular reassessment. Progress depends on carefully monitoring whether the animal is improving, remaining stable, or showing signs of increased stress. If fear or reactivity escalates, the pace of exposure is exceeding the animal's coping capacity and the plan must be adjusted by increasing distance, reducing intensity, or slowing the process. Effective counterconditioning and desensitization prioritize the animal's emotional safety over speed, ensuring progress remains humane and sustainable.

9.4 Differential Rate of Reinforcement (Schedules of Reinforcement)

When training shelter pets, it is essential to recognize that rewards change in value over time. Animals may lose interest if they become satiated, fatigued, stressed, or distracted by competing stimuli in the environment. To remain engaging – often described by trainers as staying *"sexier than the squirrel"* – handlers must not only choose effective reinforcers but also deliver them at the right time and frequency.

The differential rate of reinforcement, also known as schedules of reinforcement, refers to how often and when a reinforcer is delivered following a behavior (see Table 9.1).

These schedules strongly influence motivation, persistence, and resistance to distraction (Kelleher and Gollub 1962; Mazur 2013).

Table 9.1 Comparison of Reinforcement Schedules (Adapted from Forkman 2002; Mazur 2013)

Schedule	How Reinforcement Is Delivered	Typical Response Pattern	Shelter-Relevant Considerations
Fixed Interval (FI)	Reinforcement available only after a set amount of time has passed	Low response rate initially Increased responding just before reinforcement ("scalloping")	May cause frustration or agitation Limited usefulness in shelter training
Fixed Ratio (FR)	Reinforcement after a fixed number of responses (e.g. every 10 sits)	High, steady responding, followed by a brief pause after reward	Useful for building fluency once behavior is learned Risk of frustration if ratio increases too quickly
Variable Interval (VI)	Reinforcement available after varying time intervals	Steady, moderate response rate	Helpful for maintaining calm, consistent behaviors in distracting environments
Variable Ratio (VR)	Reinforcement after an unpredictable number of responses	Very high, persistent responding Most resistant to extinction	Produces durable behaviors Should be introduced gradually after behavior is well established

9.4.1 Relevance in Shelter Environments

A critical principle is that higher rates of reinforcement produce stronger behaviors that are more reliable, resilient, and resistant to distraction. For shelter pets exposed to constant noise, movement, and novelty, maintaining a sufficiently high reinforcement rate is key to successful training and daily management.

By strategically adjusting reinforcement schedules, trainers can sustain motivation, compete with environmental distractions, and help shelter pets remain engaged despite stress and change. This flexibility is especially important when animals are handled by multiple caregivers with varying experience levels.

9.4.1.1 Key Takeaway

Strategic use of reinforcement timing and frequency keeps learning strong, motivation high, and shelter pets are more able to cope with an unpredictable environment.

9.5 Differential Reinforcement of Alternative Behaviors (DRA)

Differential Reinforcement of Alternative Behaviors (DRA) is a humane behavior-modification strategy that replaces undesirable behaviors with appropriate alternatives. It has been adapted to use in animals; DRA relies on positive reinforcement to increase appropriate behaviors, making it especially suitable for stressed shelter animals. Rather than punishing unwanted behavior, the pet is taught a desirable behavior that earns reinforcement, while the unwanted behavior is no longer rewarded and gradually fades through extinction. For example, a dog that jumps on the kennel door is reinforced for sitting when people approach. Over time, sitting replaces jumping as the dog's default response.

Whenever possible, DRA should be applied proactively through redirection before the unwanted behavior occurs. For instance, reinforcing a dog for walking calmly at the handler's side prevents leash pulling or engaging cats with toys before entering a room reduces grabbing or defensive behavior.

If the pet is already performing the unwanted behavior, a neutral, nonaversive distractor may be used to interrupt the behavior, followed immediately by redirection to the alternative behavior and reinforcement. The distractor must be strong enough to gain attention but not so intense that it causes fear or anxiety.

Through consistent reinforcement of the alternative behavior, the undesirable behavior loses reinforcement and gradually diminishes (Martin et al. 2011). The use of DRA teaches shelter pets what to do, not just what to avoid, supporting learning, wellbeing, and safer handling.

9.6 Applying Learning Theory to Individualized Behavior Treatment Planning

Understanding how animals learn is essential when designing behavior modification and training plans for shelter pets. Just as medical treatment requires accurate diagnosis and a tailored care plan or architectural design begins with a blueprint, effective behavior intervention depends on a solid foundation in learning theory. Without this understanding, attempts to change behavior risk being ineffective or unintentionally adding fear to an already stressful environment.

Knowledge of learning processes allows caregivers to intentionally guide behavior from undesirable to desirable, shape new skills progressively, and select humane, science-based techniques that support welfare. These principles are critical when developing Individualized Behavior Treatment Plans (see Chapter 5), particularly for pets with complex emotional or behavioral needs.

Behavioral treatment – whether implemented in a home or shelter setting – follows a structured, multifaceted approach built around five core components:

1) Management
2) Interactions and environment
3) Tools
4) Reintroduction
5) Medications and/or nutraceuticals

Completion of a full plan typically takes six to eight weeks, though timelines vary based on the individual pet, severity of the concern, and available resources. While shelters may not be able to implement all five steps completely, Steps 1–3 are foundational and should be understood and applied whenever possible, as they establish the conditions necessary for learning and behavior change.

This framework is intentionally flexible. Steps may be applied independently or in combination, depending on case specifics, shelter capacity, and handler expertise. This subchapter provides an overview of the treatment framework; detailed guidance on designing and implementing each step is provided in Chapter 5. Treatment frameworks for specific behavior conditions can be found in Chapter 11.

In summary, learning depends on emotional safety. Chronic stress in shelter pets impairs attention, memory, and flexibility, making behavior change difficult and strengthening fear-based responses. Because animals are always learning; every interaction matters. Positive reinforcement is the safest and most effective approach, promoting motivation and resilience, while punishment carries significant welfare risks. Stress reduction and enrichment should come first, creating the foundation for humane, effective care trajectory strategy (CTS). Grounding behavior plans in learning theory ensures individualized, welfare-centered care that improves outcomes and adoptability.

References

Arnsten, A.F.T. (2009). Stress signalling pathways that impair prefrontal cortex structure and function. *Nature Reviews Neuroscience* 10 (6): 410–422. https://doi.org/10.1038/nrn2648.Stress

Berridge, K.C. and Robinson, T.E. (1998). What is the role of dopamine in reward: hedonic impact, reward learning, or incentive salience? *Brain Research Reviews* 28: 309–369.

Fahmie, T.A., Iwata, B.A., and Jann, K.E. (2015). Comparison of edible and leisure reinforcers. *Journal of Applied Behavior Analysis* 48 (2): 331–343. https://doi.org/10.1002/jaba.200.

Forkman, B.A. (2002). Learning and cognition. In: *The Ethology of Domestic Animals: An Introductory Text*, 1e (ed. P. Jensen), 51–64. Wallingford: CAB International https://doi.org/10.1079/9781786391650.0062.

Herron, M.E., Shofer, F.S., and Reisner, I.R. (2009). Survey of the use and outcome of confrontational and non-confrontational training methods in client-owned dogs showing undesired behaviors. *Applied Animal Behaviour Science* 117 (1–2): 47–54. https://doi.org/10.1016/j.applanim.2008.12.011.

Hiby, E.F., Rooney, N.J., and Bradshaw, J.W.S. (2004). Dog training methods: their use, effectiveness and interaction with behaviour and welfare. *Animal Welfare* 13 (1): 63–69.

Joëls, M., Pu, Z., Wiegert, O. et al. (2006). Learning under stress: how does it work? *Trends in Cognitive Sciences* 10 (4): 152–158. https://doi.org/10.1016/j.tics.2006.02.002.

Kelleher, R.T. and Gollub, L.R. (1962). A review of positive conditioned reinforcement. *Journal of the Experimental Analysis of Behavior* 5 (S4): 543–597. https://doi.org/10.1901/jeab.1962.5-s543.

Keller, N.E., Hennings, A.C., and Dunsmoor, J.E. (2020). Behavioral and neural processes in counterconditioning: past and future directions. *Behaviour Research and Therapy*. Elsevier 125 (July 2019): 103532. https://doi.org/10.1016/j.brat.2019.103532.

Kwan, J.Y. and Bain, M.J. (2013). Owner attachment and problem behaviors related to relinquishment and training techniques of dogs. *Journal of Applied Animal Welfare Science* 16 (2): 128–183. https://doi.org/10.1080/10888705.2013.768923.

Lupien, S.J., McEwen, B.S., Gunnar, M.R., and Heim, C. (2009). Effects of stress throughout the lifespan on the brain, behaviour and cognition. *Nature Reviews Neuroscience* 10 (6): 434–445. https://doi.org/10.1038/nrn2639.

Martin, A.L., Bloomsmith, M.A., Kelley, M.E. et al. (2011). Functional analysis and treatment of human-directed undesirable behavior exhibited by a captive chimpanzee. *Journal of Applied Behavior Analysis* 44 (1): 139–143. https://doi.org/10.1901/jaba.2011.44-139.

Mazur, J.E. (2013). *Learning and Behavior*, 7e. Boston: Pearson.

McEwen, B.S. and Morrison, J.H. (2013). The brain on stress: vulnerability and plasticity of the prefrontal cortex over the life course. *Neuron*. Elsevier Inc. 79: 16–29. https://doi.org/10.1016/j.neuron.2013.06.028.

Roozendaal, B., McEwen, B.S., and Chattarji, S. (2009). Stress, memory and the amygdala. *Nature Reviews Neuroscience* 10 (6): 423–433. https://doi.org/10.1038/nrn2651.

Schapiro, S.J., Bloomsmith, M.A., and Laule, G.E. (2003). Positive reinforcement training as a technique to alter nonhuman primate behavior: quantitative assessments of effectiveness. *Journal of Applied Animal Welfare Science* 6 (3): 175–187.

Schultz, W. (2016). Dopamine reward prediction error coding. *Dialogues in Clinical Neuroscience* 18 (1): 23–32. https://doi.org/10.31887/dcns.2016.18.1/wschultz.

Williams, B.A. (1991). Marking and bridging versus conditioned reinforcement. *Animal Learning & Behavior* 19 (3): 264–269. https://doi.org/10.3758/BF03197885.

10

The Role of Natural Supplements and Behavioral Psychopharmacology for Shelter Pets

Ideally the shelter environment is only a temporary home for most animals. However, precisely because of its transient nature and the challenges of confinement, this environment can be highly stressful for many dogs and cats. Animals entering shelters often experience fear, anxiety, and stress, which can significantly reduce their welfare and, consequently, their adoptability. Stress-related signs may manifest as behavioral changes, such as withdrawal, hypervigilance, or aggression, and physical symptoms, including sleep disturbances, anorexia, gastrointestinal (GI) upset, or compromised immune function.

It is not sufficient to ask whether behaviors are purely neurotypical or dysregulated. In reality, they are deeply interconnected. Emotional distress can alter physiology, and biological imbalances can amplify behavioral changes. Therefore, assessing and addressing the overall wellbeing of each individual animal is essential. Accurately assessing stress in shelter dogs and cats is a crucial first step toward improving welfare and guiding effective behavioral or medical interventions (see Chapter 7). Because animals vary greatly in how they express distress, it is important to evaluate behavioral, physiological, and environmental indicators together when considering treatment plans, particularly those involving psychoactive medications. Stress assessment should be ongoing, not a one-time event done only upon admissions or a specific date. Tracking changes over time is needed and provides valuable information about how an animal responds to enrichment, training, and medication(s). Documentation and collaboration between veterinary, behavior, and caregiving teams in a coordinated manner is a must.

It is critical to evaluate whether the presenting condition stems primarily from psychological factors, environmental stressors, or underlying biochemical disturbances. This comprehensive assessment guides evidence-based decision-making and ensures that interventions target both the mind and body to support each pet's wellbeing and long-term success.

When considering psychoactive (also referred to as psychotropic) or behavior-modifying medications for shelter pets, the primary factor to evaluate is whether the animal's needs are best met through short-term or long-term pharmacologic support or a combination of both. These medications may be indicated for the management of anxiety-related, fear-based, or aggressive behaviors, all compromising the animal's wellbeing, safety, or adoptability. A variety of medications and nutraceutical supplements are available, each with potential benefits and drawbacks. Therefore, the decision to medicate must be individualized, based on a thorough behavioral and medical assessment.

It is important to recognize that the current scientific evidence supporting psychoactive medication use in shelter settings is limited. While these medications can improve wellbeing and facilitate behavior modification, they should not be used routinely or preventatively; for example, they should not be administered at the time of admissions as a matter of policy, in the same way vaccines are.

In summary, psychoactive medications and supplements can be valuable tools to reduce suffering and support rehabilitation when used judiciously. However, they should never replace comprehensive evaluation, environmental enrichment, or behavior modification efforts. Prescribers must consider the broader physiological and welfare impacts, not solely the behavioral changes. The goal is always to enhance the overall quality of life (QOL) for the individual pet, ensuring that medical, behavioral, and environmental needs are addressed in an integrated manner.

10.1 When to Use Psychoactive Medications in Shelter Pets?

Psychopharmacologic intervention can play an important role in alleviating fear, anxiety, and related behavioral distress in shelter pets. It is crucial to reserve their use for cases with evident clinical signs of emotional suffering, rather than employed as a preventative measure.

Medications should be considered when a shelter pet exhibits persistent or severe anxiety, fear, or aggression despite adequate environmental management or behavior modification alone and as such compromising welfare, health, or adoptability. If the pet is deemed not adoptable due to safety reasons, compassionate euthanasia should be discussed as part of the care trajectory strategy (CTS), rather than a long-term plan with medications that may prolong suffering in the shelter.

Once medications are initiated, regular assessment is essential to determine whether the medication plan remains appropriate. This includes evaluating:

- The effectiveness of the drug in reducing the target signs.
- The presence of side effects or adverse reactions.
- Evaluation, whether dose, frequency of administration, or combination with other medications or supplements requires adjustment.

Unlike antibiotics or other medical treatments with standardized mg/kg dosing, psychoactive medications often require a more individualized approach. Dosing ranges are typically broad, and each animal's response, tolerance, and clinical progress should guide the decision to increase, taper, switch, or discontinue a given medication.

Ultimately, the goal of psychopharmacologic use in shelter pets is to reduce suffering, facilitate learning, and improve wellbeing, while always balancing the benefits against potential risks. These medications are most effective when used as part of comprehensive CTS, including behavior and wellbeing protocols that include environmental enrichment, training, and appropriate social interaction.

The use of psychoactive medications (with some being controlled substances) in animals requires a veterinary prescription and a clinician with appropriate behavioral pharmacology knowledge. Successful implementation depends heavily on collaboration between the veterinary and animal care teams. Consistent feedback from team members and volunteers regarding an animal's behavior, appetite, energy level, and side effects is essential to evaluate efficacy and safety. All this needs to be regularly documented in the Problem-Oriented Veterinary Behavior Record (POVBR), and progress should be tracked with the help of the Behavior Health Assessment Staging (BHAS) (see Chapter 5).

Therefore, it may be more feasible and practical in some circumstances to use nutraceuticals or natural supplements as part of a behavior support plan. Such products include L-theanine, alpha-casozepine, tryptophan, omega-3 fatty acids, or pheromone therapy. They can provide mild calming and anti-anxiety effects, support stress reduction, or improve overall wellbeing, especially when used early on in the treatment process. While the effects of nutraceuticals may be less potent or less immediately observable than those of prescription psychoactive medications, they may still serve as a valuable adjunct or alternative, particularly because they tend to carry fewer side effects and lower safety risks when used appropriately. Even with supplements, however, their use should be thoughtful and evidence-informed, with regular assessment to determine benefits and avoid unnecessary costs.

Supplements and nutraceuticals are a valuable adjunct or alternative when:

- A veterinarian is not immediately available to prescribe medication.
- The pet's signs are mild to moderate.
- The shelter environment limits or inhibits long-term pharmacologic monitoring.
- There are concomitant medical issues or drug interactions.

10.2 How Do Natural Supplements Work?

The term "nutraceuticals" refers to a blend of "nutrition" + "pharmaceutical" and are dietary supplements, functional ingredients, or special diets that go beyond basic nutrition and aim to influence health, behavior, or physiological functioning. In 1996 the Center for Veterinary Medicine, a subset of the U.S. Food and Drug Administration (FDA), declared animal products to be exempt from this term, hence, the term has no longer regulatory meaning. Nutraceuticals are now regulated as food products, not drugs, despite their ability to modify an animal's health beyond meeting nutritional needs. Nutraceuticals contain various different ingredients and some products contain a combination of these ingredients. It is therefore crucial to understand the mechanism of action of the various ingredients before implementing them. Nutraceuticals and diets can be prescribed in combination with psychopharmacologic agents, but it is critical to pay attention to potential adverse interactions.

The most recent research includes products that modulate the gut–brain axis. The gut microbiome, via neural, endocrine, and immune signaling, has been shown to be capable to influence mood, stress reactivity, behavior, and cognition (Zheng et al. 2016; Boehme et al. 2023; Fan et al. 2023; Khan and Ullah 2024). Nutraceuticals (such as special probiotics, prebiotics, Omega-3 fatty acids) may influence that axis (Bosch et al. 2007; Ephraim et al. 2022). There are tested dog and cat products available on the market. The onset of the benefits for some of these substances may take weeks.

Better understood are supplements and diets that work as neurotransmitters on neuroendocrine modulation. One of the key ways nutraceuticals and natural supplements are thought to influence behavior and emotional regulation in animals is through modulation of neurotransmitters and neuroendocrine function (Fan et al. 2023). These systems regulate how the brain perceives and responds to stress, fear, and environmental challenges, all factors particularly relevant for animals living in shelter environments. Some studies show changes in serotonin, dopamine, β-endorphin, noradrenaline, and cortisol in dogs given nutraceutical diets or supplements (Araujo et al. 2010; Sechi et al. 2017) (see Table 10.1).

Serotonin (5-HT) plays a major role in mood stability, anxiety regulation, and impulse control.

- Nutraceuticals such as the serotonin precursor L-tryptophan and L-theanine can enhance serotonergic signaling in the central nervous system (CNS).
- Research has shown that diets enriched with tryptophan lead to increased central serotonin synthesis and reduced aggression and reactivity in dogs (DeNapoli et al. 2000; Bosch et al. 2009).
- The enhancement of serotonergic tone can promote emotional balance, improved tolerance of confinement, and reduced stress responses in shelter settings.

Table 10.1 List of Natural Supplements

Supplement/Ingredient	Proposed Mechanism of Action	Evidence Level	Intended Use/Effects	Key Considerations for Shelter Use
L-Theanine (e.g. *Anxitane*)	Increases GABA, serotonin, and dopamine activity; promotes alpha-wave brain activity (calming without sedation)	Moderate (several canine studies show reduced fear/anxiety) (Michelazzi et al. 2015; Pike et al. 2015; Alagawany et al. 2020; Stillo et al. 2021)	Situational anxiety, fear of noise, or mild separation distress	Safe, nonsedating; start several days before stressful events. Minimal side effects. Cost can be a factor for large shelters.
Alpha-Casozepine (e.g. *Zylkene*)	Milk-derived peptide binding GABA receptors, mimicking benzodiazepine-like calming	Moderate; small RCTs in dogs/cats show mild anxiolytic effects (Beata et al. 2007a,b)	Mild anxiety, adaptation to new environments	Well-tolerated, good for short-term transitions (intake, foster, transport). Mild effect; works best for low-level anxiety.
Tryptophan (e.g. *Composure* Treats, Diet Additive)	Precursor of serotonin; may enhance mood and reduce aggression in stress-prone pets	Moderate for dogs; limited feline data (DeNapoli et al. 2000; Fan et al. 2023)	Mild aggression, anxiety, or irritability	Should not be combined with SSRIs or TCAs without veterinary oversight. Benefit may depend on baseline serotonin status.
Omega-3 Fatty Acids (eicosapentaenoic acid [EPA]/Docosahexaenoic acid [DHA])	Anti-inflammatory, supports neuronal membrane fluidity, may modulate neurotransmission	Strong evidence for general health; moderate for cognitive/behavioral effects (Bosch et al. 2007; Ephraim et al. 2022)	Cognitive health, stress resilience, and anti-inflammatory support.	Safe for long-term use; may improve coat and joint health. Use fish oil from reputable sources to avoid oxidation.
S-Adenosyl-L-Methionine (SAMe)	Involved in methylation, neurotransmitter synthesis, and antioxidant defense	Moderate for cognitive support; limited behavioral studies (Araujo et al. 2012)	Cognitive dysfunction, age-related anxiety, mood stabilization.	Generally well tolerated; use veterinary formulations for consistent dosing.
Probiotics (e.g. *Enterococcus faecium*, *Lactobacillus*, *Bifidobacterium* strains)	Influence gut–brain axis through serotonin production and immune modulation	Emerging; several canine studies show reduced stress markers (Diez-Gutiérrez et al. 2020; Boehme et al. 2023; Khan and Ullah 2024; Zhang et al. 2025)	Mild anxiety, GI-associated stress, overall wellbeing.	May aid gut health and improve stool quality – important in shelters. Monitor for individual response.
Pheromone Therapy (e.g. *Adaptil*, *Feliway*)	Synthetic analogues of species-specific pheromones providing reassurance	Strong for short-term calming; well studied in shelters (Pageat and Gaultier 2003)	Noise phobia, adaptation to kennels, and co-housing stress.	Easy to use (diffusers, sprays, and collars). Cost-effective for communal spaces.
Herbal Blends (e.g. Valerian, Chamomile, Magnolia, Phellodendron)	GABA modulation, serotonergic and sedative plant compounds	Variable; limited high-quality data (DePorter et al. 2012; Ağan et al. 2022)	Mild calming; sleep support.	Potential variability in product quality and potency. Avoid unknown-source products.
Medium-Chain Triglycerides (MCTs)	Provide ketone bodies as alternative brain energy source; neuroprotective effects	Strong for canine cognitive dysfunction; mild behavioral benefit (Pan et al. 2018b; Pan 2021; McGrath et al. 2024)	Senior animals with cognitive decline or anxiety	Best used in diet formulation or specific supplements; monitor for GI upset.

Dopamine influences motivation, learning, and reward-seeking behavior.

- Diets supplemented with amino acids, omega-3 fatty acids, and antioxidants may increase dopaminergic activity, supporting improved focus and engagement (Bosch et al. 2007).
- In stressed or under-stimulated dogs, balanced dopamine function may encourage positive exploratory behavior and enhance responsiveness to enrichment or training.

β-Endorphins act as natural opioids within the brain, mediating comfort, pain, and stress relief.

- In studies involving nutraceutical diets, increased β-endorphin levels were observed alongside improved behavioral stability (Sechi et al. 2017).
- Elevated β-endorphin activity is associated with greater relaxation and reduced distress, which can improve welfare for dogs coping with shelter-related anxiety or sensory overstimulation.

Noradrenaline (Norepinephrine [NE]) regulates arousal and vigilance as part of the "fight or flight" system.

- Nutraceuticals that modulate the hypothalamic–pituitary–adrenal (HPA) axis can reduce noradrenergic activity, tempering excessive arousal.
- A controlled study documented a significant reduction in circulating noradrenaline levels in dogs receiving a nutraceutical. This suggests a more stable sympathetic regulation (Sechi et al. 2017).
- It helps animals recover more quickly after stress and maintain calmer behavior in noisy, unpredictable environments.

Cortisol is the primary stress hormone. Circulating increased levels are used in many studies to measure stress response, in particular to monitor chronic persistent stress.

- Several studies have demonstrated that nutraceuticals such as L-theanine can reduce cortisol secretion during stressful events and speed recovery after exposure (Araujo et al. 2010).
- Lower cortisol levels correspond with improved welfare, better immune function, and enhanced adaptability to the shelter environment.

This modulation can explain the observed benefits of nutraceutical diets and supplements. While these effects are typically milder and potentially slower than those of prescription psychotropic drugs, they can provide meaningful support to shelter animals, especially in conjunction with enrichment, behavior modification programs, and in some cases psychoactive medications.

Other supplements include substances with anti-inflammatory or antioxidant effects, such as omega-3 fatty acids. Chronic stress, behavioral disorders, and cognitive decline are often associated with oxidative stress, neuroinflammation, and immune changes, and nutraceuticals containing antioxidants or plant extracts may help reduce some of these underlying processes (Palestrini et al. 2010; Orlando 2018).

In addition, for aging pets in the shelter, the support of cognitive function and brain health may be beneficial as stress can have a detrimental effect on aging. Enriched diets or supplements such as medium-chain triglycerides (MCTs), omega-3-fatty acids, and *S*-adenosyl-L-methionine (SAMe), have shown promise in delaying cognitive decline and improving executive function (Rème et al. 2008; Pan et al. 2010, 2018a,b).

Pheromones and other modifiers provide the message of constant security, safety, and reassurance and are species-specific (Pageat and Gaultier 2003). They can be adequate for mild behavioral issues or as adjuncts to training and medication and may assist shifting baseline arousal, supporting relaxation, and improving resilience. Applications include spray, diffuser, or collar.

Here are some of the key research findings (and caveats) relevant to companion animals:

- A controlled study in 69 dogs with behavioral disorders found that after 45 days on a specific nutraceutical diet, dogs had increased levels of serotonin, dopamine, and β-endorphin and decreased levels of noradrenaline, cortisol, and oxidative-stress markers compared to a control diet (Sechi et al. 2017).
- A recent systematic review on enriched diets and nutraceuticals in aged dogs and cats including 30 studies reported that omega-3 fatty acids showed evidence of cognitive benefit (Blanchard et al. 2025). Other ingredients such as MCTs, SAMe, and antioxidants showed promise, but the evidence is variable.
- A review article on the use of nutraceuticals in dogs and cats indicates that nutraceuticals *can* contribute to wellness via gut–brain axis, immune modulation, and antioxidant effects (Orlando 2018; Fan et al. 2023). However, the quality of evidence is limited, and many studies are small, non-randomized, or industry funded.

10.2.1 Key Takeaways for Application in Shelters

- Nutraceuticals are appropriate:
  - For animals with mild to moderate behavioral/fear/anxiety issues, not severe aggression.
  - As adjuncts to enrichment, behavior modification, and environment improvement.
  - For animals where long-term pharmaceutical behavior medication may be less feasible (e.g. due to costs, monitoring constraints, or medical conditions).
- They are not a substitute for:
  - A comprehensive behavior assessment, environmental modifications, enrichment, socialization, and training.
  - Veterinary behaviorist involvement when there is a serious risk such as aggression, high fear, or welfare compromise.
- Due to the variable evidence base:
  - Choose veterinary-formulated or peer-review-supported brands.
  - Monitor the individual animal's response (behavioral changes, side effects, and interactions with other medications).
  - Use them as part of a plan, not a "set and forget" add-on.
  - Be cautious about claims; check for quality control and transparency from manufacturers.
- Practical considerations:
  - Introduce slowly and monitor carefully. Some animals may respond and some may not (nonresponders).
  - Document baseline behavior, materials used, timeframe, and changes for at least four to eight weeks to assess efficacy.
  - Consider costs, shelf-life, potential side effects, and interactions with other medications.
  - Use supplements and veterinary guidance rather than frequent experimentation with unknown products.

10.2.2 Limitations and Risks

- Supplements are not regulated; issues of quality, dose accuracy, and purity exist.
- The positive effects are often small or moderate. It may not substitute for pharmacologic medication when animals are in severe distress.
- Some animals may show no response (nonresponders).
- Because of this variability, evaluating cost-benefit is important in shelter settings with limited resources.
- Overreliance on supplements could result in delayed proper intervention using behavior modification, environmental change, or medication in animals who need it.
- Avoid combining serotonin-enhancing supplements (L-theanine, tryptophan) with prescription selective serotonin reuptake inhibitors (SSRIs) or tricyclic antidepressants (TCAs) unless directed by a veterinarian.

10.3 How Do Psychoactive Medications Work?

Psychoactive medications are used in veterinary medicine to modify neurochemical signaling in the brain, helping us to regulate emotional states, reduce maladaptive behaviors, and improve an animal's ability to cope with stress and environmental demands.

10.3.1 The Neurobiological Basis of Emotion and Behavior

In both dogs and cats, emotions and behavioral responses arise from interactions among several key regions of the brain (McEwen and Morrison 2013):

- Amygdala: processes fear and threat perception.
- Hippocampus: involved in memory and contextual learning.
- Prefrontal cortex: modulates impulse control and decision-making.
- HPA axis: coordinates hormonal stress responses.

In shelter pets, chronic stress, noise, confinement, and unpredictability can activate the amygdala and HPA axis, causing persistent hypervigilance, reactivity, or anxiety. With time, this can lead to neurochemical imbalances (e.g. low serotonin, high cortisol, and noradrenaline), impaired learning, and decreased welfare (Arnsten et al. 2015).

Selecting the right medication(s) that target-specific neurotransmitters or pathways is critical in implementing a multimodal plan that also includes behavior modification, enrichment, and welfare assessment. When applied thoughtfully, psychopharmacology can restore neurochemical balance, promote emotional recovery, and significantly improve the QOL and adoptability of shelter animals.

The effective and ethical use of psychopharmacology in shelter animals requires a solid grasp of neurophysiology and neurotransmission. Particularly because there are *NO* FDA-approved drugs to treat generalized anxiety and phobia in pets. All current medications used to treat behavioral disorders in pets are "*off label.*" "Off-label" or "extra-label" use in veterinary medicine is the use of an approved drug in a manner not specified by its label (see Table 10.2). It is legal and often necessary to prescribe, provided it is prescribed by a veterinarian, justified by clinical needs, and carefully monitored. This practice expands treatment options for

Table 10.2 Off-Label/Extra-Label Use

Consideration	Explanation
Safety and Efficacy	Off-label does not mean unsafe, but dosing, side effects, and duration may differ from label information. Close monitoring is essential.
Informed Consent	Clients or caretakers should be informed that the use is off-label and why it's being prescribed.
Species Differences	Metabolism and receptor sensitivity can vary greatly between species; extrapolation from human data can lead to errors if not done carefully.
Documentation	The rationale for off-label use, dosage, and observed outcomes should be recorded in the medical record.
Welfare Focus	The intent of off-label use must always be to improve the animal's health or welfare, never for convenience or sedation without medical justification.

conditions like fear, anxiety, and behavioral disorders, especially in shelter and behavior medicine, where only very few drugs are specifically approved for use.

Medications approved by the FDA include the following:

- Reconcile® and Clomicalm® for dogs with a clinical diagnosis of separation anxiety.
- Sileo® for dogs with a clinical diagnosis of noise aversion.
- Anipryl® for canine cognitive dysfunction.
- Bonqat for feline transportation and anxiety concerns.

Psychoactive medications now play a vital role in enhancing the welfare, emotional stability, and adoptability of shelter animals with the condition that they are used judiciously and guided by an understanding of neurophysiology, specifically, how the brain's electrical and chemical signaling systems influence emotion and behavior. Psychoactive medications act on the CNS to modify brain chemistry and neuronal communication. The goal is not to sedate animals, but to normalize emotional regulation, reduce maladaptive anxiety or fear, and facilitate learning, particularly in stressful environments like shelters.

10.3.2 Neuronal Communication and Its Role in Psychopharmacology

Understanding neuronal communication is critical when using psychoactive medications as it allows clinicians to choose medications that target the correct neurotransmitter system. Furthermore, it will avoid inappropriate drug combinations that could cause adverse interactions (e.g. serotonin syndrome). Realistic expectations can only be set when there is acknowledgment that structural changes in the brain take time (weeks, not days). With this understanding, combining pharmacologic support with training, socialization, and enrichment to reinforce adaptive behavior can certainly optimize outcomes.

All behavior originates in the brain through electrical and chemical communication among neurons. Electrical activity occurs within each neuron. Nerve impulses (action potentials) are generated by changes in voltage across the cell membrane, allowing ions such as sodium (Na^+), potassium (K^+), and calcium (Ca^{2+}) to flow in and out of the neuron (Stahl 2013a). Chemical activity occurs between neurons at synapses (see Figure 10.1). When an electrical impulse reaches the

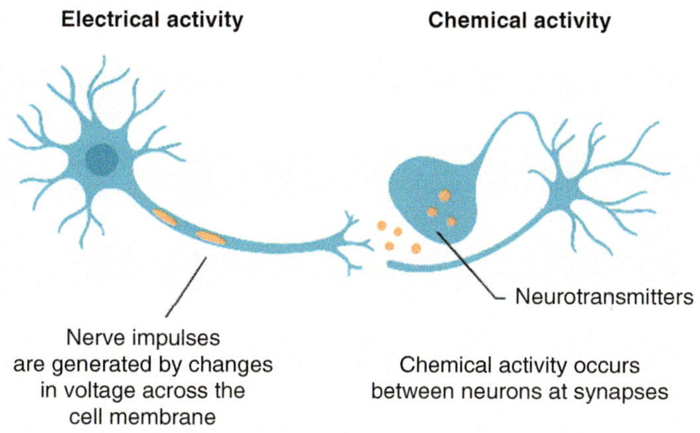

Figure 10.1 Electrical and Chemical Communication Among Neurons

Table 10.3 Key Neurotransmitters and Their Roles

Neurotransmitter	Primary Function	When Dysregulated
Serotonin (5-HT)	Regulates mood, impulse control, and calmness	Low levels → anxiety, aggression, impulsivity
GABA (Gamma-Aminobutyric Acid)	Main inhibitory neurotransmitter; reduces excitability	Low activity → hyperarousal, panic
Norepinephrine	Mediates arousal and "fight or flight"	Excess → hypervigilance, fear, restlessness
Dopamine	Motivation, reward, and focus	Imbalance → compulsive behaviors, agitation
Glutamate	Main excitatory neurotransmitter	Reactivity → stress-related neural sensitization

axon terminal, it triggers the release of neurotransmitters, which are chemical messengers that cross the synaptic cleft and bind to receptors on the next cell (Stahl 2013b).

The balance and function of these neurotransmitters determine whether the brain circuits, governing fear, anxiety, reward, and learning, are reactive and stressed or responsive and stable.

Key neurotransmitters include glutamate and gamma-aminobutyric acid (GABA) as well as monoamine/neuropeptide modulators, which include dopamine, NE, and serotonin, as well as epinephrine, melatonin, and histamine (Stahl 2013a) (see Table 10.3). Glutamate and GABA are amino acids that are classified as excitatory or inhibitory based on the responses evoked and are generally fast acting; GABA-γ, synthesized from glutamate, is the major inhibitory neurotransmitter. They have important functions in the CNS. Monoamine/neuropeptide modulators are generally considered slower acting. In the mammalian brain, serotonergic neurons are located in the limbic system, hence, their involvement in anxiety-related disorders.

Serotonin (5-HT) is synthesized from tryptophan obtained by dietary intake; hence, dietary levels of tryptophan can significantly alter brain serotonin levels (Murray 2019b). There are serotonin receptors throughout the body, and consequently, serotonin plays a role in the control of mood, impulsivity, anxiety and panic, satiety, cognition, aggression, sex drive, sleep, pain, and even thermoregulation.

NE is made from dopamine and plays a role in control of emotions, arousal, and the reward systems. Some emphasis should be placed on the α_2-adrenergic receptors, given their crucial role in modulating NE activity (Murray 2019c). α_2-Agonists, including xylazine, dexmedetomidine, and clonidine, act by inhibiting the release of NE from presynaptic neurons, resulting in sedation, analgesia, muscle relaxation, and, at lower doses, anxiolytic (anxiety-reducing) effects. In contrast, α_2-antagonists such as yohimbine, atipamezole, and amphetamines block α_2 receptors, thereby increasing the release of NE. This mechanism underlies their use as reversal agents for α_2-agonist-induced sedation and their stimulant properties in some contexts.

Acetylcholine (Ach) is the only neurotransmitter not directly synthesized from an amino acid. It is synthesized by linking choline with acetyl coenzyme A (acetyl CoA) (Murray 2019c). It is involved in signal transmission for postganglionic parasympathetic synapses (muscarinic), autonomic ganglia (nicotinic n), and neuromuscular junctions (nicotinic m). Anticholinergic effects such as dry mouth, dry eyes, urine retention, constipation, mydriasis, and increased heart rate can occur with medications that affect this neurotransmitter, such as TCAs. This neurotransmitter's effect at the muscarinic receptors can play a role in memory. Due to its effect on the nicotinic-n receptors in the brain, adrenal medulla, and autonomic ganglia, acetylcholine contributes to learning and memory. Nicotine also binds these receptors, activating the reward and dependence systems, but also improving mental alertness and memory. Degeneration of cholinergic pathways is implicated in learning and memory decline, as occurs in Alzheimer's disease.

The same principles that guide the use of any medication apply equally to behavior-modifying (psychoactive) medications. When selecting a psychoactive drug for shelter dogs or cats, one of the primary considerations is whether a short-term, long-term, or combined approach will best address the animal's anxiety-related or fear-based behaviors.

Another key factor influencing drug selection is the animal's predicted length of stay (LOS). In shelters, the goal is always to optimize welfare while minimizing LOS through timely behavioral stabilization, fast-tracking adoptions, or placement into foster care. Therefore, medication plans should be tailored to both the individual animal's behavioral needs and the practical realities of the shelter environment.

A variety of psychoactive medications can be used in shelter pets, but the advantages and disadvantages of each drug class must be carefully evaluated. Selecting the most appropriate medication depends on several factors, including the target neurotransmitter system, the desired clinical effect, the latency to onset of action, and the potential for adverse effects. As discussed, most of these medications are used "off-label" in shelter medicine. According to the U.S. FDA, extra-label drug use is defined as the *"actual or intended use of a drug in an animal in a manner that is not in accordance with the approved labeling."*

Off-label/Extra-Label Use Requires

- A valid Veterinarian–Client–Patient Relationship (VCPR).
- A licensed veterinarian with the authority to prescribe.
- A documented diagnosis and justified need for pharmacologic intervention.
- Accurate medical records detailing dosage, duration, and rationale for drug selection.
- Proper labeling and communication of instructions to caregivers or staff.

10.4 A Framework for Psychoactive Medication Selection in Shelters

This careful, structured approach ensures that psychoactive medications are used ethically, legally, and effectively to improve animal wellbeing, while maintaining professional standards in shelter practice. When implementing behavior-modifying or psychoactive medications in a shelter setting, practical considerations surrounding administration are crucial for success and animal welfare.

10.4.1 Frequency of Administration

Before prescribing, assess whether the organization has adequate staffing and time to administer medications multiple times a day. In general, lower-frequency dosing schedules (e.g. once daily) promote better compliance and minimize disruption to daily operations.

10.4.2 Route of Administration

Most psychoactive medications are administered orally, but palatability and ease of delivery can vary. Whenever possible, choose formulations that are easy to administer and minimally invasive, reducing stress for both pets and team members.

To improve compliance, medications can often be hidden in palatable foods such as canned food, pill pockets, peanut butter, cheese, or other safe treats, which is particularly useful for dogs. Cats can be more challenging to medicate; in some cases, pheromone therapy (e.g. Feliway® sprays, wipes, or diffusers) may serve as a valuable adjunct or alternative to pharmacological interventions, helping reduce anxiety and promote calm behavior.

10.4.3 Medication Administration as a Stressor in Shelter Pets

The team must weigh the benefits of treatment against the stress caused by administration, especially for fearful or aggressive animals. For example, repeatedly forcing oral medication in a fearful cat may increase anxiety and counteract the intended therapeutic effect. In such cases, alternative approaches, such as transdermal formulations, treat-based delivery, or nutraceutical substitutes, may be more humane and effective.

10.4.4 Creative and Compassionate Strategies

10.4.4.1 Medication Administration and Selection in Shelter Animals

Using positive reinforcement, minimal restraint, and low-stress handling techniques can improve medication compliance while reducing fear. Selecting flavored or compounded formulations may further increase acceptance and create a more positive experience for both staff and animals.

10.4.4.2 Financial and Logistical Considerations

Shelters often operate with restricted budgets and limited staff, so the cost, availability, and ease of administration of psychoactive or behavior-modifying medications must be carefully evaluated. Whenever possible, medications should be affordable, readily sourced, and simple to administer within existing operational frameworks. Generic formulations or nutraceutical alternatives may offer cost-effective solutions. Consider procurement factors such as pharmacy access, shipping times, and compounding needs to avoid treatment interruptions and ensure consistent care.

10.4.4.3 Abuse and Diversion Risk

Some psychoactive medications – such as benzodiazepines (e.g. alprazolam and diazepam) or stimulants (e.g. amphetamines) – have potential for human misuse. Evaluate whether prescribed medications could pose a diversion risk among team members, volunteers, or the public. Always implement strict storage and dispensing protocols.

10.4.4.4 Legal and Regulatory Considerations

State and municipal laws may impose restrictions on the use of certain medications, even when behavioral intervention is clinically justified. It is essential to remain compliant with legal and regulatory requirements when prescribing psychoactive medications in shelter settings.

10.4.4.5 Rabies Observation Cases

Animals under rabies observation must remain behaviorally and neurologically assessable. Certain medications can produce side effects including sedation, ataxia, or altered mentation and, hence, may mimic neurological signs of rabies. In these cases, the use of psychoactive medications may be contraindicated or require consultation with public health authorities before administration.

10.4.4.6 Court-Ordered or Legal Holds

Animals held as part of legal investigations (e.g. cruelty, neglect, or bite cases) are considered evidence and must be maintained in a condition that prevents deterioration. This obligation includes not only physical health but also mental and emotional welfare.

These cases are often long-term holds, which can lead to behavioral decline due to prolonged confinement and stress. It is important to engage in open communication with law enforcement officers, attorneys, and other involved professionals to discuss welfare concerns and explore appropriate options to preserve the animal's wellbeing throughout the holding period. This may include behavioral medications, enrichment strategies, and stress-reduction measures.

When choosing a medication for fear or anxiety in a shelter animal, clinicians should consider the exposure to unpredictable stressors (noise, confinement, and social isolation). Chronic stress can cause persistent activation of fear circuits, leading to reduced serotonin and GABA activity and elevated levels of NE and cortisol.

Identify the target behavior and underlying emotional state – fear, anxiety, frustration, or aggression – as different neurotransmitter systems may be involved. Medication should be selected to address the most likely neurochemical imbalance (e.g. SSRIs for serotonin-related anxiety).

10.5 Common Psychoactive Medications for Canine and Feline Patients

This chapter introduces the major classes of psychoactive medications used in shelter dogs and cats to reduce stress, anxiety, and maladaptive behaviors.

10.5.1 Serotonin Enhancers

General Information

1) It may take several weeks to establish the full drug effect.
2) Gradual discontinuation needed.
3) Uses: Anxiety, aggression, and compulsive behavior.
4) No evidence of dependence.
5) Cleared by hepatic mechanism, excreted by kidneys.

10.5.1.1 Selective Serotonin Reuptake Inhibitors (SSRIs)

Species – Dogs and Cats

1) Medications:
   a) Fluoxetine, paroxetine, sertraline, citalopram, and fluvoxamine
2) Pharmacology (Simpson and Papich 2003; Ogata et al. 2019):
   a) Blocks reuptake of 5-HT
3) Side effects
   a) Sedation, agitation, GI disturbance, may lower seizure threshold, may alter blood glucose levels diabetes mellitus (DM), not as sedating as TCAs
4) Contraindications:
   a) Concurrent use with other SSRIs, TCAs, or monoamine oxidase inhibitors (MAOIs)
   b) Use with caution in patients with hepatic disease and renal disease

10.5.1.2 Tricyclic Antidepressants (TCAs)

Species – Dogs and Cats

1) Medications:
   a) Clomipramine and amitriptyline
2) Pharmacology (Simpson and Papich 2003; Crowell-Davis 2019):
   a) Blocks reuptake of serotonin, NE, and dopamine
   b) Blocks muscarinic cholinergic receptors (side effects)
   c) Blocks H1 histamine receptors (side effects)
   d) Blocks α1-adrenergic receptors (side effects)
3) Side effects:
   a) Sedation: H1 histamine receptor and α1-adrenergic receptor blockades
   b) Anticholinergic effects (dry eyes and mouth, constipation, urine retention, and mydriasis), decreased cardiac conduction from α1-adrenergic receptor blockage (tachycardia, arrhythmias), testicular hypoplasia, changes in blood glucose levels, and decreased seizure threshold
   c) GI disturbances
4) Contraindications:
   a) Concurrent with the use of other TCAs, SSRIs, and MAOIs
   b) Concurrent antihistamine or thyroid replacement
   c) Cardiac disease
   d) Seizure disorders
   e) Glaucoma

10.5.1.3 Serotonin Norepinephrine Reuptake Inhibitors (SNRIs)

Species – Dogs and Cats

1) Medications:
   a) Venlafaxine
2) Pharmacology (Metz et al. 2021; Mercier and Seksel 2024; Masson et al. 2025):
   a) Inhibits serotonin NE reuptake
   b) Increases the levels of the neurotransmitters serotonin (5-HT) and NE
   c) Do not block α1-noradrenergic, histaminic, or cholinergic receptors
   d) Serotonergic effects occur at low doses
   e) Noradrenergic effects are progressively enhanced as the dose is increased
3) Side effects:
   a) Sedation, depression, arousal, GI disorders, tachycardia, and hypertension
4) Contraindications:
   a) Concurrent with the use of other TCAs, SSRIs, and MAOIs
   b) Cardiac disease
   c) Seizure disorders

10.5.1.4 Serotonin Antagonist Reuptake Inhibitors (SARIs)

Species – Dogs and Cats

1) Medications:
   a) Trazodone
2) Pharmacology (Gruen and Sherman 2007; Dantas and Crowell-Davis 2019b):
   a) Serotonin 2A antagonist and reuptake inhibition, potentiates serotonin activity
   b) α1-Adrenergic antagonism
   c) Some antihistaminic properties
3) Side effects:
   a) Sedation, reduces blood pressure, GI upset, ataxia, agitation, and aggression
4) Contraindications:
   a) Do not exceed 15 mg/kg/day if giving with serotonin-enhancing medications to avoid serotonin syndrome
   b) Cardiac disease
   c) Seizure disorders

10.5.2 Azapirone

Species – Dogs and Cats

1) Medication
   a) Buspirone
2) Pharmacology (Simpson and Papich 2003; Dantas and Crowell-Davis 2019b)
   a) Serotonin 1A agonist
   b) Increases serotonin
3) Side effect:
   a) Generally mild, vomiting, diarrhea, tremors, increased anxiety, or increased irritability
   b) Increased wakefulness and decreased rapid eye movement (REM) sleep in cats

   c) Anecdotal increase in affection or aggression (cats)
   d) Anecdotal post-pill anxiety
4) Contraindications: Concurrent with the use of other TCAs, SSRIs, and MAOIs

10.5.3 GABA-Enhancing Anxiolytics

10.5.3.1 Benzodiazepine – Controlled Drug

Species – dogs and cats: Use in animals without a history of exhibiting aggressive behaviors

Cats: Use with caution in cats since they do not use glucuronic acid pathways efficiently. There are reported cases of some acute hepatic necrosis.

1) Medications: diazepam, alprazolam, clonazepam, chlorazepate, oxazepam, and lorazepam
2) Pharmacology (Dantas and Crowell-Davis 2019a; Murray 2019a):
   a) Facilitates or potentiates GABA and increases the binding affinity of the GABA receptor for GABA
   b) Hepatic biotransformation
   c) Obesity increased the accumulation of the drug in fat
   d) Potential for abuse and dependence
3) Side effects
   a) Ataxia, paradoxical reaction, interferes with learning, muscle relaxation, and disinhibition of aggression
4) Contraindications: Liver and kidney disease, hypersensitivity to benzodiazepines, and be careful when used in combination with antifungal medication due-to-drug interactions

10.5.4 Monoamine Oxidase Inhibitors (MAOIs)

Species – dogs: cognitive dysfunction, in Europe, used for anxiety and "mood" disorders

1) Medication:
   a) Selegiline
2) Pharmacology (Dantas and Crowell-Davis 2019c):
   a) Increases dopamine by suppressing breakdown
   b) Active metabolites: amphetamine relatives
3) Side effects:
   a) Agitation, anxiety, and GI upset
4) Contraindications:
   a) Concurrent with the use of other TCAs, SSRIs, and MAOIs

10.5.5 Calcium Channel Modulation Anxiolytic and Neuropathic Pain Modulator

10.5.5.1 Pregabalin – Controlled Drug

Species – Cats

1) Medications:
   a) Bonqat® is the first FDA-approved pregabalin formulation for veterinary use (approved 2023 in the United States for cats) (Lamminen et al. 2022)
   b) Given 1–1.5 hours before the anticipated event
   c) Onset typically occurs within 30–60 minutes, lasting up to 12 hours

2) Pharmacology (Crowell-Davis et al. 2019):
   a) α2δ (alpha-2-delta) subunit ligand (Offord and Isom 2016); anticonvulsant and anxiolytic agent
   b) Binds with high affinity to the α2δ subunit of voltage-gated calcium channels
   c) Does not act directly on GABA receptors, but its effects are similar to GABAergic modulation due to its influence on excitatory neurotransmission
3) Side effects:
   a) Incoordination, lethargy, decreased appetite, or mild GI upset
4) Contraindications:
   a) Cardiac disease, hypertension, renal disease, hypersensitivity to pregabalin, or severe systemic disorder
   b) Has not been evaluated in breeding, pregnant or lactating cats, and cats younger than seven months of age
   c) Use with caution in animals with renal insufficiency or when combined with CNS depressants

10.5.5.2 Gabapentin

Species – Dog and Cat

1) Medications:
   a) Gabapentin (van Haaften et al. 2017; Sinn 2018)
2) Pharmacology (Crowell-Davis et al. 2019):
   a) α2δ ligand; anticonvulsant/neuropathic pain analgesic
   b) Closes presynaptic calcium channels, resulting in the decrease in neuronal activity
   c) No direct action on GABA
3) Side effects:
   a) Sedation, incoordination, lethargy, and GI
4) Contraindications:
   a) Cardiac disease, hypertension, renal disease, or hypersensitivity to the medication

NOTE: Gabapentin has been placed on the controlled substance list in some states.

10.5.6 Central α-2A Adrenergic Receptor Agonist: Sedation and Anxiolytics

Species – Dog

1) Medication:
   a) Clonidine (Ogata and Dodman 2011), Sileo, Dexdomitor® (Sinn 2018), and Guanfacine (Freeman et al. 2015)
2) Pharmacology:
   a) NE release through activation of α-2 receptors on presynaptic neurons in the locus coeruleus
   b) Also affects α A, B, and C receptors
   c) Reduces CNS arousal and nociceptive pain at lower doses
3) Side effects:
   a) Sedation, agitation, and vomiting
4) Contraindications:
   a) Cardiovascular disease and significant neurological disease
   b) Severe hepatic or renal disease

10.5.7 Antipsychotic Agents: Phenothiazine Class

General information: Oldest behavior-modifying drug, sedation/tranquilizer with poor anxiolytic properties; it can induce aggression

Species – Dog and Cat

1) Medication:
   a) Acetylpromazine (acepromazine)
2) Pharmacology (Seibert and Crowell-Davis 2019)
   a) Dopamine antagonist: (→ prolactin increase)
3) Side effects
   a) Sedation, extrapyramidal signs, hypotension, potentiates seizures, and priapism
4) Contraindications
   a) Seizure disorders and cardiovascular problems

10.5.8 β-Adrenergic Blockers

Species – Dog and Cat

1) Medication:
   a) Propranolol (Sinn 2018)
2) Pharmacology (Ogata and Dantas 2019)
   a) β-Adrenergic blockers
   b) Reduce the physiological manifestations of stress and anxiety by blunting somatic signs such as tachycardia, tremors, and heightened arousal.
3) Side effects
   a) Sedation, bradycardia, diarrhea, lethargy, depression and vomiting.
4) Contraindications:
   a) Cardiac, respiratory or metabolic conditions

Propranolol does not directly treat fear or anxiety at the emotional level. By reducing these physical stress responses, propranolol may help some animals remain below threshold and better tolerate triggering situations. It is most often used as an adjunctive or situational medication, rather than a sole treatment, and should be combined with behavior modification and appropriate environmental management.

10.5.9 Determine if the Situation Calls for Daily or Intermittent/as Needed Medication

Daily medication should be considered when undesirable behaviors occur frequently or when the animal experiences prolonged periods of stress, anxiety, or arousal throughout the day and/or night. The goal is to stabilize the animal's emotional state and promote behavioral recovery through consistent therapeutic levels of medication. Medications can enable learning by reducing excessive arousal. Medications work best if they are integrated with behavior plans and environmental enrichment by helping to create new, positive neural pathways.

Psychoactive medications are not "one-size-fits-all." Regular monitoring and reassessment are essential to ensure the ongoing appropriateness of the medication plan.

- For short-term daily medications, evaluate the animal daily, ideally one to two hours after the therapeutic level has been reached.
- For long-term medications, determine evaluation intervals, typically every four to eight weeks.
- Use a numeric scale to track behavioral changes over time.

Once improvement is observed, maintain the medication at the lowest effective dose that continues to manage the behavior. This approach minimizes side effects while supporting welfare and adoptability.

Because of individual differences in receptor sensitivity, metabolism, and stress reactivity, each animal's dose and response must be reassessed frequently. Continuous monitoring and adjustment are critical to ensure safety, efficacy, and positive outcomes.

10.5.10 Determine if the Situation Calls for Short-Term or Long-Term Intervention or for a Combination

1) Short-term: For acute fear, handling, transportation stress, or unavoidable trigger situations
   - Dogs: → SARIs, α_2-agonists, benzodiazepines, or gabapentin
   - Cats: → gabapentin, pregabalin, SARIs, transdermal buprenorphine, and in some cases benzodiazepines
2) Long-term: For generalized anxiety, compulsive, fear-based behavior, and in some cases aggression (I feel this needs a caveat)
   - Dogs: → SSRIs, SNRIs, TCAs, MAOIs, or azapirone
   - Cats: → SSRIs, SNRIs, TCAs, or azapirone

Long-term medications should not be discontinued abruptly after being administered longer than one month as serious side effects can occur.

Appendix E Framework for a Decision Tree for Psychoactive Medication Selection Pathway in Shelters provides a step-by-step clinical algorithm for the use of short-acting oral behavior medications in dogs.

10.6 Key Considerations When Using Psychoactive Medications in Shelter Pets

A clear post-outcome plan is essential to ensure continuity of care and the long-term welfare of animals leaving the shelter, whether through adoption, transfer, or foster placement.

In some cases, it is appropriate and compassionate to include end-point discussions at the very beginning of an animal's treatment or management plan. In the CTS, early reflection on possible outcomes – including defining clear end points – allows for thoughtful, transparent, and ethically grounded, welfare-centered decision-making throughout the pet's care.

10.6.1 Responsibility for Counseling and Communication

Identify who is responsible for communicating the pet's behavioral and medical status to the next caregiver or organization. In some jurisdictions, veterinarians are legally required to provide this counseling, while in others, a qualified behavior professional or shelter representative may assume the role. Always confirm and comply with state and municipal regulations, regarding disclosure and transfer of animals on behavioral or psychotropic medications.

10.6.2 Management and Education Plan

Every pet with a behavior or medication history should be accompanied by a written management and education plan. This document should include:

- A summary of the behavioral concerns noticed and addressed in the shelter.
- Details of the current treatment plan, including medications, doses, frequencies, and any nutraceuticals or supplements used.
- Behavior modification strategies that have been implemented and proven effective or were not helpful.
- Recommendations for follow-up, including contact information for the shelter's veterinary team, a qualified behaviorist, or a recommended training organization.

10.6.3 Medication Continuity and Weaning

Medication management must be clearly documented and carefully planned during transfer:

- Complete treatment records should accompany the animal.
- Include a step-by-step plan for how and when to wean off medications, if appropriate.
- Some animals may need to be weaned prior to transfer to prevent withdrawal or confusion about ongoing treatment responsibilities.
- Conversely, if an animal is stable on medication, continuing therapy until the next veterinarian re-evaluates the case may be the best option.

10.6.4 Full Disclosure and Compassionate Communication

Full disclosure of the pet's behavioral history and treatment needs is not only an ethical obligation but also essential for successful long-term placement. Information should be presented in a thoughtful but objective way. Educating the new caregivers on past experiences includes emphasizing the progress made, listing the strategies that have worked and the resources available for continued support.

10.6.5 Transfer Considerations

In some cases, certain animals may not be appropriate for transfer, particularly if their behavioral or medical needs exceed the receiving organization's capacity for care. Such decisions should always prioritize animal welfare, ensuring that any transition supports stability, safety, and the animal's emotional wellbeing.

10.6.6 Quality-of-Life Evaluation and Humane End Points

Reflective end-point assessments are structured discussions that consider the complex ethical, emotional, and clinical factors surrounding an animal's welfare. These conversations provide a framework for evaluating QOL, prognosis, and treatment response, while ensuring decisions are made in the best interest of the animal.

Such assessments also support the emotional wellbeing of veterinary professionals, teams, leadership, volunteers, and the broader community, helping them process the difficult decisions, the event itself, and the emotional aftermath. Integrating compassion fatigue awareness and post-event debriefing into these processes promotes both ethical integrity and team resilience within the shelter environment.

Evaluation of QOL provides a structured, compassionate framework for determining when continued treatment or housing is no longer in the best interest of the pet. This process involves reflecting on the entire journey of the pet's care and assessing all medical, behavioral, emotional, and welfare factors that contribute to their overall wellbeing.

Reflective decision-making encourages collaboration among veterinarians, behaviorists, caregivers, and leadership, guaranteeing informed, ethical, and humane final decisions that are aligned with the pet's welfare needs. A humane end point is defined as the point at which an animal's pain, distress, or suffering can no longer be adequately alleviated and euthanasia becomes the most compassionate option. The aim is to safeguard animals from unnecessary suffering while upholding the quality of care and staying true to the organization's mission. Establishing and adhering to clear, measurable end points ensures ethical stewardship, emotional accountability, and humane treatment for every animal under care.

In this context, the term "end point" refers to the conclusion of care for an individual animal based on one or more of the following:

- Physical signs (e.g. body weight loss, medical conditions, and poor coat condition)
- Behavioral changes (e.g. decreased interaction, grooming, or exploration, lack of joy, self-mutilation)
- Clinical deterioration (e.g. unmanageable pain, organ failure, severe anxiety, or aggression impairing welfare)

In summary, the use of psychoactive medications in shelter pets should neither be feared nor misused. These medications are not intended to sedate animals, suppress normal behavior, or compensate for inadequate housing, enrichment, or handling practices. Rather, when thoughtfully selected and carefully monitored, they should be regarded like any other medical intervention – such as antiparasitics, antibiotics, or analgesics – and used judiciously to treat behavioral conditions that compromise wellbeing. When combined with appropriate environmental management, behavior modification, and humane care, psychoactive medications can significantly improve emotional stability, learning capacity, and overall wellbeing. However, their use requires structured oversight. The pet's behavioral and emotional status should be assessed before, during, and after initiating or adjusting any medication or dosage. Establishing a clear baseline and using a consistent scoring system to track changes over time allows teams to identify improvement, side effects, paradoxical responses, or welfare decline early, ensuring timely adjustments while prioritizing safety and wellbeing.

References

Ağan, U.B., Raouf, S.H., Uzun, B., and Meral, Y. (2022). The hidden potential of herbal remedies and neutraceuticals in canine and feline behavioural disorders. *Van Veterinary Journal* 33 (1): 36–41. https://doi.org/10.36483/vanvetj.955081.

Alagawany, M., Abd El-Hack, M.E., Saeed, M. et al. (2020). Nutritional applications and beneficial health applications of green tea and l-theanine in some animal species: a review. *Journal of Animal Physiology and Animal Nutrition* 104 (1): 245–256. https://doi.org/10.1111/jpn.13219.

Araujo, J.A., de Rivera, C., Ethier, J.L. et al. (2010). Anxitane reduces fear of humans in a laboratory study in dogs. *Journal of Veterinary Behavior*. Elsevier Inc. 5 (1): 32. https://doi.org/10.1016/j.jveb.2009.10.023.

Araujo, J.A., Faubert, M.L., Brooks, M.L. et al. (2012). NOVIFIT® (NoviSAMe®) tablets improve executive function in aged dogs and cats: implications for treatment of cognitive dysfunction syndrome. *International Journal of Applied Research in Veterinary Medicine* 10 (1): 90–98.

Arnsten, A.F.T., Raskind, M.A., Taylor, F.B., and Connor, D.F. (2015). The effects of stress exposure on prefrontal cortex: translating basic research into successful treatments for post-traumatic stress disorder. *Neurobiology of Stress*. Elsevier Inc. 1 (1): 89–99. https://doi.org/10.1016/j.ynstr.2014.10.002.

Beata, C., Beaumont-Graff, E., Coll, V. et al. (2007a). Effect of alpha-casozepine (Zylkene) on anxiety in cats. *Journal of Veterinary Behavior: Clinical Applications and Research* 2 (2): 40–46. https://doi.org/10.1016/j.jveb.2007.02.002.

Beata, C., Beaumont-Graff, E., Diaz, C. et al. (2007b). Effects of alpha-casozepine (Zylkene) versus selegiline hydrochloride (Selgian, Anipryl) on anxiety disorders in dogs. *Journal of Veterinary Behavior* 2 (5): 175–183. https://doi.org/10.1016/j.jveb.2007.08.001.

Blanchard, T., Eppe, J., Mugnier, A. et al. (2025). Enhancing cognitive functions in aged dogs and cats: a systematic review of enriched diets and nutraceuticals. *GeroScience*. Springer International Publishing 47 (3): 2925–2947. https://doi.org/10.1007/s11357-025-01521-z.

Boehme, M., Rémond-Derbez, N., Lerond, C. et al. (2023). *Bifidobacterium longum* subsp. longum reduces perceived psychological stress in healthy adults: an exploratory clinical trial. *Nutrients* 15 (14): 3122.

Bosch, G., Beerda, B., Hendriks, W.H. et al. (2007). Impact of nutrition on canine behaviour: current status and possible mechanisms. *Nutrition Research Reviews* 20 (02): 180–194. https://doi.org/10.1017/S095442240781331X.

Bosch, G., Beerda, B., Beynen, A.C. et al. (2009). Dietary tryptophan supplementation in privately owned mildly anxious dogs. *Applied Animal Behaviour Science* 121 (3–4): 197–205. https://doi.org/10.1016/j.applanim.2009.10.003.

Crowell-Davis, S.L. (2019). Tricyclic antidepressants. In: *Veterinary Psychopharmacology*, 2e (ed. S.L. Crowell-Davis, T.F. Murray, and L.M.d.S. Dantas), 231–256. Hoboken, NJ: Wiley Blackwell https://doi.org/10.1002/9781119226253.

Crowell-Davis, S.L., Irimajiri, M., and Dantas, L.M.d.S. (2019). Anticonvulsants and mood stabilizers. In: *Veterinary Psychopharmacology*, 2e (ed. S.L. Crowell-Davis, T.F. Murray, and L.M.d.S. Dantas), 147–156. Hoboken, NJ: Wiley Blackwell https://doi.org/10.1002/9781119226253.

Dantas, L.M.d.S. and Crowell-Davis, S.L. (2019a). Benzodiazepines. In: *Veterinary Psychopharmacology*, 2e (ed. S.L. Crowell-Davis, T.F. Murray, and L.M.d.S. Dantas), 67–102. Hoboken, NJ: Wiley Blackwell https://doi.org/10.1002/9781119226253.

Dantas, L.M.d.S. and Crowell-Davis, S.L. (2019b). Miscellaneous serotonergic agents. In: *Veterinary Psychopharmacology*, 2e (ed. S.L. Crowell-Davis, T.F. Murray, and L.M.d.S. Dantas), 129–146. Hoboken, NJ: Wiley https://doi.org/10.1002/9781119226253.

Dantas, L.M.d.S. and Crowell-Davis, S.L. (2019c). Monoamine oxidase inhibitors. In: *Veterinary Psychopharmacology*, 2e (ed. S.L. Crowell-Davis, T.F. Murray, and L.M.d.S. Dantas), 185–199. Hoboken, NJ: Wiley Blackwell https://doi.org/10.1002/9781119226253.

DeNapoli, J.S., Dodman, N.H., Shuster, L. et al. (2000). Effect of dietary protein content and tryptophan supplementation on dominance aggression, territorial aggression, and hyperactivity in dogs. *Journal of the American Veterinary Medical Association* 217 (4): 504–508.

DePorter, T.L., Landsberg, G.M., Araujo, J.A. et al. (2012). Harmonease Chewable Tablets reduces noise-induced fear and anxiety in a laboratory canine thunderstorm simulation: a blinded and placebo-controlled study. *Journal of Veterinary Behavior: Clinical Applications and Research* 7 (4): 225–232. https://doi.org/10.1016/j.jveb.2011.05.024.

Diez-Gutiérrez, L., Vicente, L.S., Barrón, L.J.R. et al. (2020). Gamma-aminobutyric acid and probiotics: multiple health benefits and their future in the global functional food and nutraceuticals market. *Journal of Functional Foods*. Elsevier 64 (November 2019): 103669. https://doi.org/10.1016/j.jff.2019.103669.

Ephraim, E., Brockman, J.A., and Jewell, D.E. (2022). A diet supplemented with polyphenols, prebiotics and omega-3 fatty acids modulates the intestinal microbiota and improves the profile of metabolites linked with anxiety in dogs. *Biology* 11 (7): 1–18. https://doi.org/10.3390/biology11070976.

Fan, Z., Bian, Z., Huang, H. et al. (2023). Dietary strategies for relieving stress in pet dogs and cats. *Antioxidants* 12 (3): https://doi.org/10.3390/antiox12030545.

Freeman, Z.T., Rice, K.A., Soto, P.L. et al. (2015). Neurocognitive dysfunction and pharmacological intervention using guanfacine in a rhesus macaque model of self-injurious behavior. *Translational Psychiatry*. Nature Publishing Group 5 (5): e567–e567. https://doi.org/10.1038/tp.2015.61.

Gruen, M.E. and Sherman, B.L. (2007). Use of trazodone as an adjunctive agent in the treatment of canine anxiety disorders: 56 cases (1995–2007). *Journal of the American Veterinary Medical Association* 233 (12): 1902–1907.

van Haaften, K.A., Eichstadt Forsythe, L.R., Stelow, E.A., and Bain, M.J. (2017). Effects of a single preappointment dose of gabapentin on signs of stress in cats during transportation and veterinary examination. *Journal of American Veterinary Medical Association* 251 (10): 1175–1181.

Khan, M.F. and Ullah, N. (2024). Impact of microbiome engineering on gut-brain axis modulation and behavioral disorders in canines: a precision veterinary medicine perspective. *Agricultural and Biotechnological Reflections* 2 (1): 79–102.

Lamminen, T., Doedée, A., Hyttilä-Hopponen, M., and Kaskinoro, H.J. (2022). Pharmacokinetics of single and repeated oral doses of pregabalin oral solution formulation in cats. *Journal of Veterinary Pharmacology and Therapeutics* 45 (4): 385–391. https://doi.org/10.1111/jvp.13061.

Masson, S., Metz, D., Bleuer-Elsner, S., and Schwobthaler, F. (2025). Retrospective study on the use of venlafaxine in 176 cats diagnosed with behavioral disorders. *Journal of Veterinary Behavior* 77: 1–10. https://doi.org/10.1016/j.jveb.2024.11.004.

McEwen, B.S. and Morrison, J.H. (2013). The brain on stress: vulnerability and plasticity of the prefrontal cortex over the life course. *Neuron*. Elsevier Inc. 79: 16–29. https://doi.org/10.1016/j.neuron.2013.06.028.

McGrath, A.P., Horschler, D.J., and Hancock, L. (2024). Feline cognition and the role of nutrition: an evolutionary perspective and historical review. *Animals* 14 (13): 1967.

Mercier, P. and Seksel, K. (2024). Territorial aggression in a German Shepherd treated with venlafaxine. *Journal of Veterinary Behavior*. Elsevier 73: 66–70. https://doi.org/10.1016/j.jveb.2024.03.004.

Metz, D., Medam, T., and Masson, S. (2021). Double-blind, placebo-controlled trial of venlafaxine to treat behavioural disorders in cats: a pilot study. *Journal of Feline Medicine and Surgery* https://doi.org/10.1177/1098612X211036792.

Michelazzi, M., Berteselli, G.V., Talamonti, Z. et al. (2015). Efficacy of l-theanine in the treatment of noise phobias in dogs: preliminary results. *Veterinária* 29 (2): 1–7.

Murray, T.F. (2019a). Amino acid neurotransmitters: glutamate, GABA and the pharmacology of benzodiazepines. In: *Veterinary Psychopharmacology*, 2e (ed. S.L. Crowell-Davis, T.F. Murray, and L.M.d.S. Dantas), 11–20. Hoboken, NJ: Wiley Blackwell https://doi.org/10.1002/9781119226253.

Murray, T.F. (2019b). Biogenic amine neurotransmitters: serotonin. In: *Veterinary Psychopharmacology*, 2e (ed. S.L. Crowell-Davis, T.F. Murray, and L.M.d.S. Dantas), 21–28. Hoboken, NJ: Wiley Blackwell https://doi.org/10.1002/9781119226253.

Murray, T.F. (2019c). Biogenic amine transmitters: acetylcholine, norepinephrine, and dopamine. In: *Veterinary Psychopharmacology*, 2e (ed. S.L. Crowell-Davis, T.F. Murray, and L.M.d.S. Dantas), 29–42. Hoboken, NJ: Wiley Blackwell https://doi.org/10.1002/9781119226253.

Offord, J. and Isom, L.L. (2016). Drugging the undruggable: gabapentin, pregabalin and the calcium channel α2δ subunit. *Critical Reviews in Biochemistry and Molecular Biology* 51 (4): 246–256. https://doi.org/10.3109/10409238.2016.1173010.

Ogata, N. and Dantas, L.M.d.S. (2019). Sympatholytic agents. In: *Veterinary Psychopharmacology*, 2e (ed. S.L. Crowell-Davis, T.F. Murray, and L.M.d.S. Dantas), 157–169. Hoboken, NJ: Wiley Blackwell https://doi.org/10.1002/9781119226253.

Ogata, N. and Dodman, N.H. (2011). The use of clonidine in the treatment of fear-based behavior problems in dogs: an open trial. *Journal of Veterinary Behavior: Clinical Applications and Research*. Elsevier Inc. 6 (2): 130–137. https://doi.org/10.1016/j.jveb.2010.10.004.

Ogata, N., Dantas, L.M.d.S., and Crowell-Davis, S.L. (2019). Selective serotonin reuptake inhibitors. In: *Veterinary Psychopharmacology*, 2e (ed. S.L. Crowell-Davis, T.F. Murray, and L.M.d.S. Dantas), 103–128. Hoboken, NJ: Wiley Blackwell https://doi.org/10.1002/9781119226253.

Orlando, J.M. (2018). Behavioral nutraceuticals and diets. *Veterinary Clinics of North America: Small Animal Practice*. Elsevier Inc. 48 (3): 473–495. https://doi.org/10.1016/j.cvsm.2017.12.012.

Pageat, P. and Gaultier, E. (2003). Current research in canine and feline pheromones. *Veterinary Clinics of North America: Small Animal Practice* 33 (2): 187–211. https://doi.org/10.1016/S0195-5616(02)00128-6.

Palestrini, C., Minero, M., Cannas, S. et al. (2010). Efficacy of a diet containing caseinate hydrolysate on signs of stress in dogs. *Journal of Veterinary Behavior: Clinical Applications and Research*. Elsevier Inc. 5 (6): 309–317. https://doi.org/10.1016/j.jveb.2010.04.004.

Pan, Y. (2021). Nutrients, cognitive function, and brain aging: what we have learned from dogs. *Medical Sciences* 9 (72): https://doi.org/10.3390/medsci9040072.

Pan, Y., Larson, B., Araujo, J.A. et al. (2010). Dietary supplementation with medium-chain TAG has long-lasting cognition-enhancing effects in aged dogs. *British Journal of Nutrition* 103 (12): 1746–1754. https://doi.org/10.1017/S0007114510000097.

Pan, Y., Kennedy, A.D., Jönsson, T.J., and Milgram, N.W. (2018a). Cognitive enhancement in old dogs from dietary supplementation with a nutrient blend containing arginine, antioxidants, B vitamins and fish oil. *British Journal of Nutrition* 119 (3): 349–358. https://doi.org/10.1017/S0007114517003464.

Pan, Y., Landsberg, G., Mougeot, I. et al. (2018b). Efficacy of a therapeutic diet on dogs with signs of cognitive dysfunction syndrome (CDS): a prospective double blinded placebo controlled clinical study. *Frontiers in Nutrition* 5 (December): 1–10. https://doi.org/10.3389/fnut.2018.00127.

Pike, A.L., Horwitz, D.F., and Lobprise, H. (2015). An open-label prospective study of the use of l-theanine (anxitane) in storm-sensitive client-owned dogs. *Journal of Veterinary Behavior*. Elsevier Inc. 10 (4): 324–331. https://doi.org/10.1016/j.jveb.2015.04.001.

Rème, C.A., Dramard, V., Kern, L. et al. (2008). Effect of S-adenosylmethionine tablets on the reduction of age-related mental decline in dogs: a double-blinded, placebo-controlled trial. *Veterinary Therapeutics* 9 (2): 69–82.

Sechi, S., Di Cerbo, A., Canello, S. et al. (2017). Effects in dogs with behavioural disorders of a commercial nutraceutical diet on stress and neuroendocrine parameters. *Veterinary Record* 180 (1): 18. https://doi.org/10.1136/vr.103865.

Seibert, L. and Crowell-Davis, S. (2019). Antipsychotics. In: *Veterinary Psychopharmacology*, 2e (ed. S.L. Crowell-Davis, T.F. Murray, and L.M.d.S. Dantas), 201–215. Hoboken,NJ: Wiley Blackwell https://doi.org/10.1002/9781119226253.

Simpson, B.S. and Papich, M.G. (2003). Pharmacologic management in veterinary behavioral medicine. *Veterinary Clinics of North America: Small Animal Practice* 33: 365–404.

Sinn, L. (2018). Advances in behavioral psychopharmacology. *Veterinary Clinics of North America: Small Animal Practice*. Elsevier Inc. 48 (3): 457–471. https://doi.org/10.1016/j.cvsm.2017.12.011.

Stahl, S.M. (2013a). Chemical neurotransmission. In: *Stahl's Essential Psychopharmacology*, 4e, 1–27. New York: Cambridge University Press.

Stahl, S.M. (2013b). Transporters, receptors, and enzymes as targets of psychopharmacological drug action. In: *Stahl's Essential Psychopharmacology*, 28–51. New York: Cambridge University Press.

Stillo, T., Norgard, R.J., Stefanovski, D. et al. (2021). The effects of Solliquin administration on the activity and fecal cortisol production of shelter dogs. *Journal of Veterinary Behavior*. Elsevier Inc. https://doi.org/10.1016/j.jveb.2021.05.001.

Zhang, R., Hu, W., Zhong, S. et al. (2025). Impact of *Enterococcus faecium* kimate-X on reducing stress in dogs through gut microbiota modulation. *Veterinary Sciences* 12 (5): 1–15. https://doi.org/10.3390/vetsci12050412.

Zheng, P., Zeng, B., Zhou, C. et al. (2016). Gut microbiome remodeling induces depressive-like behaviors through a pathway mediated by the host's metabolism. *Molecular Psychiatry* 21 (6): 786–796. https://doi.org/10.1038/mp.2016.44.

11

Addressing Specific Behavioral Issues

It is important to acknowledge that not every shelter has the resources, staffing, or specialized expertise to implement a comprehensive behavior modification program for every animal in their care. This reality is not a failure of commitment, it reflects the scope of sustainability (SoS) unique to each organization. Staffing levels, funding, admissions volume, facility design, and access to qualified behavior professionals vary widely and expectations must be aligned with what is realistically achievable. This chapter is written with that understanding at its core.

The guidance presented here is intended primarily for shelters that do have access to behavior teams or trained personnel and are working from problem lists generated through problem-oriented veterinary behavior records (POVBR). As outlined in Chapter 5, POVBRs are a critical foundation for ethical, defensible, and effective behavior intervention. They allow teams to identify priorities, track progress, communicate consistently, and design treatment plans that are proportional to the animal's needs and the organization's capacity.

At the same time, we recognize that many shelters care for pets with behavioral challenges without a dedicated behavior team. While the behavior plans described in this chapter are presented as structured approaches, they are not intended to be all-or-nothing. Even without specialized teams, most organizations can find components that are practical, feasible, and beneficial to use. In some settings, trained volunteers – or volunteers with prior experience – may be able to implement portions of these plans under supervision. In others, small changes in handling, enrichment, and communication can still meaningfully improve welfare. Our hope is that both pets and people benefit, regardless of organizational size or resources.

In the next nine subsections, we address the most common behavior challenges observed in shelter pets and provide focused behavior-modification plans for each. These plans are intentionally concise and practical, designed as clear, step-by-step starting points that teams can implement immediately after admission to the shelter. They are not meant to replace individualized assessment or professional judgment, but rather offer structure, consistency, and direction.

Each plan must be adapted to fit the individual pet, the facility, and the resources available. While the overarching principles remain consistent, specific interventions should ideally be developed and refined. This requires guidance from a qualified behavior team or trainer whenever possible.

Successful implementation relies on the integration of multiple components:

- A detailed care trajectory strategy (CTS) discussed in Chapter 1
- Standardized assessment tools such as the POVBR, Behavior Health Assessment Staging (BHAS), Risk assessment check list, Bite severity classification (BSC) discussed in Chapter 5
- Safe handling and intervention techniques outlined in Chapter 9
- Enrichment strategies presented in Chapter 8

When appropriate, thoughtful use of natural supplements or pharmacological support discussed in Chapter 10

This chapter has one overarching goal: to provide shelters with usable, repeatable frameworks that support safer handling, improved welfare, and better outcomes across a wide range of behavioral conditions while honoring the realities of sustainability, capacity, and compassion that define modern sheltering.

For this approach to be effective, a separate behavior plan should be created for each individual pet. The plan becomes an integral part of the CTS and POVBR and should be reviewed and updated regularly as the pet progresses through care. Equally important, a lack of progress must also be documented. When expected improvement is not observed, the plan should prompt reassessment, modification of interventions, or reconsideration of goals. This structured, iterative process supports consistency, accountability, and clear tracking of each pet's behavioral trajectory over time.

11.1 Behavior Treatment Plan Framework: A Flexible, Multistep Approach

As outlined in **Chapter 5,** behavioral challenges are addressed through a structured **five-step process framework** (Bergman and Gaskins 2013). Behavior treatment plans are not an all-or-nothing process, but a flexible, multistep approach. Much like a puzzle, the more pieces that can be thoughtfully implemented – especially early on – the clearer the picture and the more effective the intervention becomes. Recognizing that shelters vary widely in resources, staffing, and expertise, this framework is designed to be adaptable rather than prescriptive.

Every behavior treatment plan should include the following foundational elements:

- Signalment: Species, breed (or suspected breed), age, sex, and unique identifying features
- Shelter information: Facility name or location, animal ID number, and admissions details
- Admissions date
- Behavior modification program timeline:
  - Start date
  - Planned progress checkpoints
  - Defined endpoints or reevaluation criteria, when applicable
  - Prognosis and Risk assessment documentation if applicable

And it **begins with a clearly defined problem statement:**

- For example: Behavior problem: Jumping on people when greeting and biting the leash when being walked outside

Establishing and adopting this core structure ensures that behavior plans are transparent, measurable and adaptable. This supports both animal wellbeing and informed decision-making within the organization.

These plans are designed to serve as starting points that can be tailored to individual pets, facilities, staffing models, and available resources. Importantly, these approaches have been implemented successfully – using the same stepwise framework – with thousands of owned and shelter pets by the authors, providing strong confidence that the structure of this model is both practical and effective. When a plan is not producing the expected results, this should not be viewed as a failure of the framework. Instead, it signals the need to return to the problem list and reassess whether a key issue has been missed, whether the team is addressing the wrong primary concern, whether the pace of progression exceeds the pet's ability to learn and cope, and whether underlying medical or psychological conditions require different or additional interventions.

Ultimately, regular check-ins, reassessment and plan adjustments are essential components of any successful behavior program. Continuous evaluation ensures that interventions remain aligned with the pet's needs, wellbeing, and capacity for learning and supports more sustainable, humane outcomes in both shelter and home settings. Using the **BHAS**, a structured monitoring system developed by the author as described in Chapter 5 supports objective, consistent decision-making for shelter pets with behavioral concerns.

When describing any bite, shelters should use standardized bite-severity scales. Sophia Yin's Bite Scale and Ian Dunbar's Dog Bite Scale are widely used in clinical and shelter settings. The authors have proposed an alternative approach – the **BSC** – which evaluates the *level of contact* rather than the complexity of the injury. This approach minimizes the need for team members or even volunteers to assess wound depth or tissue damage. This makes the BSC more practical, reliable, and consistent for shelter use. However, regardless of which system is chosen, shelters should adopt one scale and apply it consistently across the organization and all cases. The concepts of the behavior treatment framework was discussed in Chapter 5. Chapter 11 applies this framework to the specific behavioral conditions most commonly encountered in shelter pets. The goal is to provide practical treatment plan examples that support implementation across a wide range of shelter settings. To that end, we have adapted a standardized format for behavior challenges that require both short- and long-term management in the shelter environment, allowing for consistent communication.

11.2 Five Steps of the Behavior Framework

Steps 1–4 of the behavior treatment framework are outlined below and addresses each behavioral condition individually. While Step 5 applies universally across all conditions and focuses on communication and documentation.

11.2.1 Step 5: Communication and Documentation

Clear communication and thorough documentation are essential to ensure continuity, accountability, and ethical decision-making throughout the behavior modification process.

Key components include:

- **Comprehensive treatment notes** have to be recorded in the **POVBR, BHAS, BSC, and Risk assessment** (see Chapter 5). Daily assessment sheets should be reviewed and incorporated into ongoing evaluations to guide timely adjustments to the treatment plan and the CTS.
- **Regularly scheduled rechecks and follow-ups**, ideally on a weekly basis, with frequency adjusted according to how often the pet is being worked with, case complexity and medication use. Pets starting fast-acting medications should be reassessed daily and to monitor early response and adverse effects, whereas long-term or maintenance medications often require weekly or even monthly evaluations to reliably assess therapeutic impact and adjust treatment as needed.

- **Clear, consistent instructions** for team and volunteers to guarantee uniform handling and training approaches.
- **Adopter and foster education**, including written handouts and in-person demonstrations when appropriate.
- **Documentation of adopter or foster consent and understanding**, ensuring transparency and shared expectations for the behavior condition.

This standardized approach supports consistent care across teams, improves tracking of progress, and strengthens outcomes for both pets and caregivers.

11.3 Arousal-Driven Contact Behavior (ADCB) – Dog

11.3.1 Definition

Arousal-Driven Contact Behavior (ADCB) refers to dogs that exhibit overexcited, highly aroused greeting behaviors and attempts to make physical contact with people or the leash. These dogs often display a **Motor–Oral Disinhibition Pattern**, characterized by jumping up on people, grabbing at clothing or objects, and using the mouth during interactions.

Jumping up is a behavior in which the dog's front paws leave the ground during greetings with escalated social interactions. This behavior is not a sign of dominance; it is most commonly a social greeting, an effort to gain attention or an arousal-driven response.

Mouthing describes the use of the mouth to grab or bite hands, clothing, leash, or other objects during play or interaction – especially common in young or adolescent dogs. On the **BSC**, mouthing typically falls within **Level 2–3**, indicating contact without intent to injure, however, with potential for escalation if left unmanaged. In homes, some caregivers may find these types of challenges overwhelming or difficult to manage, which can contribute to relinquishment. Once surrendered, these same challenges often persist and may be exacerbated in the shelter environment.

11.3.2 Explanation of the Condition

These two behaviors often go hand in hand. These common problems become especially challenging in adolescent large breed dogs. Although a normal part of puppy development and social exploration, these behaviors can turn problematic if they are persistent, overly rough or have been reinforced unintentionally.

ADCB can pose safety risks, disrupt appropriate interactions, and reduce adoptability without proper training and consistency. Shelter volunteers and team members often reduce interactions with these dogs due to the handling challenges, which can inadvertently exacerbate the condition. Often these dogs have longer than average length of stay (LOS), especially if the behavior results in more serious bites (BSC > 3). Consequently, these dogs need to be placed under a mandatory bite quarantine. During this time, they cannot be made available to the public, which further delays adoption and can contribute to the worsening of their behavior.

11.3.3 What Can Cause the Condition? – Motivation

- Underlying medical problems are less likely, but an oral exam is recommended to rule out oral pain.
- Greeting ritual, specifically to interact with humans.

- Learned behavior or reinforcement history.
- Environmental or social stressors
- Lack of mental and physical stimulation

11.3.4 Behavior Treatment Plan Framework for the ADCB Dog

11.3.4.1 Management

Strategies prioritize safety, predictability, and stress reduction for dogs, team members, volunteers, and adopters. These include supervision protocols, individualized handling and guided walk plans, environmental adjustments, avoidance and redirection strategies, and routine-based care. Effective management reduces rehearsal of unwanted behaviors and creates the conditions necessary for learning and emotional regulation.

- Safety measures:
  - Supervision (one handler and ideally one helper to assist moving dog through the shelter)
  - Multiple short visits —two to three per day (documentation in exposure log outside the room)
  - Design a safe individualized walk and handling plan
  - Shelter setup adjustments; use visual and physical barriers
- Avoidance strategies:
  - In-kennel interactions with barriers
  - Redirection to keep all four paws on the ground
  - Redirection away from handler
- Environmental modifications:
  - Create calming environment
  - Change location of housing
  - Increased in-kennel enrichment
  - Routine for feeding, walking, and play

11.3.4.2 Behavior Modification Steps

Behavior modification focuses on teaching alternative behaviors and reshaping emotional responses through evidence-based methods such as counterconditioning, desensitization, and positive reinforcement. Plans emphasize step-by-step progression, threshold management, and the avoidance of punitive techniques, which can increase fear, anxiety, and aggression.

- Threshold management
  - Calm greetings when coming and leaving
  - Multiple short in-kennel visits, always end on a calm note
- Positive reinforcement of alternative behaviors and substitute emotional response
  - Sit for all greeting
  - Pick up a ball or toy for greetings
- Teach basic foundational skills
  - Sit, down, stand, stay, go to mat, stand on mat, four paws on the ground, loose leash walking
- Focus cues
  - Look, touch a target, find it, get your toy
- Counterconditioning and desensitization
  - Step-by-step behavior shaping plans
- Modification of the behavior
  - Remove attention for unwanted behaviors (negative punishment)

Turn away until the pet is calm, and then reward (positive reinforcement)
In some cases, handler has to walk away or leave the enclosure

- Do not physically or verbally punish the behavior (can lead to increase in anxiety or even aggression)
- Leave a leash on the dog and step on the leash so the dog cannot jump higher than a few inches of the ground with the front feet (negative reinforcement); as soon as the front feet touch the ground reward with attention, food, and or toys (positive reinforcement) (for learning see Chapter 9)

11.3.4.3 Training Aids and Tools

Practical tools that support implementation of both the management and behavior modification strategies – including food rewards, toys, enrichment devices, handling equipment, visual barriers, and calming aids. Selection of tools should be humane and individualized to the dog, the specific behavior concern and the shelter environment.

Examples include treats, toys, clickers, long lines, double leashes, target sticks, exposure logs, calming wraps or caps (e.g. ThunderShirt®, ThunderCap®), pheromones, supplements, head halters, harnesses, mats, crates, basket muzzles, visual and physical barriers, feed-dispensing toys, and interactive toys.

11.3.4.4 Pharmacological and Supplemental Support

Pharmacologic support is not required in most cases of dogs with **ADCB** and should never replace management or training. In some cases, medications or supplements may be appropriate as adjuncts to behavior modification, particularly when fear, anxiety, pain, or underlying medical factors contribute to the behavior. When used, considerations include short- vs. long-term use, appropriate dosing, monitoring for side effects and coordination with foster or adoption transitions, including pre-adoption weaning, or post-adoption support when indicated. Medication selection and implementation should follow the guidance outlined in Chapter 10, with treatment plans individualized to the animal's emotional state, medical status and the shelter's capacity for monitoring and follow-up.

Prior to initiating a natural supplement or psychoactive medication in a shelter animal, establish a baseline behavior score. This score should be assigned on a 1–10 scale, with 10 representing the highest level of agitation or most severe response to identified trigger(s). Once the natural supplement or medication has been initiated, assign a behavior score at each subsequent evaluation. These follow-up scores constitute the medication response score and allow for objective monitoring of treatment efficacy over time. An effective intervention should result in a medication response score that is lower than the established baseline. If follow-up scores do not demonstrate meaningful improvement relative to baseline, the treatment plan – including dosing, medication selection, adjunct therapies, or environmental modifications – should be reassessed and adjusted accordingly.

For ADCB dogs: start with serotonin antagonist reuptake inhibitors (SARIs) or α_2-agonists. Consider selective serotonin reuptake inhibitors (SSRIs) if anticipated longer LOS.

Key Considerations Include

- **Short-term vs. long-term use** should be considered early in the CTS.
  - Short-term medications may be appropriate for immediate relief and stress reduction.

Dogs with an anticipated LOS < 30 days – start on short-term medications, such as SARIs or α_2-agonists

- Long-term medications require planning around expected LOS, time to therapeutic effect and post-adoption needs.
- Key questions include whether the pet is likely to remain in the shelter long enough for long-term medications to take effect (often four to six weeks), whether ongoing medication will be needed in a home setting or whether the pet may instead benefit from expedited adoption or foster placement. Addressing these questions early supports appropriate medication selection and improves continuity of care.
- Appropriate dosing and titration
  - Start with one medication and evaluate response.
  - Short term medications

Evaluate the shelter pet's response after two and seven days.

- Monitoring and side-effect tracking
- Provide the medication response score.
  - Record the Baseline Wellbeing (see Chapter 7) and Behavior score prior to starting on the natural supplement or medication.
  - Track the Daily Wellbeing and Medication response score once the pet has been started on medication.
- There should be at minimum a weekly reevaluation. If there is no improvement, then medication and treatment plan needs to be adjusted.
- If there is no change after the second week, then the CTS for the shelter pet needs to be revisited and modified.
  - Coordination with adoption or foster transitions, including pre-adoption weaning plans or post-adoption continuation and support.

11.3.5 Communication and Documentation

Education for adopter or foster to ensure transparency and continued training support utilizing handouts, training videos, and in-person demonstration.

11.4 Barking and/or Pulling Behavior – Dog

11.4.1 Definition

Pulling on leash is a common problem behavior in which a dog creates sustained tension on the leash, often moving ahead of the handler during walks. This behavior is not a sign of dominance; rather, it typically reflects a lack of training in loose-leash walking or difficulty regulating arousal in stimulating environments. When the dog is large or physically strong, pulling can pose a significant safety risk to handlers.

Leash pulling accompanied by barking at other dogs, people, vehicles, or environmental stimuli is one of the most commonly reported behavior challenges – both in private homes and in shelter settings. These behaviors often intensify in shelters, where dogs arrive from a wide range of backgrounds and are suddenly placed into compact, high-stimulus environments. In such settings, exposure to triggers is frequent, unpredictable, and difficult to avoid, making such challenges more likely to emerge or escalate.

Barking and other vocalizations are normal canine communication behaviors, with motivation varying by context and individual dog. Vocalization becomes a problem when it is excessive, persistent, or occurs outside of an appropriate context, particularly when it interferes with handling, housing, or public interactions.

These behaviors may or may not be signs of "aggression." They could be driven by:

- **Overstimulation** from the busy shelter setting.
- **Frustration** due to barrier restrictions and limited outlets for energy.
- **General arousal or excitability** as the dog adapts to a new, unpredictable environment.
- **Fear-based,** where the dog attempts to create distance from perceived threats.

Understanding the underlying motivation helps teams and volunteers respond appropriately with management. Controlled exposure, enrichment, and leash training rather than interpreting the behavior as aggression or hopelessness will help prevent escalation.

Owners find these behaviors often overwhelming or difficult to manage. This can ultimately lead to relinquishment, placing the animal (back) in a shelter setting where existing challenges frequently continue or even intensify.

11.4.2 Explanation of the Condition

Pulling and barking behaviors are common in dogs of all ages, sexes, and breeds. When they occur together, they can create challenging and potentially unsafe situations. Pulling may stem from excitement, distraction, or a strong motivation to explore the environment. Barking may be driven by excitement, attention-seeking, boredom, fear, territorial responses, or reactivity to environmental stimuli. When barking occurs alongside pulling *away* from triggers, it may indicate fear or anxiety.

Dogs that pull and bark intensely and fail to recover even after the stimulus has passed, often exhibit dysregulated interaction patterns. These dogs react to their environment with escalating, poorly controlled behaviors and struggle to modulate arousal, making it difficult for them to return to a calmer emotional state without support. These dogs are frequently non-responsive to handlers, cues, or treats in the moment because their emotional arousal overrides their ability to process information or engage in learned behaviors.

Without consistent training and appropriate management, combined pulling and barking behaviors can pose safety risks, disrupt safe handling and social interactions, and reduce adoptability. As a result, shelter teams and volunteers may limit outings due to handling concerns, leading to increased confinement. Prolonged confinement can contribute to the development or worsening of additional behavioral challenges and is often associated with extended LOS for these dogs.

11.4.3 What Can Cause the Condition? – Motivation

- Underlying medical problems are less likely.
- Excitement, desire to explore, or reach someone or something.
- Rule out fear related behavior problems.
- Learned behavior or reinforcement history.
- Environmental or social stressors.

11.4.4 Behavior Treatment Plan Framework

Management strategies focused on predictability, and reducing exposure to triggers that cause the barking. This is achieved through supervision, environmental adjustments, structured routines, and avoidance of high-risk situations.

- Safety measures:
  - Supervision (one handler and ideally one helper to assist moving dog through the shelter)
  - Multiple short, calm walks —two to three per day (documentation in trigger log outside the room).
  - Shelter setup adjustments; avoid blind corners.
  - Use well-fitted humane no-pull equipment (Harness or head halters) and no longer than 6 ft leashes.
  - If a dog is particularly reactive, it can be helpful to use a clear external signal - such as a vest or marker worn by the dog or handler - to alert others to maintain appropriate distance and avoid triggering situations.
- Avoidance strategies:
  - Walks in low traffic environments and during low traffic times (early morning/late at night).
  - Transporting the dog for walks outside the shelter environment to a quiet area.
  - Redirection to carrying a toy and/or focus on the handler instead of the surroundings.
- Environmental modifications:
  - Create a calming walking environment.
  - Set routine times and protocols for all interactions including feeding and walking.
  - Be the first dog (and not last dog) to the dog play area, etc.

Behavior Modification Steps that emphasize counterconditioning, desensitization, and reinforcement of quiet behaviors, while avoiding punitive techniques that may increase fear, anxiety, or aggression.

- Threshold management
  - Calmly arrival at destinations, when approaching people, dogs; when coming and leaving to the dog park area for example.
  - Multiple short calm walks.
- Positive reinforcement of alternative behaviors and substitute emotional response
  - "*Red light – Green light*" exercises – (Green: walk when not pulling; Red: Stop or turn when pulling).
  - Reward loose leash walking consistently (don't take for granted).
  - Carry a toy or ball – may limit barking.
  - Walk slow and calm toward the dog play area, be the first one to arrive, turn when pulling or barking, perform sit, and look at the handler before turning loose in the park, sit before leashing and leaving the park
- Teach basic foundational skills
  - Heel, sit, down, stand, and stay.
  - Teach to carry a ball or toy.
- Focus cues
  - Look, touch a target stick or hand, find it (focus on the ground in front of the handler and slow down the walk).

- Counterconditioning and desensitization
  - Step-by-step behavior shaping plans.
- Modification of the behavior
  - When the dog pulls and or barks, turn in the opposite direction of where the dog wants to go.
  - Do not physically or verbally punish the behavior (can lead to increase in anxiety or even aggression).

Training aids and tools to support dogs that pull and bark should be selected to promote humane handling, effective learning, and stress reduction for both the animal and the handler. These tools may also include enrichment strategies and environmental supports, such as noise-canceling or sound-dampening devices, to help reduce overstimulation.

Examples include head halters, front-clip or double-buckle harnesses, indicator vests for dogs and/or handlers, mirrors placed in blind corners within the shelter, treadmills or swimming for controlled physical outlets, nosework exercises and scent-based enrichment resources, treats or special diets, treat pouches, toys, clickers, target sticks, calming wraps or caps (e.g. ThunderShirt®, ThunderCap®), pheromones, supplements, basket muzzles, and visual or physical barriers.

11.4.4.1 Pharmacological and Supplemental Support

In general, dogs that exhibit pulling and barking behaviors do not require psychoactive medication. Pharmacological and supplemental considerations should be used judiciously and only when clinically indicated, as adjuncts to behavior modification, not as replacements for training or management. However, some cases may be more challenging, particularly when triggers cannot be reliably avoided in the shelter environment or when fear or anxiety significantly contributes to the behavior.

Antianxiety medications, analgesics, or supplements may be considered when anxiety-related behaviors are present and interfere with learning or welfare. Key considerations include short- vs. long-term use, appropriate dosing and monitoring for side effects. This has to be assessed in coordination with adoption or foster transitions, including pre-adoption weaning or post-adoption support when appropriate.

Key Considerations Include

- **Short-term vs. long-term use** should be considered early in the treatment trajectory.
  - Short-term medications may be appropriate for immediate relief and stress reduction.

Dogs with an anticipated LOS < 30 days – start on short-term medications, such as SARIs or α_2-agonists

- Long-term medications require planning around expected LOS, time to therapeutic effect, and post-adoption needs.
- Key questions include whether the dog is likely to remain in the shelter long enough for long-term medications to take effect (often four to six weeks), whether ongoing medication will be needed in a home setting, and whether the pet may instead benefit from expedited adoption or foster placement. Addressing these questions early supports appropriate medication selection and improves continuity of care.
- Appropriate dosing and titration
  - Start with one medication and evaluate response.
  - Short-term medications

Evaluate the shelter dog's response after two and seven days.

- Monitoring and side-effect tracking
- Provide the medication response score.
  - Record the Baseline Wellbeing (see Chapter 7) and Behavior score prior to starting on the medication.
  - Track the Daily Wellbeing and Medication response score once the pet has been started on medication.
- There should be at minimum a weekly reevaluation. If there is no improvement, then medication and treatment plan needs to be adjusted.
- If there is no change after the second week, then the CTS for the shelter pet should be revised.
  - Coordination with adoption or foster transitions, including pre-adoption weaning plans or post-adoption continuation and support.

When indicated, clinicians should refer to **Chapter 10**.

For dogs that display persistent barking and/or pulling related to heightened arousal, reactivity, or dysregulated interaction patterns, pharmacologic support may be helpful. Consider the use of short acting medications: SARIs, α_2-agonists, and calcium-channel modulators. *Gabapentin* is a calcium-channel modulator and can also be used situationally for short-term calming in select cases. Start on SSRIs or serotonin norepinephrine reuptake inhibitors (SNRIs) if the pet will have a longer anticipated LOS.

In some situations, low-dose acepromazine may be considered as a short-term adjunct, with careful monitoring of individual response. Regardless of the medication chosen, decisions should prioritize the animal's welfare, safety, and ability to participate meaningfully in behavior modification sessions.

11.4.5 Communication and Documentation

Education for adopter or foster to ensure transparency and continued training support utilizing handouts, training videos, and in-person demonstration.

11.5 Environmental Sensitivity and Fear-Related Behavior – Dog and Cat

11.5.1 Definition

Fear-related behavior in dogs and cats refers to a set of physiological and behavioral responses triggered by a real or perceived threat. These responses are survival-based and may manifest as flight, fight, freeze, or fidget behaviors. Common fear-related body language includes cowering, trembling, backing away, tail tucking, ears held down or back, avoidance, freezing, or attempts to escape.

When fear is persistent or intense, it can significantly interfere with an animal's overall welfare. Highly fearful animals may be difficult to handle safely and often require timely, targeted intervention to prevent further deterioration in emotional state or wellbeing.

Fear-related behaviors are very common in shelter environments for both dogs and cats. Fear is a normal and adaptive response to unfamiliar or potentially threatening stimuli and animals entering shelters are abruptly confronted with new people, other animals, loud noises, confinement, and unpredictable routines. This sudden exposure can heighten fear responses, especially in pets already struggling with stress, uncertainty, or limited coping skills.

Several factors influence how pets respond to this transition:

- Animals arrive from diverse backgrounds and fear responses vary based on temperament, prior experiences, and individual coping strategies.
- For some animals, fear diminishes over time as they habituate and begin to feel safer after several days.
- For others, fear may escalate into anxiety, resulting in sustained distress, handling challenges, or reduced adoptability.

Importantly, fear in shelter pets should not automatically be interpreted as abnormal or permanent. In most cases, it reflects the stress of a major life transition. Providing predictability, patience, gentle handling, and environmental support is critical to helping animals regain a sense of safety and security. In some situations, foster placement or expedited pathways to adoption may be appropriate strategies to reduce stress and support recovery.

11.5.2 Explanation of the Condition

Fear is a normal emotional response and is essential to survival. Therefore, it can be observed in both species (canines and felines), as well as in all breeds, at any ages and both sexes. Fear behaviors are often influenced by lack of socialization, past negative experiences, or trauma or genetic factors and are heavily context-dependent. It's possible for a dog or cat to get scared when they encounter an otherwise benign situation (a person, dog, sound, object, or place), which then triggers significant distress, panic, or anxiety. In instances where a pet is unable to calm quickly or becomes fearful in anticipation, anxiety develops, resulting in a decrease in wellbeing. It is therefore important to treat fear and anxiety in dogs and cats proactively. Whether an animal escalates to exhibiting defensive aggression, depends on many factors, including temperament.

Fear is a very common condition in shelter pets, leading to moderate-to-severe behavior problems including anxiety or even aggression. Without proper management and behavior modification, fear can pose safety risks, disrupt appropriate interactions, and reduce adoptability. As a result, shelter volunteers and teams may not want to spend time with these animals. Consequently, other medical or behavioral problems may arise putting these pets at risk for longer than average LOS.

11.5.3 What Can Cause the Condition? – Motivation

- Underlying medical problems can be a reason or consequence of the behaviors and need to be ruled out first. Pain, disease, and injury can mimic fear or make fear worse.
- Lack of socialization and positive early exposure.
- Traumatic experience and changes in routine and environment.
- Pets from hoarding situations.
- Pets born in a free-roaming population.
- Genetics and temperament.
- Environmental or social stressors.

11.5.4 Behavior Treatment Plan Framework

11.5.4.1 Management

See Table 11.1.

Table 11.1 Management Categories for Fearful Dog or Cat in the Shelter

Category	Dogs	Cats
Calm Interaction	Calm in-kennel interactions Sitting quietly or reading aloud	Quiet presence Sitting nearby without direct interaction
Visit Structure	Multiple short, quiet visits 2–3× daily (document in trigger log)	Same: short, predictable visits with minimal disruption
Handling Approach	Closely observe fear body language; avoid sudden reaching or looming over	Do not reach for fearful cats Allow approach on the cat's terms
Movement and Transport	Use well-fitted, humane equipment Crates for transport	Use carriers or covered transfer methods
Distance and Signage	Fear or "Do Not Pet/In Training" vests to create distance	Clear signage at housing to cue "go slow"
Housing	Single housing if fearful of other animals Quiet areas or foster	Single housing if needed Quiet placement preferred
Social Considerations	Social dogs may benefit from calm group housing (social facilitation)	Selective group housing only if the cat is clearly social
Avoidance	Walk during low-traffic times/areas (early morning or late night)	Use wand toys Let the cat initiate interaction
Environment	Predictable routines Quiet spaces	Predictable routines Quiet, low-traffic housing
Enrichment and Support	Prioritize enrichment to support coping	Prioritize enrichment Ensure access to hide
Resources	Crates and areas to hide	Litter box and food accessible while remaining hidden
Adjuncts	Species-specific pheromones	Species-specific pheromones
Trajectory Strategy	Prioritize for foster or adoption when appropriate	Prioritize for foster or adoption when appropriate

11.5.4.2 Behavior Modification Steps

Threshold management prioritizes preventing the shelter pet from being overwhelmed by reducing exposure to fear-eliciting stimuli until the pet is emotionally able to learn and cope safely (see Table 11.2).

- Substitute emotional response
  - Relaxation behaviors are desirable.
  - Improve coping strategies by rewarding calm behaviors consistently.
- Positive reinforcement of alternative behaviors can be applied to dogs and cats
  - Clicker training, if not afraid of noise, otherwise a calm marker tone or word can be used.
  - Teach desirable behaviors in the absence or safe distance of a fear trigger(s).
- No punishment for fear behavior
  - Do not physically or verbally punish the behavior (can lead to increase in anxiety or even aggression).
- Teach relaxation behaviors
  - Down, mat exercises, go to mat (or cat tree), head down.

Table 11.2 Dog–Cat Behavior Modification

Category	Dogs	Cats
General Principles	Do not force social interactions Respect thresholds	Do not force interaction Allow choice and control
Timing of Training	Delay counterconditioning and desensitization until anti-anxiety medications or supplements (if used) have taken effect	Same principle applies
Fear of People	Limit handling to a small number of familiar people Instruct others to ignore the dog initially Avoid approaching, touching, or staring Walk during low-traffic times and in quiet areas Foster/adoptive homes may need to limit visitors temporarily or provide a safe retreat	Limit handling to a few familiar caregivers Avoid reaching or forced interaction Allow the cat to initiate contact Ensure access to hiding places away from people
Fear of Dogs	Avoid dog parks, playgroups, and daycare Prevent close approaches from other dogs Reduce exposure to specific trigger dogs Walk during low-traffic times in low-traffic areas	Not applicable
Fear of Cats	Not applicable	Provide quiet housing Single-cat housing when needed Avoid visual contact with other cats Use visual barriers between enclosures
Sound Sensitivity	House in the quietest possible area Add white noise, fans, or calming music Use sound-dampening strategies when available	Same strategies apply
Object or Place Fear	Avoid known triggers when possible If unavoidable, reduce exposure by covering objects, rerouting paths, or relocating the dog to a quieter area or foster home	Same strategies apply

- Teach basic foundational skills
  - Sit, stand, stay – dogs.
  - Go to mat – cats.
  - Teach to find a ball or toy – dogs and cats.
- Focus cues
  - Look, touch a target stick or hand, look at that in a relaxed manner, find it (focus on something positive).
- Counterconditioning and desensitization
  - Step-by-step behavior shaping plans.

(See Table 11.3.)

11.5.4.3 Pharmacological and Supplemental Support

Pharmacological and supplemental support is often indicated for overly fearful animals that do not habituate to the shelter environment or for pets that develop anxiety. The latter show signs of fear

Table 11.3 Training Aids and Tools for Fearful Dogs and Cats

Category	Dogs	Cats
Handling and Movement	Head halters, front-clip or double-buckle harnesses, long lines	Harnesses (when appropriate), carriers
Identification and Communication	Indicator vests (e.g. *"I am fearful," "In training," "Do not approach"*)	Labeled rooms or signage indicating fearful cats / go slow
Food and Reinforcement	Treats or special diets, treat pouches	Treats or special diets, treat pouches
Training Tools	Toys, clickers, target sticks	Toys, clickers, target sticks
Enrichment and Activity	Nosework resources, treadmills, controlled swimming	Interactive toys, vertical exploration (cat trees)
Calming and Emotional Support	Calming aids (e.g. ThunderShirt®, ThunderCap®), pheromones, supplements	Pheromones, supplements
Sensory Management	Noise-reducing devices, relaxation music	Noise-reducing devices, relaxation music
Environmental Control	Visual and physical barriers	Visual and physical barriers
Safety and Retreat	Crates, designated hiding or rest areas	Hiding places, cat trees, covered beds, crates
Housing and Space Use	Quiet areas, predictable pathways	Quiet rooms, single-cat housing when needed

responses that intensify over time, remain constant or become overwhelming, and interfere with daily functioning. For these pets, fear is no longer an adaptive response, but a welfare concern that impairs learning, handling, and quality of life.

Antianxiety medications, analgesics, and/or supplements may be necessary to reduce fear, lower emotional arousal, and allow the animal to engage meaningfully in behavior modification. Ideally, pharmacological interventions should be used as adjuncts – not replacements – for management and training strategies. However, in many shelter environments, environmental stressors cannot be fully controlled and even with optimal handling and enrichment, some animals struggle to cope. In these cases, psychoactive medications – most commonly anxiolytics – may play a critical role in reducing distress and improving wellbeing and, therefore, enabling the pet to better tolerate daily care and participate in behavior modification.

Key Considerations Include

- **Short-term vs. long-term use** should be considered early in the treatment trajectory.
  - Short-term medications may be appropriate for immediate relief and stress reduction.

Dogs with an anticipated LOS < 30 days – start on short-term medications, such as SARIs, odiazepines or α_2-agonists. For cats, consider the use of nutraceuticals and pheromones.

- Long-term medications require planning around expected LOS, time to therapeutic effect and post-adoption needs.
- Key questions include the following: if the animal is likely to remain in the shelter long enough for long-term medications to take effect (often four to six weeks), will ongoing medication be

needed in a home setting or may the animal benefit instead from expedited adoption or foster placement. Addressing these questions early supports appropriate medication selection and improves continuity of care.

- Appropriate dosing and titration
  - Start with one medication and evaluate response.
  - Short-term medications.

Evaluate the shelter pet's response after two and seven days.

- Monitoring and side-effect tracking.
- Provide the medication response score.
  - Record the Baseline Wellbeing (see Chapter 7) and Behavior score prior to starting on the medication.
  - Track the Daily Wellbeing and Medication response score once the pet has been started on medication.
- There should be at minimum a weekly reevaluation. If there is no improvement, then medication and treatment plan needs to be adjusted.
- If there is no change after the second week, then the CTS for the shelter pet should be revised.
  - Coordination with adoption or foster transitions, including pre-adoption weaning plans or post-adoption continuation and support.

For pets with fear and/or anxiety, consider the most commonly used anxiolytic classes: SARIs, calcium-channel modulator (delta ligands), and benzodiazepines. Consider SSRIs, tricyclic antidepressants (TCAs), or SNRIs if you anticipate the pet will have a longer LOS. Medication selection should be guided by the specific presentation, safety considerations, medical history, and the animal's ability to participate in behavior-modification work.

11.5.5 Communication and Documentation

Education for adopter or foster to ensure transparency and continued training support utilizing handouts, training videos, and in-person demonstration.

11.6 Overstimulation – Dog and Cat

11.6.1 Definition

Overstimulation refers to a state in which an animal reacts *disproportionately* or *excessively* to levels of sensory or social input that most animals would tolerate or recover from easily. In other words, the stimulus itself is normal, but the pet's response is amplified, rapid, or even dysregulated.

Feline: This type of problem behavior refers to a state in which a cat becomes overly agitated or aroused. This can happen during petting or play, leading to sudden behavioral changes such as hissing, biting, swatting, tail lashing, or escape attempts. This response typically occurs in otherwise friendly cats when physical interactions exceed the cat's tolerance threshold.

Canine: This behavior indicates a state of heightened stimulation triggered by excessive excitement, sensory input, or prolonged activity. This behavior challenge often leads to additional behavior concerns such as jumping, biting, barking, pulling, spinning, and uncontrolled urination or difficulties settling.

It is important to recognize these behaviors as stress responses influenced by early experiences, personality, and current environment. It is critical to understand when the threshold for overstimulation is reached by identifying early warning signs including pupillary dilation, tail flicking, skin twitching, ears flattening, and sudden tension. Stopping interaction before escalation is crucial and helps keep both the pet and handler safe. If unmanaged, these behaviors can escalate, making the pet harder to handle and potentially reducing adoption chances. With appropriate management, careful monitoring during handling, and deliberate teaching of calm, predictable interactions, pets can be well-supported during their shelter stay and set up for long-term success.

11.6.2 Explanation of the Condition

11.6.2.1 Overstimulation in Cats

Overstimulation is a common and complex behavior challenge in shelter cats. It most frequently occurs during human interaction – especially petting – and can be confusing to handlers. A cat may initially solicit attention, rubbing, or leaning into touch, but once their tolerance threshold is exceeded, behavior can rapidly escalate to swatting, scratching, or biting. This pattern is correctly termed petting-induced aggression.

Overstimulation in cats may also present as overgrooming, sometimes leading to hair loss or skin irritation. These behaviors are often linked to underlying anxiety, temperament, or deficits in coping strategies, though medical issues such as pain can lower a cat's ability to tolerate normal interactions.

This behavior can occur in cats of any age, sex, or breed, though some breeds or individuals may naturally have lower thresholds for tactile stimulation. Common triggers include:

- Brushing or grooming.
- Prolonged or repetitive petting.
- Touching sensitive body regions.
- Inconsistent handling from multiple caregivers.

Recognizing early warning signs is essential to prevent escalation. These may include:

- Twitching or rippling skin.
- Dilated pupils.
- Ears shifting down or backward.
- Tail twitching.
- Sudden restlessness or tenseness.

Understanding and respecting a cat's thresholds supports safer handling, reduces stress, and helps maintain adoptability.

11.6.2.2 Overstimulation in Dogs

Overstimulation is also a common issue in dogs, particularly within the high-arousal, unpredictable shelter environment. Overstimulation is more likely in young or high-energy dogs, regardless of breed or sex. It may be exacerbated by excessive handling or exaggerated physical interactions, such as petting instead of stroking. Often due to limited opportunities for exercise, enrichment, and rest. Dogs may become overstimulated during:

- Play
- Social interactions; loud or high-pitched voices, exaggerated petting
- Training sessions, physical corrections
- Exposure to busy or noisy environments

Overstimulation often lowers the threshold for a range of problem behaviors, including:

- Barking
- Jumping
- Biting
- Fearful outbursts in certain situations

Overstimulation itself is not a disorder, but if unaddressed, it can interfere with learning, self-regulation, and impulse control, all of which are critical for a dog's success in both shelter and home settings. Dogs unable to settle or rest appropriately are at risk of escalating to more serious concerns such as anxiety or arousal (see Sections 11.3 and 11.4).

Supporting dogs through structured exercise, predictable routines, calm interactions, and appropriate enrichment helps reduce overstimulation and improves both welfare and adoptability.

11.6.3 What Can Cause the Condition? – Motivation

- Medical rule-outs
  - Cats: hyperthyroidism and hypersensitivities (e.g. flea allergy dermatitis)
  - Dogs: hypersensitivities (e.g. food hypersensitivities and flea allergy dermatitis)
  - Both species: consider other skin diseases, pain-related neurological conditions
- Emotional motivations: lack of mental and physical stimulation, fear, anxiety, and frustration
- Learned behavior or reinforcement history
- Environmental or social stressors

11.6.4 Behavior Treatment Plan Framework

11.6.4.1 Management

11.6.4.1.1 For Dogs

Overstimulation often presents as high-arousal behaviors – jumping, biting, barking, etc. – and worsens in shelter environments with inadequate outlets. Early intervention, structured exercise, and calm, predictable interactions are essential.

11.6.4.1.2 For Cats

Overstimulation is frequently tactile and can rapidly escalate, if early warning signs are missed. Respecting thresholds, minimizing touch, prioritizing predictable routines, and hiding opportunities protect both wellbeing and safety.

Recognizing early warning signs is critical in this condition, as overstimulation can escalate quickly and compromise both animal wellbeing and handler safety (see Table 11.4).

Below is a side-by-side management table for overstimulation in dogs and cats, organized under Safety Measures, Avoidance Strategies and Environmental Modifications (see Tables 11.5–11.7).

Table 11.4 Body Language Escalation Warning Signals

Dogs	Cats
Increasing vocalization (barking, whining)	Skin twitching/rippling
Heightened arousal: jumping, spinning, pacing	Tail flicking or lashing
Dilated pupils, stiffening, freezing for a moment	Ears flattening or rotating backward
Grabbing clothing, biting (BSC level 2–3)	Sudden tension or body stillness
Low growl or sudden shift from playful to frantic	Dilated pupils, rapid head turning
Difficulty settling, inability to rest	Swatting, biting, "lightning-fast" grab
	Overgrooming or licking when stressed

Table 11.5 Management and Handling Safety Tips Side-by-Side Dog/Cat Summary

A. Safety Measures

Dogs	Cats
Provide a controlled, safely confined area for interactions	Limit or avoid physical interactions such as petting until thresholds are known
Use short, calm sessions to prevent escalation	Always provide accessible hiding spaces (boxes, covered beds)
Use leashes, gates, or crates to maintain safe distance when needed	Monitor subtle changes in body language closely
Prioritize early foster placement for overly stimulated dogs if applicable	Single housing may reduce arousal from visual or social stressors
Handling Tips (Dogs):	**Handling Tips (Cats):**
Keep movements slow and predictable	Allow the cat to initiate all contact
Reward calm behavior frequently	Avoid restraining or picking up fearful/overstimulated cats
Avoid wrestling-style play, frequent or rough petting	Use hands-off engagement (wand toys, brushes, and reading aloud)
If arousal spikes, pause and allow a cooldown period	Stroke only briefly and stop before the body language escalates

11.6.4.2 Behavior Modification Steps

- Threshold management
  - Reduce or limit physical interactions
  - Use tools (pompom or brushes) rather than hands
  - Calm voices (no high-pitched voices)
  - Multiple short visits
- Substitute emotional response
  - Relaxation behaviors are desirable
  - Improve settling and calming strategies

Table 11.6 Avoidance Strategies Safety Tips Side-by-Side Dog/Cat Summary

Dogs	Cats
Limit exposure to known triggers (high-energy play and chaotic rooms) Avoid high-traffic or noisy areas whenever possible Keep interactions brief, calm, and predictable Replace high-arousal play with structured, low-intensity activities (sniff walks and treat scatter games)	Avoid touching sensitive body areas (belly, tail base, and overstimulated zones) Avoid or limit fast or repetitive touching – which tends to trigger escalation Maintain predictable routines and low-stimulation visits Allow cats to fully disengage when they choose
Handling Tips (Dogs): If arousal increases, calmly redirect to a familiar cue ("sit" and "find it") Stop interactions before arousal peaks Use distance and time-outs – never physical or verbal punishment	**Handling Tips (Cats):** Use enrichment (food toys and scent items) to redirect energy Do not touch cats showing early warning signs Let cats rest uninterrupted when overstimulated Use distance and time-outs – never physical or verbal punishment

Table 11.7 Environmental Modifications Tips Side-by-Side Dog/Cat Summary

Dogs	Cats
Move to a quieter wing or low-stimulation housing area Use visual barriers to block view of other dogs Create predictable routines alternating calm time and controlled exercise Prioritize daily enrichment (sniffing, puzzle feeders, and decompression walks)	Relocate to quieter rooms or cat-only areas Use curtains or barriers to block visual access to other cats/people Maintain a predictable routine for feeding, cleaning, and interaction Provide species-appropriate enrichment (vertical space, hiding spots, and puzzle feeders)
Handling Tips (Dogs): Provide scheduled rest periods in a quiet room Use calming music or white noise to dampen sound triggers	**Handling Tips (Cats):** Offer multiple resting options and high perches Keep lighting soft and avoid sudden movements or noise Use pheromone diffusers (Feliway) to support calm behavior

- Teach relaxation behaviors
  - Placement exercises: dog: go to mat; cat: go to cat tree or crate
  - Sit, lie down, roll over
  - Teach to chase, find or hold a toy
- Focus cues
  - Look, touch a target stick or hand, find it (focus on something positive)
- Modification of the behavior
  - Time outs for escalating behaviors
  - Do not physically or verbally punish the pet (can lead to increase in anxiety or even aggression)
- Counterconditioning and desensitization
  - Step-by-step behavior shaping plans toward calm behavior

11.6.4.3 Training Aids and Tools

Head halters, front or double buckle harness, treadmill, swimming, nosework exercises and resources, indicator vests for dog and or handlers, treats or special diet, treat pouches, toys, clicker, brushes, pompom, target stick, calming aids (e.g. ThunderShirt®, ThunderCap®, pheromones, and supplements), basket muzzles, visual and physical barriers, brushes, wand toys, interactive cat toys, food dispensing toys, hiding boxes, cat trees, etc. (see Table 11.8).

11.6.4.4 Pharmacological and Supplemental Support

For pets exhibiting overstimulation, underlying medical conditions should be ruled out before initiating psychoactive medication. Antianxiety medications, analgesics, or supplements may or may not be indicated but should be considered when conditions are dysregulated, medical contributors, and/or true anxiety disorders can be identified. Key considerations include short- vs. long-term use, appropriate dosing, monitoring and side-effect tracking, and coordination with adoption or foster transitions, including pre-adoption weaning or post-adoption support when appropriate.

Key Considerations Include

- **Short-term vs. long-term use** should be considered early in the CTS.
  - Short-term medications may be appropriate for immediate relief and stress reduction.

Dogs with an anticipated LOS < 30 days – start on short-term medications, such as SARIs or α_2-agonists. For cats, consider the use of nutraceuticals and pheromones.

Most pets will initially start on a short-term (situational) medication, especially during early assessment or when immediate safety and welfare needs must be addressed.

- Long-term medications (e.g. SSRIs, TCAs, and SNRIs) require planning around expected LOS, time to therapeutic effect, and post-adoption needs.

Table 11.8 Training Aids and Tools for Dogs and Cats with Overstimulation Behavior

Category	Dogs	Cats
Handling and Movement	Head halters, front-clip or double-buckle harnesses, long lines	Wand toys, Pom–Pom, Carriers
Food and Reinforcement	Treats or special diets, treat pouches	Treats or special diets, treat pouches
Training Tools	Toys, clickers, target sticks	Toys, clickers, target sticks
Enrichment and Activity	Nosework resources, treadmills, controlled swimming	Interactive toys, vertical exploration (cat trees)
Calming and Emotional Support	Calming aids (e.g. ThunderShirt®), pheromones, supplements	Pheromones, supplements
Sensory Management	Relaxation music ThunderCap®, Doggles® or RexSpecs® to limit vision Happy Hoodie®, Mutt Muffs®, RexSpecs Ear Pro®	Relaxation music, soft brushes

These medications help stabilize underlying anxiety or emotional dysregulation, improving wellbeing, and supporting progress over time.

- Key questions include whether the animal is likely to remain in the shelter long enough for long-term medications to take effect (often four to six weeks), whether ongoing medication will be needed in a home setting, and whether the animal may instead benefit from expedited adoption or foster placement. Addressing these questions early supports appropriate medication selection and improves continuity of care.
- Appropriate dosing and titration
  - Start with one medication and evaluate response before considering any additions.

Begin with a low-to-moderate dose and monitor behavior, side effects, and the animal's ability to engage in behavior-modification work.

- Short-term medications

Evaluate the shelter pet's response after two and seven days.

- Monitoring and side-effect tracking
- Provide the medication response score.
  - Record the Baseline Wellbeing (see Chapter 7) and Behavior score prior to starting on the medication.
  - Track the Daily Wellbeing and Medication response score once the pet has been started on medication.
- There should be at minimum a weekly reevaluation. If there is no improvement, then medication and treatment plan needs to be adjusted.
- If there is no change after the second week, then the CTS for the shelter pet should be revised.
  - Coordination with adoption or foster transitions, including pre-adoption weaning plans or post-adoption continuation and support.

Consider using SSRIs, SNRIs, or gabapentin, with clonidine as an option for dogs and pregabalin for cats, depending on the animal's underlying emotional state and clinical needs.

11.6.5 Communication and Documentation

Education for adopter or foster to ensure transparency and continued training support utilizing handouts, training videos, and in-person demonstration.

11.7 Play – Dog and Cat

11.7.1 Definition

Play behavior is a normal and healthy activity in which dogs and cats engage for developmental, social, and emotional reasons. In puppies and kittens, play is essential for social development, motor skill practice, and learning appropriate bite inhibition. Importantly, play behavior often persists into adulthood, particularly in domesticated animals. This persistence is largely attributed to neoteny, a byproduct of domestication in which juvenile traits, including playfulness, are retained into adulthood. As a result, many adult dogs – and some adult cats – continue to engage in play behaviors well beyond maturity.

Play-related behaviors commonly include chasing, pawing, pouncing, play bowing, biting, stalking, or ambushing. These behaviors are typically exaggerated, reciprocal, and interspersed with pauses or self-handicapping – a deliberate reduction in strength, speed, or intensity that allows animals to play without causing harm or escalating conflict. When expressed appropriately, play supports physical fitness, social learning, emotional regulation, and bonding.

However, when play needs are unmet or poorly directed, play behaviors can escalate into destructive actions, uninhibited biting or scratching, or interactions that appear aggressive – especially in high-stress environments such as shelters. Social play has an important learning component: animals develop bite inhibition, self-handicapping, and the ability to read and respond to social cues through repeated, appropriate play experiences. When an animal has not had the opportunity to learn these skills, or has had limited or chaotic social play, their arousal may rise too quickly and their behavior may escalate, not out of aggression but because they lack the developmental tools to regulate themselves.

11.7.1.1 Play Behavior in the Shelter Environment

Many pets entering shelters are young, energetic, and developmentally primed for play. Unfortunately, shelter environments often restrict normal play outlets due to:

- Solitary or confined housing.
- Infectious disease prevention.
- Limited opportunities for physical and mental stimulation.
- Constant exposure to triggers (other animals, foot traffic, noise, and visual stimulation).

This mismatch between a strong internal drive to play and limited opportunities to express it appropriately can result in the escalation of normal play into problem behaviors, including:

- Jumping and BSC 2–3 (grabbing clothing, hands, leashes).
- Overstimulation or reactive behaviors (barking, lunging, and swatting).
- Frustration-related behaviors (destruction, vocalization, and agitation).

Providing appropriate play outlets is therefore a welfare intervention, not a luxury. Adequate play opportunities reduce frustration, support emotional wellbeing, and increase adoptability by preventing normal play from being mislabeled as problematic behavior.

11.7.1.2 Play Behavior in Dogs

In dogs, play commonly involves:

- Chasing and being chased
- Play bows
- Biting (BSC 1–3)
- Wrestling and body contact

Dogs deprived of appropriate play outlets may redirect play energy toward people or objects, resulting in jumping and/or biting behavior, leash grabbing, or barking and lunging. These behaviors are often misinterpreted as disobedience or aggression when they instead reflect unmet developmental, play, and exercise needs.

11.7.1.3 Play Behavior in Cats

In cats, play closely mirrors predatory sequences and often includes:

- Stalking
- Pouncing
- Batting or swatting
- Chasing moving objects
- Biting (BSC 2–4)

When play needs are unmet, cats may redirect play toward people, leading to ankle swatting, grabbing hands, or play-related biting. In confined or overstimulating environments, this can escalate into injury or be misclassified as aggression.

11.7.2 Explanation of the Condition

Play is a normal, essential behavior in dogs and cats across life stages (see Table 11.9). In shelter environments, failure to provide appropriate play outlets can cause normal play to escalate into behaviors that compromise welfare, safety, and adoptability. Meeting play needs through species-appropriate enrichment and structured activities is a foundational strategy for preventing problem behaviors and supporting successful outcomes.

11.7.2.1 When Play Becomes a Problem (Dogs and Cats)

Play behavior can become problematic when it becomes overly rough, intense, or poorly regulated, escalating into uninhibited biting, scratching, growling, or unsolicited attacks. This is most commonly seen in:

Table 11.9 Play Behavior Side-by-Side Dog/Cat Summary

Function	Dogs	Cats
Practice of Natural Behaviors	Simulate chase, herding, and hunting behaviors through running, wrestling, and play bows	Rehearse predatory sequences such as stalking, pouncing, grabbing, and batting
Social Development	Learn appropriate interaction through mock fighting, chasing, and play Develop bite inhibition, boundaries, and communication Play strengthens bonds with other dogs and humans	Learn boundaries and communication primarily through play with littermates Play may be social or solitary Strengthen bonds with humans through interactive play
Physical Exercise	Provides essential aerobic activity that builds strength, coordination, and endurance	Supports coordination, agility, and muscle tone through short bursts of high-intensity movement
Cognitive Enrichment	Encourages problem-solving, impulse control, and curiosity (e.g. puzzle toys, structured chase games)	Stimulates hunting-related cognition and problem-solving (e.g. stalking moving toys, and food puzzles)
Stress Relief and Emotional Outlet	Releases pent-up energy, reduces boredom, and helps regulate arousal and can reduce anxiety and fear-related behaviors	Reduces stress and frustration Provides emotional regulation, especially in confined or stimulating environments

- Puppies or kittens that have not learned appropriate bite inhibition.
- Pets with limited socialization or few appropriate play outlets.
- Shelter pets experiencing confinement, frustration, or chronic overstimulation.

Unlike true aggression, play aggression lacks intent to cause harm, but it can still be painful, frightening, or unsafe for people and other animals. Dogs and cats that struggle to disengage from play or self-regulate arousal may require behavior modification to learn appropriate play skills. Without intervention, these patterns can contribute to more serious concerns such as anxiety, arousal, or aggression (see Sections 11.3 and 11.4).

11.7.3 What Can Cause the Condition? – Motivation

- Normal physiological behaviors.
- Environmental and emotional motivations (lack of mental and physical stimulation, exploration, and frustration).
- Orphans or hand-reared kittens and puppies.
- Underlying medical problems are less likely – rule out orthopedic or oral pain or neurological conditions such as seizures/epilepsy and congenital conditions such as portosystemic shunt.
- For dogs with destruction in the kennel, rule out separation or confinement distress
  - Determine if torn bedding is ingested or not.

  Not ingested: Continue to provide bedding.

  Ingested: Provide safe food dispensing enrichment for oral stimulation, other forms of safe resting places and rule out gastrointestinal (GI) medical conditions.

11.7.4 Behavior Treatment Plan Framework

Appropriate Outlets for Dogs Include

- Daily opportunities for safe, well-managed social play (when appropriate)
- Structured physical activities (walks, sniffing, training games, etc.)
- Interactive enrichment and problem-solving tasks (agility, treadmills, swimming, etc.)
- Group housing with compatible dogs

Appropriate Outlets for Cats Include

- Motion-activated or wand-style toys
- Feed-dispensing and puzzle toys
- Vertical spaces such as cat trees and shelves
- Enrichment that stimulates hunting and play sequences
- Group housing in compatible groups

11.7.4.1 Management

- Safety measures: Only needed when play becomes aggressive.
  - Schedule daily play time.
  - Can often be effectively managed with appropriate play.
  - Reduce chase or rough play by redirecting the behavior to toys. If toys elicit aggression, then remove the toys. Another option is to provide an abundance of toys to reduce competition over toys.
  - Provide controlled play environment and appropriate play mates (similar age, size, and play-style; in some cases, a calmer adult dog present can help).

  - Prioritize for fast track adoptions, housing in compatible pairs.
  - Basket muzzle for dogs when needed for safe handling or training. Basket muzzles should *not* be used to allow aggressive dogs to play with other dogs; if a dog displays aggression, inter-dog play should be avoided altogether for safety.
  - Reduce or limit physical interactions, increase the use of object play, or create smaller play groups.
  - Provide safe retreat spaces for all dogs in the play group.
  - Watch closely for changes in body language – high arousal should be reduced by implementing short breaks for all dogs in the play group.
- Avoidance strategies:
  - Engage in learning opportunities and obedience training.
  - De-escalate with regular short play breaks.
  - Provide appropriate play mates.
  - Limit exposure to high excitement situations.
  - Fewer, shorter and more predictable play sessions.
- Environmental modifications:
  - Consider appropriate group housing.
  - Prioritize and increase in- and out of kennel enrichment (play time).
  - Alternate strict predictable routine between calming time and exercise.
  - Dedicated enclosed enrichment spaces such as enrichment or scent rooms, play areas, catios, and similar facilities.

11.7.4.2 Behavior Modification Steps

- Threshold management
  - Frequent play with short play breaks, avoid escalation.
- Providing appropriate play and exercise
  - Social play.
  - Object play (toy, rope, ball, and chew).
  - Interactive toys.
  - Food dispensing toys.
  - Chase or fetch play.
  - Other form of exercise.
- Substitute emotional response
  - Relaxation time in between play is important.
  - Improve settling and calming strategies.
- Positive reinforcement of alternative behaviors
  - Clicker training.
  - Target training.
- Modification of the behavior
  - Time outs for escalating play behaviors.
  - Stop all play and remove yourself, and then ask the dog to sit before restarting play.
  - Do not physically or verbally punish the pet (can lead to increase in anxiety or even aggression).
- Teach new skills and cues
  - Stand, stay, sit, down, loose leash walking exercises, and mat exercises.
  - Teach to find a ball or toy.
- Focus cues
  - Look, touch a target stick or hand, find it (focus on something positive).

11.7.4.3 Tools and Enrichment for Supporting Healthy Play

11.7.4.3.1 Dogs

Play, Training, and Enrichment Tools

- Toys: balls, tug toys, soft toys
- Target stick, clicker
- Long lines for controlled outdoor play
- Treats or special diets and treat pouches
- Food-dispensing toys (puzzle feeders and snuffle mats)
- Agility or exercise equipment (tunnels, jumps, and cavaletti)
- Nosework exercises and supplies (scent hides, containers, and search games)
- A flirt pole is an interactive dog toy consisting of a long handle or pole with a rope or cord attached, ending in a soft lure (such as a faux fur toy or fabric strip) provides vigorous aerobic exercise, builds coordination and engages natural chase play behaviors in a controlled way

Handling and Management Equipment

- Head halter
- Front-clip or double-buckle harness
- Visual and physical barriers for arousal management
- Long lines for safer distance play or decompression walks
- Indicator or message vests ("In Training" or "Give me Space")

Environmental and Physical Exercise Resources

- Hide-and-seek boxes for toys/treats
- Playgroup or group housing if appropriate
- Treadmills (for controlled movement)
- Swimming opportunities where appropriate
- Enrichment yards or fenced outdoor areas
- Relaxation spaces for cooling down after play

11.7.4.3.2 Cats

Play, Training, and Enrichment Tools

- Wand toys (feather toys and fishing-pole toys)
- Interactive toys (motion-activated toys, balls, and chase toys)
- Food-dispensing toys (puzzle feeders and rolling feeders)
- Clicker and target stick (for shaping low-arousal play and manners)
- Boxes, paper bags, and hide-and-pounce containers
- Cat trees, perches, and climbing shelves
- Tunnels for chase and hide-and-seek
- Agility-style equipment (small jumps and weave poles)

Environmental and Management Resources

- Visual and physical barriers to reduce overstimulation
- Group housing
- Quiet play spaces away from dogs or high traffic
- Multiple vertical spaces to allow safe retreat
- Comfortable resting areas for post-play decompression

Box 11.1

It is true that many kittens benefit from being adopted in pairs, especially when an older adult cat is already in the home, as an appropriate playmate can prevent play-related problems with people or the resident cat. However, pair-only adoption policies should not be applied rigidly. In some cases, adopting out one kitten is far better than adopting out none, and many homes can provide excellent lifelong care for a single kitten but are not prepared to take on two. Strict two-kitten requirements, when applied without flexibility, can unintentionally hinder welfare by limiting adoption opportunities rather than improving outcomes.

11.7.4.4 Pharmacological and Supplemental Support

Antianxiety medications, analgesics, and supplements are generally not needed.

11.7.5 Communication and Documentation

Education for adopter or foster to ensure transparency and continued training support utilizing handouts, training videos, and in-person demonstration.

Clear education on species-typical play behavior helps teams and adopters distinguish normal play from problematic arousal, reducing risk, and supporting better outcomes.

11.8 Repetitive Behaviors – Dog and Cat

11.8.1 Definition

Repetitive behavior, also called *stereotypy,* is a repetitive, persistent behavior pattern that appears to have no clear purpose or function. They are referred to as canine compulsive disorder (CCD) or feline compulsive disorder (FCD) rather than obsessive compulsive disorder (OCD). It is a behavioral pattern in pets that requires them to do the same thing repeatedly and persistently, sometimes out of context but generally as a series of behaviors derived from routine maintenance. They are often performed in a ritualized manner out of context.

While relatively uncommon, these behaviors present significant challenges when they occur in a shelter or home environment. They are often associated with genetics, stress, anxiety, frustration, or insufficient mental and physical stimulation. Without intervention, repetitive behaviors can intensify over time, making the animal more difficult to place and ultimately reducing their likelihood of adoption. Early recognition and proactive management – through enrichment, stress reduction, and, when appropriate, medical or behavioral support – are essential for improving both animal welfare and adoptability.

11.8.2 Explanation of the Condition

In a shelter, these behaviors can be very difficult to manage. If there is a specific trigger identified that can easily be avoided, the prognosis is good. If the cause for the behavior is more complex, the prognosis is generally poor. Repetitive or compulsive behaviors in the human population was estimated to be around 2% (Overall and Dunham 2002). One study on the pet population found that the prevalence rate for compulsive behavior was 16% but 8.1% involved licking a body part (Dinwoodie et al. 2019). Some dogs and cats already had the problem in the previous home, others can develop them during an extended period in the shelter. The repetitive and compulsive behaviors develop as coping strategies due to increased environmental stressors.

These types of behavior patterns tend to interfere with normal daily function and may become worse over time. They impair quality of life, cause self-injury, or disrupt normal eating, sleeping, and social interaction.

Repetitive or compulsive behaviors may be caused by chronic stress, frustration, conflict, or genetic predispositions in dogs and cats. In some instances, repetitive behaviors start out as normal (e.g. grooming), but then become abnormal as they become excessive, difficult to interrupt, or harmful (e.g. self-injury). Any repetitive behavior should occur in the absence of any primary dermatologic, neurologic, or other medical conditions. Hence, a systematic rigorous medical diagnostic approach is needed for any repetitive behaviors prior to reaching a diagnosis of CCD/FCD. However, extensive medical work-up is often not feasible, especially in the shelter.

11.8.2.1 Common Examples

Dogs

- Tail chasing or spinning
- Flank sucking or licking
- Shadow or light chasing
- Pacing, circling, or fence running
- Excessive licking leading to acral lick dermatitis ("lick granuloma")

Cats

- Tail chasing or pouncing
- Wool-sucking or fabric-chewing
- Vocalizing repetitively without a clear cause
- Excessive grooming (sometimes leading to bald spots or skin trauma)

11.8.3 What Can Cause the Condition? – Motivation

- Medical conditions (dermatological, neurological, ocular, general or neuropathic pain, metabolic, neoplastic, gastrointestinal and other)
- Genetics (some animal or breeds can be predisposed)
- Emotional motivations (lack of mental and physical stimulation, confinement, fear, anxiety, and frustration)
- Learned behavior or reinforcement history
- Environmental or social stressors

11.8.4 Behavior Treatment Plan Framework

Medical evaluation: For repetitive behaviors in dogs and cats, it is essential to have a veterinarian rule out and address any underlying medical conditions first. Many repetitive or "compulsive-like" behaviors can be driven by general pain, seizure activity, neuropathic pain along the tail or spine, ocular abnormalities (especially in cases involving chasing or light-tracking behaviors), or underlying inflammatory processes. Video recording episodes is highly valuable, as it allows the medical team to evaluate frequency, context, and subtle neurologic or pain-related signs that may not be apparent during an exam.

11.8.4.1 Management

- Safety measures
  Dogs:
  - Provide controlled and safely confined environment
  - Multiple brief calm interactions
  - Prioritize for foster placement

  Cats:
  - Provide controlled and safely confined environment
  - Multiple brief calm interactions
  - Single housing can help decrease arousal levels, while group housing can provide enrichment for social cats
  - Prioritize for foster placement
- Avoidance strategies:
  - Remove or manage access to triggers
  - Avoid or limit exposure to high excitement situations
  - Fewer, shorter, and more predictable routine visits and interactions
  - Calm physical and verbal human interactions; this can include sitting with or near the pet, reading to the pet
- Environmental modifications:
  - Change location of housing to a calmer area of the shelter
  - Visual barriers to other pets can be helpful
  - Alternate strict predictable routine between calming time and exercise
  - Prioritize and increase in- and out-of-kennel enrichment (play time)

11.8.4.2 Behavior Modification Steps

- Threshold management
  - Reduce or limit physical interactions
  - Calm voices (no high-pitched voices)
  - Multiple short visits
  - Monitor body language closely and redirect before the behavior start to alternative behavior

  Cats to appropriate toys
  Dogs to stationary behaviors

- Substitute emotional response
  - Relaxation behaviors are desirable
  - Improve settling and calming strategies
- Positive reinforcement of alternative behaviors
  - Clicker training
  - Target training
  - Teach desirable behaviors
- Modification of the behavior
  - Time outs for escalating behaviors if the behavior is triggered by arousal
  - Do not physically or verbally punish the pet (can lead to increase in anxiety or even aggression)
- Teach basic foundational skills
  - Stand, stay, sit, down, loose leash walking exercises, mat exercises
  - Teach to find a ball or toy

- Focus cues
  - Look, touch a target stick or hand, find it (focus on something positive)
- Counterconditioning and desensitization
  - Step-by-step behavior shaping plans

11.8.4.3 Tools and Enrichment for Supporting Pets with Repetitive Behavior: See Tools for Healthy Play

11.8.4.3.1 Pharmacological and Supplemental Support

Antianxiety medications, analgesics, and supplements should be considered when repetitive behaviors are driven or exacerbated by underlying medical conditions or true anxiety disorders. Many animals with repetitive behavior conditions require long-term pharmacologic management and close monitoring. When multiple medications are used, careful side-effect tracking is essential. Ongoing post-adoption support is critical to ensure medication adherence, monitor response, and adjust treatment plans as needed over time.

Key Considerations Include

- **Short-term vs. long-term use** should be considered early in the treatment trajectory.
  - Short-term medications may be appropriate for immediate relief and stress reduction.

Start on short-term medications., such as SARIs, gabapentin, benzodiazepines or α_2-agonists.

- Long-term medications require planning around expected length of stay, time to therapeutic effect, and post-adoption needs.
- Key questions include whether the animal is likely to remain in the shelter long enough for long-term medications to take effect (often four to six weeks), whether ongoing medication will be needed in a home setting, and whether the animal may instead benefit from expedited adoption or foster placement. Addressing these questions early supports appropriate medication selection and improves continuity of care.
- Appropriate dosing and titration
  - Start with one medication and evaluate response.
  - Short term medications

Evaluate the shelter pet's response after two and seven days.

- Monitoring and side-effect tracking
- Provide the medication response score.
  - Record the Baseline Wellbeing (see Chapter 7) and Behavior score prior to starting on the medication.
  - Track the Daily Wellbeing and Medication response score once the pet has been started on medication.
- There should be at minimum a weekly reevaluation. If there is no improvement, then medication and treatment plan needs to be adjusted.
- If there is no change after the second week, then the CTS for the shelter pet should be revised.
  - Coordination with adoption or foster transitions, including pre-adoption weaning plans or post-adoption continuation and support

Consider SSRIs, TCAs, SNRIs; long-term medication is often needed for repetitive behavior problems[1].

11.8.5 Communication and Documentation

Education for adopter or foster to ensure transparency and continued training support utilizing handouts, training videos, and in-person demonstration.

Education is especially critical for pets adopted with repetitive behaviors, as these conditions often require lifelong management and, in many cases, ongoing medication. Clear, transparent discussions with adopters about expectations, long-term care needs, and available support are essential. Thorough documentation ensures continuity of care, informed consent, and realistic planning for both the animal's welfare and the adopter's capacity over time.

11.9 House-Soiling/Undesirable Elimination (UE) – Dog and Cat (Adult)

11.9.1 Definition

House-soiling is defined as urinating or defecating in locations that are undesirable. For dogs any area inside the home is generally unacceptable, unless the animal is trained and uses a dedicated elimination area and surface. For cats any areas outside the litterbox are generally unacceptable.

House-soiling is one of the most frequent reasons for surrender to shelters in both dogs and cats. While frustrating for owners, it is often a manageable and reversible issue once the underlying cause is understood. House-soiling or kennel-soiling is a complex but solvable behavior challenge. With attention to medical rule-outs, proper housing, routine, and supportive care, most dogs and cats can regain appropriate elimination habits and thrive in adoptive homes.

11.9.2 Explanation of the Condition

11.9.2.1 Dog

A female dog typically urinates in a squatting position, while a male dog may or may not lift his leg when urinating. Both male and female dogs may urinate inside the home for a variety of reasons. The first step in evaluating inappropriate elimination is determining whether the dog has ever been successfully housetrained. This can be difficult in a shelter setting, as pets often arrive with little or no behavioral history.

Generally, a period of three months without accidents in a home is considered reliable housetraining. It is important to remember, however, that even fully housetrained dogs may have accidents when they move to a new environment. As a result, most adopted dogs – including adults – will require some degree of housetraining or refresher training.

For dogs who were previously housebroken, regular outdoor access is essential, as many will not eliminate in their kennel. Kennel-soiling does not always reflect how a dog will behave in a home. Fully housetrained dogs who are unable to void outside of their kennel may experience stress, and dogs who urinate in their kennel may simply lack sufficient opportunities for outdoor relief. Environmental changes can also temporarily disrupt housetraining in any dog.

While managing housetraining needs can be challenging in the shelter environment, these issues are typically temporary and should not prevent a dog from being considered adoptable.

---

1 If animals show self-injurious behaviors despite other attempts and can not be removed from the shelter sedatives such as ace can be considered.

11.9.2.2 Cat

Both male and female cats squat to urinate, and most cats reliably use a litterbox when one is available. A cat that is marking typically stands with its tail upright and sprays small amounts of urine on vertical surfaces while still using the litterbox for normal elimination. Some cats are highly particular about their litterbox setup, including the type of litter, the cleanliness of the box, its location, and how many other cats they must share it with.

The best way to reestablish litterbox use in a cat who is eliminating outside the box is to identify and address the issue early and recreate the cat's "ideal" litterbox environment. Undesirable urination or defecation is a complex behavior with multiple potential causes, including stress, substrate preference, poor litterbox management, household conflict, or underlying medical conditions that must be ruled out.

A six-year retrospective study of surrendered cats with a history of inappropriate elimination were successfully rehabilitated in the shelter environment. Confinement paired with proper litterbox setup often helps reestablish consistent elimination habits. This study found that cats with inappropriate elimination (periuria) had outcomes similar to the general shelter population when medical and behavioral interventions were applied, challenging the assumption that such cats are intrinsically poor adoption candidates (Liu et al. 2021).

Because cats surrendered to shelters generally lack access to their preferred substrate from home, they frequently resume using the litterbox reliably in the shelter. In this way, the shelter setting can serve as a reset, helping cats reestablish appropriate elimination patterns and supporting a smoother transition into a new home.

11.9.3 What Can Cause the Condition? – Motivation

- Medical – medical reasons always need be ruled out first for any case (UE (urinary tract infection [UTI], feline interstitial cystitis, crystals, bladder stones, bladder masses, prostatitis (intact male dog)), and metabolic disease (diabetes, renal failure, gastrointestinal disease with inappropriate defecation, hormonal incontinence, and osteoarthritis).
- Behavioral (incomplete housetraining, marking, anxiety, cognitive dysfunction, and inter-cat aggression).
- Combination (medical issue complicating behavior or vice versa).

11.9.4 Behavior Treatment Plan Framework

Medical evaluation: Always rule out and address underlying medical conditions first. Findings from Liu et al. (2021) demonstrated that undesirable elimination (UE) cases that failed to resolve frequently had unrecognized medical conditions; identifying these issues early can prevent prolonged shelter stays and conserve valuable resources.

Bladder health and stress are closely linked, such as in feline idiopathic cystitis (FIC). Other medical causes such as Cushing's disease, UTIs, bladder stones may drive or worsen inappropriate elimination. At minimum, a urinalysis should be performed for all pets presenting with urinary concerns.

11.9.4.1 Management

Dog

- Environmental modifications: Changes to the daily routine, kennel/home setup, provide dedicated elimination area, and supervision
- Confinements, crates, x-pens, barriers, and tethers

- Regular timed outings to the dedicated elimination location (initially every two to three hours)
- Avoid or remove triggers (especially if marking)

Cat

- Environmental modifications: Changes to routine, crate/home setup, supervision
- Adequate number of litter box, type, and litter type ideally multiple, large-sized, uncovered, easy access litterboxes in multiple locations (especially in the previously soiled areas)
- Litter choices (fine granulated, non-scented, clay-based litters are generally preferred)
- Separation between litterbox and food, ideally 6–10 feet – in shelter: offer different compartments in the kennel area, add a hiding box to provide a physical barrier between litterbox and food
- Confinement to small room with litterbox access when not supervised
- Avoid high traffic areas or loud noises in the location of litterboxes

11.9.4.2 Behavior Modification Steps

- Positive reinforcement for litterbox use and elimination in desired area
- Gradually extend unsupervised time
- Litter type, location, and litterbox preference testing (offer two choices side by side for 5 days)

11.9.4.3 Training Aids and Tools

- Training aids (barriers, crates, clicker, treats, various litterboxes, and litter types)
- Cameras for supervision of elimination behaviors (especially helpful for cats)
- Routine changes (increased enrichment and exercise)
- Calming aids (e.g. pheromones and supplements) may be useful during confinement

11.9.4.4 Pharmacological and Supplemental Support

- Treat underlying medical conditions
- May be considered for animals with underlying anxiety-related conditions
- Useful in some cases of marking behaviors (dog and cat): SSRI and TCAs

Key Considerations Include

- **Short-term vs. long-term use** should be considered early in the treatment trajectory.
  - Short-term medications may be appropriate for immediate relief and stress reduction.

  Start on short-term medications if determined to be anxiety related, such as SARI,benzodiazepines, gabapentin or α_2-agonists. For milder cases, consider the use of nutraceuticals and pheromones.

- Long-term medications require planning around expected length of stay, time to therapeutic effect, and post-adoption needs.
- Key questions include whether the animal is likely to remain in the shelter long enough for long-term medications to take effect (often four to six weeks), whether ongoing medication will be needed in a home setting, and whether the animal may instead benefit from expedited adoption or foster placement. Addressing these questions early supports appropriate medication selection and improves continuity of care.
- Appropriate dosing and titration
  - Start with one medication and evaluate response.
  - Short-term medications

Evaluate the shelter pet's response after two and seven days.

- Monitoring and side-effect tracking
- Provide the medication response score.
  - Record the Baseline Wellbeing (see Chapter 7) and Behavior score prior to starting on the medication.
  - Track the Daily Wellbeing and Medication response score once the pet has been started on medication.
- There should be at minimum a weekly reevaluation. If there is no improvement, then medication and treatment plan needs to be adjusted.
- If there is no change after the second week, then the CTS for the shelter pet should be revised.
  - Coordination with adoption or foster transitions, including pre-adoption weaning plans or post-adoption continuation and support

11.9.5 Communication and Documentation

Education for adopter or foster to ensure transparency and continued training support utilizing handouts, training videos, and in-person demonstration.

Education around house-soiling is critical, as misunderstandings in this area are a common reason for pets being returned to shelters. Successful management requires clear expectations and adherence to species-specific needs.

For cats, litter box setup is often central to success. Many cats require specific litter types, box sizes, box locations, and numbers of boxes. Adopters must be willing to follow shelter recommendations closely. Deviating from these guidelines – such as changing litter substrates, relocating boxes, or reducing box access – can quickly result in inappropriate elimination.

For dogs, adopters must be prepared to dedicate time and consistency, particularly during the initial transition period. Dogs that were previously house-trained may experience temporary setbacks due to stress, environmental change, or disrupted routines. Other dogs may have never been fully house-trained. Regardless of prior history, most dogs require a period of re-establishing house-training when entering a new home. Adopters should understand that this is normal and expected and that success depends on patience, supervision, and consistent routines rather than punishment.

Clear education, realistic expectations, and early support can prevent frustration, reduce returns, and help both dogs and cats succeed in their new homes.

11.10 Separation and/or Confinement Behavior Problems – Dog

11.10.1 Definition

Separation and confinement problems are behavior disorders in which a pet shows distress, anxiety, or undesirable behaviors when left alone, confined, or prevented from accessing people, preferred spaces, or freedom of movement. These cases often involve destructive behavior, vocalization, house-soiling, escape attempts, or self-injury and are driven by fear, frustration, or attachment-related anxiety – not disobedience.

Realistically, most shelters are not equipped to manage these conditions effectively. Prolonging a stay for an animal with separation or confinement distress, while waiting for an adopter, foster, or a treatment plan the shelter cannot consistently implement, can pose significant welfare concerns. What may appear to be a "mild" or routine issue is often, in reality, a complex and chronic behavioral disorder – one that is difficult to treat even in a stable home environment and especially challenging within the constraints of a shelter setting.

Therefore, rapid and accurate diagnosis is critical. Once identified, shelters should prioritize alternate trajectory plans, such as placing the animal into a qualified foster home, transferring to an organization with appropriate behavioral resources, or providing support that allows the pet to remain in their original home. Early redirection of the case can reduce suffering, prevent deterioration, and ensure that the animal's needs are met in the most humane and sustainable way possible.

Separation and/or confinement issues are a significant challenge in shelter animals, especially in dogs. These behaviors can be particularly distressing for adopters because they limit daily freedom, complicate routines, and can quickly erode the human–animal bond. As a result, separation-related problems are among the more common reasons for return or surrender, making early identification and clear adopter education essential.

While separation-related behaviors are less commonly recognized in cats, confinement stress can present a substantial challenge, particularly in shelter environments where cats are often housed in small, restricted spaces. Many shelter cats enter as strays rather than owner surrenders and may be accustomed to roaming freely; for these individuals, sudden confinement can be especially distressing and may contribute to fear, anxiety, or stress-related behaviors.

Cats housed in restricted spaces – whether in the shelter or at home – may struggle with limited control, reduced environmental choice, and insufficient outlets for normal behaviors. In cats, confinement stress often manifests indirectly through fear, anxiety, overstimulation, play-related escalation, or repetitive behaviors. Because feline "separation distress" does not typically present the same way it does in dogs, the treatment strategies for cats experiencing confinement-related issues are embedded within those topic areas. For cats with confinement-related behaviors, it is critical to create an enriching environment to maximize the use of the space. While it is ideal to be able to invest in an enrichment room, this is not feasible in all shelters. Safe outdoor space or group housing with compatible felines is used successfully in some shelters. Visits and play sessions with staff or volunteers in a routine fashion should also be encouraged.

There has been some research on separation concerns in cats, but this has been understudied and not well understood. More commonly in shelters the fact of being confined to a small area is the challenge. This may dissipate once the animal has free range in a home environment.

Given these species differences, this chapter focuses primarily on dogs, where separation-related problems are more clearly defined and more commonly reported by adopters. Hence, they are likely to influence adoption outcomes and shelter return rates.

Separation and confinement issues are complex, multifaceted problems that require early recognition, environmental support, enrichment, training and, when necessary, medical intervention. When left unaddressed, they may result in self-injurious behaviors and create serious welfare concerns. Management can range from simple interventions – such as providing enrichment when caretakers are absent – to more comprehensive plans that require structured behavior-modification strategies and in many cases, medication. Addressing these needs is essential not only for improving welfare during the shelter stay but also for supporting successful, long-term adoptions.

11.10.2 Explanation of the Condition

There is a wide range of separation-related behavior problems in dogs, and they must be distinguished from confinement-related distress. Separation anxiety is a specific medical and psychological diagnosis and represents only one subset of these problems.

A key question is:

- Dog is distressed only when confined, regardless of whether people are present, or
- Dog is distressed when a specific person leaves, whether or not the dog is confined.

Dogs experiencing both can escalate quickly, especially when left alone in a crate. This can sometimes result in serious self-injuries such as fractured nails or even teeth. Each issue must be addressed separately; placing a destructive dog inside a crate may prevent damage to the home but can severely compromise the dog's welfare.

In shelters, distinguishing these conditions is challenging because most dogs are confined and people are frequently present. Jumping, barking, or agitation in the kennel may reflect attention-seeking, confinement distress, separation distress, or a combination. Some dogs will be calm in confinement as long as people are present, suggesting separation-related issues. Others show stress whenever confined, regardless of human presence, suggesting confinement-related distress. Video surveillance can help differentiate the two.

Dogs may also develop separation-related behavior after adoption as they adjust from a busy shelter environment to periods of being alone. Because signs can be subtle – or mistaken for other conditions – separation and confinement problems are often misdiagnosed. Some dogs are labeled with separation anxiety for any vocalization or destruction, while others are missed entirely if they do not show classic signs.

For these reasons, careful assessment is essential. When concerns arise, a veterinarian with training in behavior or a veterinary behaviorist should be consulted to distinguish true separation anxiety from other behavioral or medical causes. Accurate diagnosis supports targeted treatment, improves welfare, and increases the likelihood of long-term success both in the shelter and in the home.

Separation-related behavior problems can vary in dogs and include some or all of the following:

- Self-injury
- Refusal to eat
- Escape behavior
- Excessive vocalization
- Excessive drooling or licking
- Pre-departure distress or aggression
- Shaking, restlessness, pacing, panting, and hiding
- "*Velcro dog*" – excessively following a person
- Very exuberant greeting behavior upon return
- Urination, defecation (diarrhea) or vomit problems
- Destructiveness, especially near doors and windows

11.10.3 Risk Factors

- Single owner
- Neutered males
- Environmental or social stressors
- Dogs previously surrendered or stray dogs
- Learned behavior or reinforcement history

- Emotional motivations (comorbidity with anxiety, especially noise phobia)
- Medical rule-outs (urinary, oral or other pain, gastrointestinal or urinary, neurological)

11.10.4 Behavior Treatment Plan Framework

Medical and behavioral evaluation: Medical problems – including urinary and gastrointestinal conditions – should always be considered when house-soiling is reported and underlying medical issues must be addressed first. For dogs that show destructive behavior when left alone, it is essential to consider motivations beyond separation anxiety, such as lack of environmental enrichment, insufficient alone-time training, or simple exploratory behavior. Video monitoring is extremely helpful, as it allows the team to assess the dog's body language during owner absence: anxious dogs display signs of distress and are unable to relax or rest, whereas non-anxious dogs may appear calm and simply engage with the environment – treating furniture as an object to chew rather than reacting emotionally to solitude. Differentiating these motivations is critical, as dogs experiencing true distress suffer when left alone, while others may simply need training, enrichment, and structure.

11.10.4.1 Management

Avoiding alone time is one of the greatest challenges in managing separation-related conditions, yet minimizing it is also one of the most effective ways to reduce distress and prevent escalating anxiety. Shelters often have long periods without staff on site, making this difficult, but reducing both the frequency and intensity of alone-time distress is essential. This is also a significant challenge for adopters as every dog will need to be left alone at some point, and it is not realistic to expect otherwise. Preparing families for this reality is an important part of counseling and support.

Group housing with compatible dogs may be helpful for some individuals, as some dogs show markedly less distress when housed or homed with another dog. Video surveillance during unattended hours is extremely valuable for assessing severity, identifying patterns, and evaluating intervention effectiveness in the shelter as well as in the home.

In most cases of true separation anxiety and distress, fast-onset, short-acting anxiolytics or even sedatives may be needed to help reduce acute distress and prevent self-injury. Medication effectiveness should always be monitored with video – both with and without medication.

For dogs going to adoption or foster, a clear management plan should accompany them. Caregivers should be coached to minimize time alone using strategies such as pet sitters, dog walkers, daycare, neighbors or friends, bringing the dog to work, or taking the dog along when feasible.

When the dog must be left alone, they should be placed in a safe, secure area that reduces the risk of escape attempts, self-harm, or panic escalation. Structured management, monitoring, and adopter support dramatically improve welfare and long-term outcomes.

11.10.4.2 Dogs with Confinement-Related Behavior Problems

Dogs with confinement-related behavior problems experience significant distress when restricted to small or enclosed spaces, with or without people present, similar to how a person with claustrophobia may respond to being confined. These dogs often show heightened distress when confinement is combined with being left alone and some may escalate to severe escape behaviors that can result in self-injury. Increasing the size or security of a crate or enclosure rarely resolves the problem and may, in fact, intensify panic and escalation.

Whenever possible, dogs with confinement-related distress should not be confined to crates or small spaces. In shelter environments, alternative housing options should be used, such as outdoor runs, offices, visitation rooms, or other larger, less restrictive areas.

The same general behavior treatment framework applies, but the emphasis is on reducing confinement stress through environmental modifications, predictable routines, appropriate enrichment, and gradual behavior modification.

When these dogs must be left alone, it is critical to place them in a safe, secure space that minimizes opportunities for self-harm, escape attempts, or escalating distress. A thoughtful management plan – paired with monitoring and ongoing support – can significantly improve welfare and long-term outcomes for dogs with confinement-related and separation-related behavior challenges.

11.10.4.3 Behavior Modification

Behavior modification can be implemented in the shelter, foster home, or adopter's home. The goal is to build the dog's confidence and independence through structured, gradual training.

11.10.4.4 Relaxation Mat Training

Teach the dog to relax on a designated mat (or blanket/bed). This helps reduce dependence on people and provides a portable "safe place."

- Use the mat only during training at first; put it away between sessions.
- Once the dog reliably relaxes on the mat, it can be used during brief alone-time practice.

11.10.4.5 Mat Relaxation Exercises

Choose a specific mat and use consistent cues across all trainers and caregivers.

Useful cues include: **"Sit," "Down," "Stay," "Go to Mat," "Settle on Mat."**

Training progression:

1) Start at close distance and very short durations (seconds).
2) Gradually increase **duration**, then **distance**, while the dog stays relaxed.
3) Work on **one gradient at a time,** either time or distance, not both simultaneously.
4) Over time, transfer mat skills across different people and environments.

11.10.4.6 Adjustments for Confinement-Related Problems

- For dogs with **confinement distress**, transition the mat **gradually** closer to the crate and then partially inside before expecting the dog to rest fully in the crate.
- For dogs **without** confinement issues, the crate may serve as an extension of the safe resting area.

11.10.4.7 Teaching Departures

Most shelters do not have the time or staffing to advance dogs to this step; however, foster homes may be able to work on departure training and provide valuable insights into how a dog functions in a real home. These cases are complex and progress in one environment may not fully predict behavior in the adopter's home. Every dog – and every home – is different.

11.10.4.8 Desensitization

Once the dog has built basic independence through mat work, the next step is teaching the dog to tolerate short departures. Desensitization involves introducing very low-intensity "leaving" cues and gradually working up to actual departures.

- Begin by identifying early signs of distress (e.g. scanning, dilated pupils, panting, yawning, sniffing, lip licking, pacing, and vocalizing).
- Work below threshold by practicing departure cues without actually leaving.
- Repeat until the dog ignores these cues and remains relaxed on the mat.
- If the dog escalates, return to more foundational mat exercises before progressing.

Below-threshold rule: *If the animal is showing fear, avoidance, freezing, reactivity, or refusing to accept the reward, the exposure is too intense and learning is no longer occurring.*

11.10.4.9 Confinement Training (for Dogs with Confinement Issues)

Introduce confinement **slowly and positively**:

1) Reward the dog for looking at or approaching the crate.
2) Reward for stepping in voluntarily.
3) Work toward calm entry and exit before expecting the dog to remain inside.
4) Only close the door when the dog is relaxed, engaged with a long-lasting chew, and showing no signs of distress.
5) Always open the door before anxiety increases.

11.10.4.10 Important Sidebar: Flooding vs. Habituation

Some dogs will vocalize briefly and settle if ignored, but dogs experiencing true panic or distress do not allow them to "cry it out." Flooding can worsen fear, cause self-injury, and escalate escape attempts. Dogs with genuine separation- or confinement-related distress require gradual exposure, not forced endurance.

11.10.4.11 Counterconditioning

Pair any departure or confinement event with something the dog loves (a high-value, long-lasting chew or food toy).

Exercise

- Keep departures calm and low key.
- Return when the dog is calm before they become distressed.
- Gradually increase time alone by 30–60 seconds at a time, varying intervals.
- After reaching 20 minutes, increases can be made in 5–15-minute steps.
- If distress appears, shorten the interval and rebuild more slowly.

For confinement work, counter condition the crate or confinement area by providing long-lasting chews or enrichment items whenever the dog enters or settles.

Environmental support – such as calming music, pheromones, white noise, or calming scents, such as lavender or chamomile – may help reduce arousal, but should be used as adjunctive tools, not primary treatments.

11.10.4.12 Real-World Limitations and Transferability

Training success in a shelter or foster home may not immediately transfer to an adopter's home. Each new environment requires restarting the program at the beginning and progressing gradually. There are no universal timelines; dogs must advance at their own pace.

11.10.4.13 Video Monitoring

Always use video when possible.

- Place the camera so that the exit, resting area, and enrichment items are visible.
- Review footage to determine thresholds, monitor progress, evaluate interventions, and ensure the dog does not escalate to panic.

11.10.4.14 Bottom Line

Even if shelters cannot complete all steps, every dog can learn to be more independent. Starting training and pairing it with long-lasting enrichment while in the shelter provide adopters a meaningful head start with their new dog.

11.10.4.15 Training Aids and Tools

- Training or Confinement Area: For separation-related behavior problems do not use a crate unless the dog views the crate as a safe space. Otherwise, a dog may severely panic and cause self-harm. Different ways to confine a dog is by using baby gates or an exercise pen. Wall or door guards can help protect exit doors from scratches.
- Offer Enrichment: Provide regular physical and mental stimulation and engage all five senses (dogs and cats).
  1) Ears: Play calming radio or TV sounds like classical music, blues, soft rock, talk radio, books, on tape.
  2) Eyes: TV, mobile, disco ball with lights, or mirror.
  3) Nose: Use pheromone diffusers and sprays, and dog-calming scents like chamomile, lavender. Catnip can be a useful addition for some cats.
  4) Taste: Utilize a variety of food-dispensing toys, puzzles and feeders. Place high-value, long-lasting treats around the training/ kennel area to keep the pet engaged
  5) Touch: Offer a variety of different surfaces on the floor such as carpet, plastic, card board, or fake grass. Ensure that the dog is not ingesting such items.
  6) Species specific pheromone products and anxiety wraps can help the animals feel calmer.

11.10.4.16 Pharmacological and Supplemental Support

Most dogs with true separation- and/or confinement-related anxiety or distress will require some form of pharmacologic support. Antianxiety medications, analgesics, and supplements are often useful and, in many cases, necessary in addition to enrichment, training or management.

The only FDA-approved medications for canine separation anxiety are Clomicalm® (clomipramine) and Reconcile® (fluoxetine).

Key considerations include using fast onset medications such as SARIs, benzodiazepine, $\alpha 2$-agonists or even sedation in cases of self-injurious behavior. These medications are often short acting and will have to be given frequently (q8–12 hours) to be effective. Appropriate dosage and titration, regular monitoring with side-effect tracking, and clear coordination during adoption or foster transitions are essential for these cases. This includes developing pre-adoption medication-weaning plans when appropriate, or ensuring continuation and post-adoption support when ongoing treatment is needed. The goal is that animals receive consistent and effective care.

Key Considerations Include

- **Short-term vs. long-term use** should be considered early in the treatment trajectory.
  - Short-term medications may be appropriate for immediate relief and stress reduction.

Dogs with an anticipated LOS < 30 days – start on short-term medications, such as SARIs, benzodiazepines or α_2-agonists

- Long-term medications require planning around expected length of stay, time to therapeutic effect, and post-adoption needs.
- Key questions include whether the animal is likely to remain in the shelter long enough for long-term medications to take effect (often four to eight weeks), whether ongoing medication will be needed in a home setting, and whether the animal may instead benefit from expedited adoption or foster placement. Addressing these questions early supports appropriate medication selection and improves continuity of care.
- Appropriate dosing and titration
  - Start with one medication and evaluate response.
  - Short-term medications

Evaluate the shelter pet's response after two and seven days.

- Monitoring and side-effect tracking
- Provide the medication response score.
  - Record the Baseline Wellbeing (see Chapter 7) and Behavior score prior to starting on the medication.
  - Track the Daily Wellbeing and Medication response score once the pet has been started on medication.
- There should be at minimum a weekly reevaluation. If there is no improvement, then medication and treatment plan needs to be adjusted.
- If there is no change after the second week, then the CTS for the shelter pet should be revised.
  - Coordination with adoption or foster transitions, including pre-adoption weaning plans or post-adoption continuation and support

11.10.5 Communication and Documentation

Education for adopter or foster to ensure transparency and continued training support utilizing handouts, training videos, and in-person demonstration.

Clear communication and thorough documentation are critical, especially for dogs adopted with separation- or confinement-related distress. These behaviors may or may not persist in the new home, but adopters must be prepared regardless.

All dogs should be gradually introduced to alone time after adoption, even if they showed minimal concern in the shelter or foster home. For dogs adopted while on medication, it is essential that adopters receive a clear written protocol, dosing instructions, monitoring guidelines, and information about potential side effects.

Shelters Should Provide

- A step-by-step transition plan for building independence and alone-time tolerance
- Medication guidance, including who to contact with questions
- Follow-up support, ideally within the first few days and again at one to two weeks
- Documentation in the POVBR and adopter-facing summaries to ensure continuity of care

Thoughtful communication, accurate records, and proactive follow-up significantly improve safety, welfare, and long-term adoption outcomes for dogs with separation- or confinement-related behavior concerns.

11.11 Aggression Problems – Dog and Cat

11.11.1 Definition

Aggressive behaviors in dogs and cats include threat displays such as growling, hissing, snarling and baring teeth, lunging, raised hackles or swatting, as well as physical actions such as biting, scratching, lunging, and chasing. Aggression in pets is defined as a set of threatening or harmful behaviors directed toward another individual (animal or human) with the intention of increasing distance, gaining control over a resource, protecting oneself, or inflicting harm. Aggression is not a diagnosis but a behavioral response that can arise from many motivations, including fear, anxiety, frustration, pain, territorial defense, or resource guarding. Understanding the underlying cause is essential for appropriate management and treatment.

Aggression is one of the most challenging behavior issues shelters are faced with. It is often associated with decreased welfare for both dogs and cats. It can lead to increased LOS, as animals with aggression concerns are harder to place. Multiple transfers or failed adoptions create repeated stress for the pet and may result in negative outcomes, including euthanasia, when aggression poses significant safety or liability risks.

Aggression cases frequently create controversy, as staff and stakeholders may disagree about the severity, motivation, and risk associated with the behavior. This can place significant emotional stress on shelter staff and volunteers, who want to balance compassion for the animal with safety concerns. It is important to acknowledge that aggressive animals always present safety risks for staff and volunteers and raise liability concerns for shelters placing them in the community. Protecting people, while respecting the welfare of animals, requires thoughtful and ethical decision-making.

While aggression in shelters is complex and emotionally taxing, a systematic assessment, clear communication, and professional input are essential to guide decisions that balance animal welfare, staff safety, and community responsibility.

Some pets display severe, overt, and highly predictable aggression that makes them unsafe for the community. These animals should be evaluated only by trained personnel, and decisions regarding compassionate euthanasia should not be delayed when risks are clear and unmanageable.

For pets with aggressive behaviors who are being considered for adoption, a comprehensive evaluation by a trained veterinarian – ideally a veterinary behaviorist with shelter expertise – is recommended. In most cases, it is critical to identify the underlying motivations and triggers for aggression and to establish an accurate medical and behavioral diagnosis. This supports targeted, individualized interventions and provides a realistic, defensible prognosis regarding safe adoptability.

11.11.2 Explanation of the Condition

Aggression in pets refers to a spectrum of behaviors that function to threaten, intimidate, or cause harm to another individual, human, or animal. From a clinical and behavioral perspective, aggression is a communication tool rather than a personality trait, and it often reflects an underlying emotional or medical state. Aggression in dogs as well as cats, typically occurs along an escalation ladder:

- Early warning signs: Stiff body posture, avoidance or withdrawal, freezing, tucked tail, piloerection, dilated pupils, growling, hissing, or lip lifting.
- Threat displays: Barking, snarling, lunging, swatting, and bite without contact (BSC1).
- Active aggression: Biting (BSC 2+), scratching, tackling, holding, shaking, or chasing.

Not all pets display the full range of warning signs, some escalate rapidly with little notice, while others offer multiple cues before acting. When documenting or discussing aggressive incidents, it is essential to use accurate, objective language. A bite should always be documented as a bite and not minimized with softer or ambiguous terms such as snapping, nipping, or mouthing. Clear terminology promotes accurate communication among staff, veterinarians, behaviorists, and adopters and prevents underestimating potential risks.

To describe bite severity, shelters should use standardized bite scales. Sophia Yin's Bite Scale and Ian Dunbar's Dog Bite Scale are commonly used in clinical and shelter settings. The authors have proposed an alternative approach – the BSC (Chapter 5) – which focuses on the *level of contact* rather than the complexity of injury. This reduces the need for lay staff to evaluate wound depth or tissue damage, making the tool more practical, reliable, and consistent for shelter use (see Chapter 5). Regardless of which scale is selected, shelters should adopt one method and apply it consistently.

The Risk Assessment Checklist with Scoring Weights described in Chapter 5 helps quantify both safety risk and welfare risk, guide pathway decisions, and support ethical consistency. These questions intentionally extend beyond the narrow focus of *"Is this animal dangerous?,"* a question that team members and volunteers often answer differently. Instead it provides a more comprehensive, structured evaluation of behavioral risk.

Behavioral disorders, particularly aggression, are among the most challenging cases shelters encounter and require objective, systematic assessment to determine humane and appropriate next steps. Standardized tools contribute to this process by offering clear, measurable criteria to classify incident severity and establish a defensible prognosis. Proper terminology and consistent use of these tools are essential for ensuring that aggression cases are documented accurately, managed safely, and communicated clearly across staff, volunteers, adopters, and the broader community.

11.11.3 What Can Cause the Condition? – Motivation

It is very important to understand that "aggression" is not a diagnosis, it is a behavior with multiple possible motivations. It can be offensive (assertive, controlling access) or defensive (fear-based, self-protective). Repeated aggression, or aggression without clear triggers, warrants medical and behavioral evaluation. Aggression in pets is both a welfare and safety issue. Accurate assessment of triggers, body language, medical status, and environmental factors is critical to develop a safe and effective management or treatment plan.

Forms of Aggression Include

- Fear- or anxiety-based aggression: Directed at unfamiliar people, animals, or handling.
- Territorial aggression: Triggered by perceived intrusion into an animal's space.
- Resource guarding: Directed at protecting food, toys, resting spots, or humans.
- Pain–illness-related aggression: Often sudden, unpredictable, and linked to medical conditions (pain, metabolic conditions, and neurological).
- Irritable aggression: Underlying fear, anxiety, frustration, pain, or other medical or behavioral conditions lowering the threshold.
- Petting induced aggression in cats: Fear-based, irritable, overstimulation, or medical conditions.
- Redirected aggression: When frustration or arousal toward one stimulus is redirected toward a nearby target.
- Confrontational handling experiences, learned behavior, or reinforcement history.
- Environmental or other social stressors.

11.11.4 Behavior Treatment Plan Framework – Dog and Cat

It is critical to understand that once any pet has shown signs of aggression toward people or other dogs, safety becomes the top concern. Any interactions with the aggressive pet has to be carefully managed in the shelter and often for the remainder of the pet's life. In cases with severe, unmanageable aggression compassionate euthanasia must be considered, especially if management or safe handling and training is not feasible. An aggressive animal should always be under control at all times and never be provoked or knowingly placed in trigger situations.

In any shelter or home environment, it can be challenging to safely provide appropriate exercise and training for pets exhibiting aggressive behavior, especially dogs. Creative and individualized activities may be necessary to ensure their physical and behavioral needs are met without compromising safety. When required, both dogs and cats can be trained or exercised from behind a physical barrier to reduce risk while still promoting learning and enrichment (see Table 11.10).

It is essential to keep an aggressive animal's daily life as stress-free, predictable as possible, and avoid physical punishment. Reducing arousal and underlying anxiety begins with a consistent routine, clear expectations, and calm, positive interactions from all caregivers. A structured environment supports behavioral stability and improves the pet's overall welfare and safety. Teams should use the BSC, BHAS, and a risk-assessment tool (described in Chapter 5 and provided in the Appendix) to support consistent, evidence-based evaluations.

11.11.4.1 Behavior Modification Steps

11.11.4.1.1 Environmental Management: The First Step in Treating Any Form of Aggression in Pets

At the start of any behavior-modification plan, the safest and most effective approach is environmental management. The goal is to change the pet's surroundings where aggressive behaviors are less likely to occur. This initial phase – safety and avoidance – forms the foundation of all subsequent treatment.

Table 11.10 Improving Coping Skills: Dogs vs. Cats

Skill / Exercise	Dogs	Cats
"Look" (*)	Yes	Yes
"Sit" (*)	Yes	Some cats will offer or can be shaped; optional
"Find It" (*)	Yes	Yes (especially food-motivated cats)
Loose-leash walking	Yes (short leash + front-buckle harness or head halter)	Optional (harness/leash training helpful for some cats)
"Down" (*)	Yes	Can be shaped in some individuals; optional
"Touch"/Target (*)	Yes	Yes
"Turn"	Yes	Yes (can be shaped with food or toy)
"Catch" or "Chase" a treat or toy (*)	Yes	Yes – small tossed treats or wand toys work well

(*) Can be used behind the bar – no physical contact needed with the animal.

11.11.4.1.2 Safety Measures

Safety measures are essential when handling aggressive or potentially aggressive pets. These may include:

- Basket muzzles (for dogs) or Elizabethan collars for dogs and cats.
- Physical barriers such as gates, panels, or transfer tunnels.
- Double leashes or safety clips.
- Two trained handlers present during interactions.
- Team members trained in safe animal-handling protocols.

These precautions protect teams and pets, reduce incident risk, and prevent setbacks such as mandatory bite quarantines that delay adoption and increase stress.

11.11.4.1.3 Avoidance and Environmental Modification

Avoidance strategies aim to reduce the animal's exposure to triggering situations. This may include:

- Adjusting routines or handling procedures.
- Behind the bar training.
- Modifying kennel setups or movement protocols.
- Managing access to spaces or stimuli that trigger aggression.
- Reducing unnecessary handling or interactions.

Pets should **never** be forced into trigger situations, punished for reacting aggressively or subjected to aversive techniques such as leash corrections, scolding, or repeated forced exposure. These interventions frequently worsen fear, anxiety, and aggression.

11.11.4.1.4 Early Recognition of Body Language

At the beginning of any plan, careful observation of body language is critical. While overt aggression (biting, lunging, and scratching) is obvious, earlier signals often provide the most useful information.

Early aggression- or stress-related signs may include:

- Staring, hovering, guarding, or lip lifting
- Growling, barking, hissing, or low vocalizations
- Dilated pupils, darting eyes, or furrowed brow
- Yawning, lip licking, sniffing, trembling, or panting
- Avoidance, freezing, stiffening, or seeking attention

Triggers vary by context, location, handler and even time of day. Detailed notes on what happened, where it occurred, when it occurred, and at what distance early signs appeared, are invaluable for treatment planning.

11.11.4.1.5 Species-Specific Considerations

Dogs Dogs often require more complex safety and avoidance strategies because they should be removed from their kennel for routine daily care, whenever possible.

- Double-compartment kennels with guillotine dividers are extremely useful, allowing staff to safely close one side while cleaning the other.
- Use double leashes, safety clips, or muzzle training to prevent incidents during transfers.
- Avoid situations that predictably provoke aggressive behavior (e.g. doorways, tight spaces, and kennel fronts).

- Carefully plan movement routes to minimize exposure to triggers.
- For highly fearful, aggressive, or extremely aroused dogs, sedation prior to examinations or treatments may be the safest option to avoid escalation.

Because dogs must exit kennels daily, progress may be slow or limited in a shelter setting.

Cats Cats may be easier to manage in some ways because they do not need to leave their kennel for routine care. However, they present unique challenges:

- Reaching into a kennel for cleaning or care can trigger defensive aggression.
- Double-compartment kennels are extremely useful, allowing staff to safely close one side while cleaning the other.
- Minimize handling and transportation whenever possible (e.g. use transfer cages or tunnels).
- Sedation prior to examination or procedures are often the safest and least stressful option for highly defensive or fearful cats.

Environmental predictability, hiding spaces, and visual barriers can significantly reduce stress in cats, lowering reactivity and defensive aggression.

11.11.4.1.6 Setting Animals Up for Success

Avoiding or reducing exposure to triggers does more than prevent bites; it helps decrease the underlying fear and anxiety that fuel aggressive behavior. Although shelter environments often make complete avoidance difficult, thoughtful management:

- Prevents escalation
- Supports welfare
- Improves safety
- Helps determine whether progress is feasible or whether an alternate trajectory (transfer, foster, or other plans) is more humane

11.11.5 Reward-Based Behavior Modification

In addition to environmental management, a reward-based behavior-modification program should be implemented. For aggression cases, the focus is on reinforcing calm, relaxed behavior, and rewarding the pet for staying attentive and focused on the handler or trainer.

Punishment must be avoided, as it increases fear, anxiety, and arousal – worsening aggression and undermining both safety and progress.

Many foundational coping-skill exercises can be taught through kennel bars or using transfer barriers for safety.

Leash Behavior (Dogs) Dogs should walk comfortably on a short leash using one of the following:

- A front-buckle harness
- A head halter (if appropriate and introduced gradually)

The goal is relaxed walking, reduced pulling, and consistent attention to the handler.

Teaching Relaxation (Dogs and Cats) Teach pets to remain calm and relaxed for gradually increasing periods of time. This is achieved by building duration on stationary behaviors such as "sit" or "down" (dogs) or a mat/spot behavior (both species).

Progression:

1) Reward brief calm moments.
2) Gradually increase the duration the pet remains in position.
3) Reinforce soft body language, slow breathing, and relaxed posture.

Over time, the pet learns to settle, regulate arousal and relax in the presence of triggers at safe thresholds.

Technique: Desensitization and Counterconditioning to Improve Behavior – Dog and Cat Desensitization and counterconditioning pairs low-intensity stimuli with high-level rewards. This pairing will help change the way that the pet feels about the situation that causes the aggressive behavior. It begins with threshold management and focuses on positive reinforcement of alternative behaviors such as the exercises mentioned above. It then introduces, in a step-by-step format, the potential scenarios with a specifically designed, safe behavior-shaping plan. To begin, introduce the pet to the trigger only at a very low intensity – usually at a significant distance – and keep the animal 100% focused on the trainer through structured exercises and high-value rewards. The key throughout training is to remain far enough away that the pet shows no signs of aggression, reactivity, or anxiety. Once the pet consistently demonstrates calm, appropriate behavior at that intensity level and begins to anticipate rewards without displaying unwanted responses, the difficulty can be increased gradually. Only one variable should be adjusted at a time. For example, do not decrease the distance and increase the duration of exposure simultaneously. Incremental, carefully controlled changes are essential to maintaining the pet's success and preventing setbacks. This slow, systematic progression allows the pet to build confidence, reduces stress, and ensures the behavior modification plan stays effective and safe.

This step will take time and requires a lifelong commitment to training. It is important to understand for shelters that this step cannot be finished or completed before adoption. Hopefully, the aggressive pet can be safely adopted accompanied by a detailed behavior modification plan and post adoption support. A pet with aggression toward multiple triggers, low thresholds, or accompanied medical conditions are among the most challenging pets to adopt even if the bite levels are not severe.

11.11.5.1 Training Aids and Tools

- Training aids (e.g. treats, clicker, long line, basket muzzles, and Elizabethan collars for dogs and cats)
- Calming aids (e.g. pheromones and supplements)
- Routine changes (e.g. increased enrichment and exercise)

Mental and physical enrichment is critical for aggressive pets in the shelter. These animals often suffer from anxiety and have a long LOS and are not candidates for foster placement. A great way to enrich any pet's life, but especially important for aggressive pets, is to "work" for meals and treats. Feeding all meals out of feed-dispensing toys is a positive way for a pet to have control over the environment. Changing up the toys and providing different levels of difficulties, boost the pets physical and mental enrichment. Other things to add include items like treadmills, balance boards, and balls and agility equipment. Skill solving varies with each pet, and it's important to continue to find the right challenges for the pet's ability. Is it important to monitor and ensure caloric intake and the safe removal of the empty dispensing toy needs to be guaranteed.

11.11.5.2 Pharmacological and Supplemental Support

Aggressive pets often benefit from a combination of short-acting and long-acting medications, which can significantly support a behavior modification plan. Long-term medications typically require four to eight weeks to reach full therapeutic effect, while short-term or situational medications can help reduce anxiety and make threshold management more achievable, particularly in the challenging environment of a shelter. Before initiating any behavioral medication for an aggressive pet, it is essential to collaborate with the veterinary team to ensure appropriate diagnostics, monitoring, and a clear plan for transitioning the animal to an adopter's home. This helps maintain continuity of care and sets the pet, shelter team, and potential adopters up for success.

For aggressive patients, medications must be selected with particular care. Safety-based management strategies must be in place first, with medication used to help reduce underlying emotional drivers of aggression – not to control behavior in the absence of proper handling and prevention. SSRIs may be considered when appropriate, but other drugs can lead to disinhibition, for example benzodiazepines.

Disinhibition risk refers to the possibility that certain medications may reduce fear or anxiety before they improve overall emotional regulation, which can lead some animals to display more overt or intense aggressive behaviors. In some cases, medications can lower natural bite inhibition or suppress avoidance behaviors, making aggression more likely if the animal is still exposed to triggers. This risk is especially heightened when medications are used without first implementing a robust safety, avoidance, and management plan to prevent exposure to situations the animal is not yet prepared to handle.

Things to consider include: short-term vs. long-term use, dosage, monitoring, side-effect tracking, disinhibition risk and plans for pre-adoption weaning or post-adoption support.

Key Considerations Include

- **Short-term vs. long-term use** should be considered early in the treatment trajectory.
  - Short-term medications may be appropriate for immediate relief and stress reduction.

  Start on short-term medications, such as SARIs, gabapentin or α_2-agonists

- Long-term medications require planning around expected length of stay, time to therapeutic effect, and post-adoption needs.
- Key questions include whether the animal is likely to remain in the shelter long enough for long-term medications to take effect (often four to eight weeks), whether ongoing medication will be needed in a home setting, and whether the animal may instead benefit from expedited adoption or foster placement. Addressing these questions early supports appropriate medication selection and improves continuity of care.
- Appropriate dosing and titration
  - Start with one medication and evaluate response.
  - Short term medications

  Evaluate the shelter pet's response after two and seven days.

- Monitoring and side-effect tracking
- Provide the medication response score.
  - Record the Baseline Wellbeing (see Chapter 7) and Behavior score prior to starting on the medication.
  - Track the Daily Wellbeing and Medication response score once the pet has been started on medication.

- There should be at minimum a weekly reevaluation. If there is no improvement, then medication and treatment plan needs to be adjusted.
- If there is no change after the second week, then the CTS for the shelter pet should be revised.
  - Coordination with adoption or foster transitions, including pre-adoption weaning plans or post-adoption continuation and support.

11.11.6 Communication and Documentation

Education for adopter or foster to ensure transparency and continued training support utilizing handouts, training videos and in-person demonstration.

Communication and thorough documentation are essential when managing shelter pets with aggression. This includes informed consent for adopters or fosters, regular use of a structured risk-assessment tool and early end-point discussions.

Early trajectory planning is critical. All behavioral and medical information – diagnoses, treatment plans, known risks and anticipated challenges – should be transparent and recorded in the POVBR. Care plans for aggressive animals should be individualized, ideally developed with input from a veterinary behaviorist. Progress must be tracked and welfare assessments conducted regularly before continuing care.

Humane endpoints should be established early. Clear criteria help the team recognize when ongoing intervention is no longer in the animal's best interest, ensuring that compassionate euthanasia – when indicated – is a deliberate, compassionate decision rather than a reaction to a crisis, prolonged suffering or staff injury.

In summary, not every shelter has the resources or specialized expertise to implement comprehensive behavior programs for every pet. This reflects each organization's SoS, not a lack of commitment. The frameworks presented here are designed to be flexible – supporting shelters with behavior teams while still offering practical components that any organization can apply to improve welfare, handling, and communication. Each pet should have a clearly defined problem list, documented plan and regular reassessment integrated into the CTS. Using standardized tools supports consistent, ethical and defensible decision-making. This structured yet adaptable approach promotes humane outcomes while respecting the realities of shelter capacity and sustainability.

References

Bergman, L. and Gaskins, L. (2013). Addressing any behavior problem, *NAVC Clinician's Brief* (May), pp. 79–82. Available at: https://www.cliniciansbrief.com/article/addressing-any-behavior-problem (accessed 27 May 2026).

Dinwoodie, I.R., Dwyer, B., Zottola, V. et al. (2019). Demographics and comorbidity of behavior problems in dogs. *Journal of Veterinary Behavior*. Elsevier Inc. 32: 62–71. https://doi.org/10.1016/j.jveb.2019.04.007.

Liu, S., Sung, W., Welsh, S., and Berger, J.M. (2021). A six-year retrospective study of outcomes of surrendered cats (*Felis catus*) with periuria in a no-kill shelter. *Journal of Veterinary Behavior*. Elsevier Inc. 42: 75–80. https://doi.org/10.1016/j.jveb.2020.12.002.

Overall, K.L. and Dunham, A.E. (2002). Clinical features and outcome in dogs and cats with obsessive-compulsive disorder: 126 cases (1989–2000). *Journal of the American Veterinary Medical Association* 221 (10): 1445–1452.

12

Adoption Counseling as Partnership: Creating Sustainable Pathways to Lifelong Homes

12.1 Adoption as an Outcome and an Opportunity

Adoption is the central outcome goal for most animal shelters and rescue organizations. Every successful adoption represents more than a single life changed; it creates space, time, and resources to help the next animal in need. When animals move efficiently and successfully through a shelter system, length of stay (LOS) is reduced and flow-through is healthy. As a result, the organization is able to serve more animals overall, reduce crowding, and support better wellbeing for those still in care.

Adoption counseling is not simply a customer-service transaction or an administrative step. It is a strategic, welfare-centered practice that directly influences shelter metrics, staff wellbeing, and the long-term sustainability of the organization. Thoughtful, adopter-friendly counseling helps animals leave the shelter sooner, increases adoption success, and strengthens the human–animal bond that keeps pets in homes for life.

12.1.1 There Is No Single "*Right*" Way to Adopt

Pets find new homes through many different pathways: informal rehoming, gifting, open adoptions, facilitated matches, foster-to-adopt programs, or more structured processes involving questionnaires and counseling conversations. Importantly, there is no evidence that one adoption pathway is universally superior to another. Research has not demonstrated that gifting a pet devalues the animal or increases the likelihood of relinquishment. In some cases, a gifted animal is deeply valued and cherished.

What matters most is not the rigidity of the process but the quality of communication, expectation setting, and support offered to the adopter. Adoption counseling should therefore focus less on controlling outcomes and more on sharing information, building understanding, and supporting informed, compassionate decisions.

12.1.2 Adoption Counseling as Education and Expectation Setting

At its core, adoption counseling is about partnership. It is an opportunity to provide adopters with clear, honest, and practical information about the pet they are welcoming into their home, while also learning what the adopter is truly looking for in a companion.

Effective Counseling

- Sets realistic expectations about behavior, health, and adjustment.
- Emphasizes that successful adoption is a process, not a test to pass.
- Frames challenges as manageable and normal, rather than as failures.
- Uses welfare frameworks (such as the Five Domains) to discuss quality of life in accessible, non-judgmental ways.

This educational approach benefits both the pet and the adopter. People who feel informed and supported are more likely to seek help early, remain engaged with the organization, and maintain the relationship long term (Bir et al. 2017; Holland 2019).

12.1.3 Reducing Bias: Adoption as a Conversation, Not a Judgment

One of the greatest threats to successful adoption counseling is unconscious bias. Shelters often – unintentionally – make assumptions about adopters based on age, appearance, income, housing type, or lifestyle. These assumptions can jeopardize excellent matches and prolong an animal's stay unnecessarily.

A powerful reminder comes from a case involving a high-energy black-and-white dog labeled as a "Border Collie" without genetic testing. An older, retired couple expressed interest in adopting him and were discouraged based solely on their age, under the assumption that they would be unable to meet this dog's activity needs. In reality, the couple hiked 10–20 miles daily and had lived with Border Collies their entire lives. Judging their suitability by age alone nearly cost this dog its ideal home.

Unfortunately, this type of well-intended but harmful gatekeeping happens regularly. Judging potential adopters as too young, too old, too busy, not wealthy enough, not "active-looking" enough, or any number of other subjective criteria is a dangerous practice that can directly harm shelter pets and undermine the organization's mission.

The truth is that no adoption professional can predict with certainty who will or will not provide *good* care. Even that framing is judgmental. What defines "*good care*"? Expectations vary widely across cultures, communities, and individual households.

Adoption counseling should therefore begin with *curiosity, not conclusions*. It should be a conversation rooted in listening, allowing adopters to describe their lives, experiences, and hopes, rather than a process designed to screen people out.

12.1.4 Adopter-Centered Counseling and Progressive Sheltering

Adopter-centered counseling reflects this philosophy by inviting people in rather than pushing them away. Progressive sheltering recognizes that shelters exist to serve both pets and communities. The goal is not to create barriers but to facilitate connections.

In today's world, people can purchase animals online within minutes from breeders, brokers, or puppy mills and have them delivered with supplies included. Against this reality, shelters cannot afford to position themselves as difficult, judgmental, or inaccessible. Instead, they must offer something far more valuable: *transparency, trust, education, and ongoing support*.

This shift requires reimagining the shelter not merely as an adoption facility but as a community hub – as a place that celebrates the human–animal bond, provides resources, and remains connected to adopters long after the adoption is complete.

12.1.5 Eliminating Barriers That Impede Adoption

If the goal is to move pets into homes efficiently and responsibly, shelters must critically examine their adoption processes for unnecessary barriers. Many traditional requirements discourage adopters without improving outcomes and consume valuable staff time.

Common barriers that impede adoption include:

- Mandatory fenced yards.
- Proof of home ownership.
- Adopting kittens only in pairs.
- Lease agreements verifying pet allowance.
- Prohibiting pets from being adopted as gifts.
- Home inspections conducted by shelter staff.
- Mandatory dog-to-dog meetings with resident pets.
- Requiring the name of a current veterinary hospital.
- Requiring all household members to meet the animal.
- Limiting the number of animals an adopter may meet.

These requirements often stem from a desire to ensure success, but there is little evidence that they do so. Instead, they slow down the adoption process, increase LOS, and reduce overall throughput – directly impacting the organization's impact on the number of pets it can help.

Replacing lengthy applications with smart information-gathering questionnaires shifts the tone from approval to collaboration. Trusting adopters to manage their housing situations respects their autonomy and reduces administrative burden. Each barrier removed improves flow and supports organizational efficiency and sustainability.

12.1.6 Adoption Success Supports Organizational Sustainability

Shorter LOS, efficient flow-through, and high adoption rates are not merely operational metrics, but they are welfare indicators. Animals who move quickly into homes experience less stress, fewer behavioral declines, and better long-term outcomes. Teams experience less moral distress, and resources are used more effectively.

From a sustainability perspective, successful adoptions allow organizations to:

- Improve staff retention and morale.
- Reduce overcrowding and disease risk.
- Help more pets with the same resources.
- Strengthen community trust and engagement.

Adoption counseling plays a critical role in achieving these outcomes by ensuring that placements are informed, supported, and resilient.

12.1.7 Adoption Counseling Without Dedicated Counselors

Not all organizations have the luxury of designated adoption counselors. Municipal shelters and under-resourced organizations may rely heavily on kennel cards, photos, online profiles, and brief interactions to convey a pet's story. In these settings, clear, compassionate storytelling becomes even more important.

Whether counseling is written or verbal, formal or informal, the goal remains the same: spark connection, provide honest information, and make the adoption process simple and welcoming. Once interest is established, the organization should prioritize ease of adoption while ensuring adopters understand how to support the animal's transition and wellbeing.

12.1.8 A Shared Goal: Lifelong Homes Through Partnership

Adoption counseling is not about perfection. It is about progress. It is about doing the best we can with the information we have to create matches that allow both pets and people to thrive.

When shelters focus on partnership rather than permission, education rather than exclusion, and flow rather than fear, adoption becomes what it is meant to be: *a hopeful beginning*. Each successful adoption strengthens the system, expands capacity to help others, and reinforces the shared responsibility we have to support pets and the people who love them for a lifetime.

12.2 Effective Communication with Adopters

Effective communication is the foundation of successful adoption counseling. It shapes how adopters experience the organization, how confidently they make decisions, and how well pets are matched to homes. Adoption counseling is not an interrogation or a screening exercise – it is a conversation. When done well, it feels collaborative, respectful, and supportive, creating space for honest dialogue rather than pressure or judgment. Sometimes success means discovering that it is not the right time for someone to adopt or that a different species or type of pet would be a better fit – and that is okay. The next person who meets that pet may be the right match. Adoption counseling requires the bravery to ask the right questions so that decisions truly serve both the adopter and the animal.

12.2.1 What Effective Communication Looks Like

Effective adoption communication prioritizes *open-ended* questions and active listening. Instead of asking questions designed to approve or disqualify an adopter, counselors should invite conversation:

- "What qualities are you hoping for in a companion animal?"
- "What has your experience with pets been like in the past?"
- "Tell me about what a typical day looks like in your household."

These questions allow adopters to share their lifestyle, expectations, and limitations without fear of being judged. They also give counselors critical context to help guide the match, especially when information about the animal is limited, as is often the case in shelter environments.

Effective matching begins with understanding the adopter and exploring what the adopter is truly seeking, rather than steering them toward or away from certain pets based on assumptions. Questions such as:

- "What made you decide that now is the right time to adopt?"
- "What kinds of behaviors feel manageable or challenging?"
- "What has worked well – or not so well – with pets in the past?"

Effective communication also means leaving room for uncertainty. Adoption counselors frequently work with incomplete behavioral histories and evolving medical information. Rather than presenting pets as *fixed or fully known*, counselors should communicate transparently about what is known, what is still being learned, and what support is available after adoption (Dinwoodie et al. 2022).

12.2.2 Training for Consistent, Supportive Communication

Clear, consistent communication does not happen by chance. Organizations should invest in structured training for adoption counselors, volunteers, and any team members involved in adopter interactions. This training should include:

- Use of scripts and talking points to ensure consistency.
- Strategies for managing emotional or difficult conversations.
- Role-playing exercises for common and challenging scenarios.
- Communication fundamentals (open-ended questions, reflective listening).
- Guidance on explaining organizational policies clearly and compassionately.
- Regular check-ins to ensure their messaging and decision-making remain aligned with the organization's values and mission.

Scripts and talking points are not meant to make interactions feel robotic. Instead, they provide a shared framework that ensures adopters receive accurate information while allowing counselors to adapt their style to each individual conversation. Role play is particularly valuable for new team members, helping them build confidence and emotional resilience before working independently with the public.

When volunteers are utilized as matchmakers, they should receive the same communication training as professional staff. Inconsistent messaging can confuse adopters and erode trust. Volunteers should also be empowered to recognize when a question is beyond their scope and confidently refer adopters to team members or supervisors for more detailed or complex guidance.

12.2.3 Using Available Information to Support the Match

Matching adopters with pets is one of the most complex and one of the most emotionally charged tasks in sheltering. Counselors often rely on limited snapshots of behavior, medical notes, kennel observations, and short interactions. This is where structured records such as problem-oriented veterinary behavior records (POVBR) and transparent medical documentation become invaluable tools.

These records help counselors:

- Frame expectations realistically.
- Identify known medical or behavioral needs.
- Communicate management strategies clearly.
- Match lifestyle needs with support requirements.

Even with these tools, matching is never perfect. Counselors may experience moments of doubt: *Is this really the right home? Did we miss something?* These feelings are normal and reflect the deep care counselors have for the pets. Training should normalize this emotional complexity and provide guidance on how to make thoughtful decisions without becoming paralyzed by fear of making the "*wrong*" choice.

12.2.4 Recognizing and Addressing Implicit Bias

A critical component of effective communication training is learning to recognize and mitigate implicit bias. Implicit biases are unconscious attitudes or stereotypes that influence perceptions and interactions, even when individuals consciously believe they are being fair.

In adoption counseling, implicit bias may show up as assumptions based on:

- Age (too young or too old).
- Family structure (single parents or multigenerational households).
- Appearance, clothing, or vehicles.
- Perceived socioeconomic status.
- Neighborhood or housing type.

For example, assuming an older couple cannot manage a large, energetic dog or that a single-parent household lacks adequate support to raise a puppy can lead to missed opportunities for excellent placements. No adopter wants to be judged before they have had the chance to share their story.

Training should actively address bias through discussion, reflection, and scenario-based learning. Team members should be encouraged to pause, question their assumptions, and return to curiosity. The goal is not perfection, but awareness and a commitment to approaching every adopter as an individual.

12.2.5 Trauma-Informed, Adopter-Centered Communication

A trauma-informed approach further strengthens adopter communication. Most people have experienced discrimination, housing insecurity, financial stress, or negative interactions with institutions. These experiences can influence how adopters communicate, ask questions, or respond to perceived authority.

Trauma-informed communication helps team members:

- Create a sense of psychological safety.
- Recognize stress or anxiety in adopters.
- Adjust tone and pacing of conversations.
- Avoid language that feels accusatory or dismissive.

Adopter-centered communication allows counselors to tailor their approach to each person's experience, ensuring the process feels welcoming rather than intimidating. This approach does not lower standards of care, but it improves outcomes by fostering trust and honesty.

12.2.6 The Human Side of Animal Welfare Work

Many people work or volunteer in animal shelter organizations because they love animals and want to make a difference in their lives. That passion is essential, but it is not sufficient on its own. Adoption counseling requires comfort with people, communication, and emotional complexity.

Organizations should be intentional about hiring and training individuals who enjoy working with people as much as pets. Animal welfare organizations are not only care facilities – they are community institutions. They serve as hubs for education, resources, and relationship-building.

By investing in communication training, addressing bias, and embracing adopter-centered approaches, shelters strengthen their role in the community. Effective communication does more than place animals; it builds trust, reduces returns, supports long-term success, and reinforces the shelter's mission as a partner in the human–animal bond.

12.3 Matching Pets with Adopters

Matching pets with adopters is one of the most complex and most meaningful responsibilities in sheltering. It requires balancing incomplete information, human emotion, animal wellbeing, and organizational goals. When a match succeeds and a pet goes home, it is one of the most rewarding moments in shelter work and should be celebrated. At the same time, effective matchmaking requires realism, humility, and flexibility. Not every match that looks promising in the shelter will succeed in the home – and, conversely, some matches that seem uncertain in the shelter may thrive once in a different environment. This reality must be acknowledged without blame.

A return to the shelter should never be framed as a failure. Instead, it can be understood as an *"overnight stay,"* a pause that gives the pet relief from a stressful mismatch and allows the organization to reassess and refine the placement plan. Return data should be tracked thoughtfully. While expectations of zero returns are neither realistic nor human, consistently high return rates (generally above 10%) may signal a need for additional training, improved communication, or adjustments in matchmaking practices. The goal is not perfection, but consistent, successful placements.

12.3.1 Transparency Builds Trust

Once potential matches are identified, transparency is essential. Counselors should review both medical and behavioral records with adopters, explaining what is known, what is still being learned, and how the organization is currently supporting the pet. This openness builds trust, not only in the counselor, but in the organization as a whole.

Each shelter pet should have complete, accessible medical and behavioral documentation. Standardized medical and behavior staging systems help ensure that all team members use consistent terminology and avoid confusing or emotionally loaded labels. Describing observable behaviors – rather than assigning character judgments – allows adopters to make informed decisions.

Research supports this approach. Studies have shown that adopters are more confident in their decisions when provided with detailed, accurate information about a pet's personality and behavior during counseling (Bir et al. 2017; Holland 2019). Moreover, realistic portrayals of temperament influence pet selection and long-term satisfaction.

12.3.2 Presentation Matters – But Accuracy Matters More

Online presence and in-person presentation play a significant role in adoption decisions. Attractive, honest photographs and engaging descriptions increase interest, particularly when they reflect the pet's true nature. Visual cues such as collars, size-reference objects, and active or natural backgrounds help adopters better imagine the pet in their lives (Nakamura et al. 2020).

In person, counselors should present the animal the adopter asks to see, while also offering thoughtful alternatives that may be an even better match. This is not about redirecting adopters away from their preferences, but about expanding possibilities through education and experience.

12.3.3 Avoiding Prejudgment and Challenging Myths

Matching requires counselors to actively check their own biases as well as those of adopters. Counselors should not prejudge what an adopter can or cannot handle based on age, household composition, or experience level. An older couple may be perfectly equipped to care for a large, energetic dog. A single-parent household may have an extensive support network. These realities only emerge through conversation.

This is also the opportunity to dispel common myths. Breed stereotypes, assumptions about size, or misinterpretations of past behavior often limit adoption opportunities unnecessarily. A dog who bit in a specific context – such as being pulled from a crate – may not pose the same risk when that scenario is avoided. A cat who struggled with litterbox use in a chaotic household may thrive in a quiet adult home. Context matters.

12.3.4 Showcasing the Right Qualities

Adopters vary in what draws them to a pet. Some are influenced by appearance or breed type, while others prioritize behavior, playfulness, or energy level. Counselors should select environments that allow a pet's most appealing and relevant traits to shine – whether that is play behavior, sociability, calmness, or engagement.

Studies consistently show that adopters respond to social behaviors: dogs that stay close, engage gently, or show affiliative behavior are more likely to be chosen. For cats, playfulness, vocalization, and interactive behaviors increase adopter interest. Understanding these tendencies allows counselors to structure meet-and-greet experiences more intentionally.

12.3.5 Setting Realistic Expectations

A critical part of matching is helping adopters reconcile what they *think* they want with what they can realistically manage. During meet-and-greets, counselors should seamlessly integrate discussions about daily care, activity needs, feeding routines, housetraining, and the decompression period after adoption.

Known stress-related behaviors – such as leash pulling, jumping, or kennel reactivity – should be described factually, without minimizing or dramatizing. Counselors should explain how the pet is currently being managed and invite adopters to consider whether they are able and willing to continue that plan at home.

For pets with more significant behavioral challenges, counselors should walk adopters through specific scenarios:

- "What would you do if this happens at home?"
- "Who would help you manage this situation?"
- "Does this feel doable in your environment?"

Asking adopters to summarize their understanding of the information provided ensures clarity and shared expectations.

12.3.6 Language Matters

Consistent, thoughtful language protects the pet, empowers the adopter, and supports ethical, transparent matchmaking. Counselors and volunteers must be coached on terminology. Absolute statements ("great with all dogs") and labels ("reactive" and "special needs") should be avoided. Descriptive language grounded in observable behavior is more accurate and less discouraging. Research has shown that even casually negative phrasing can significantly reduce adoption interest.

12.3.7 Celebrating Success – Allowing for Adjustment

Matching pets with adopters is both an art and a science. It is emotionally rewarding, intellectually challenging, and never perfect. Successful matches should be celebrated as milestones for the pet, the adopter, and the organization. At the same time, returns should be viewed as opportunities for learning and recalibration – not as personal or institutional failures.

By embracing transparency, open communication, bias awareness, and realistic expectations, shelters can improve match quality, reduce unnecessary returns, and support long-term success – while accepting flexibility and compassion as essential parts of responsible adoption practice.

12.4 Preparing Adopters for the Post-adoption Transition: Setting Realistic Expectations

Once adopters have made their selection, the focus of adoption counseling shifts from decision-making to preparation. This stage is critical. Thoughtful expectation setting during the post-adoption transition helps adopters feel supported, reduces anxiety, and significantly improves long-term outcomes for both the pet and the family. Adopters should leave the shelter with a clear understanding that adjustment takes time – and that challenges during the transition are normal, expected, and manageable.

12.4.1 What to Expect After Bringing a Pet Home

A commonly used framework in shelters is the *3–3–3 guideline* (ASPCA Pro 2024), which helps adopters visualize the adjustment process:

- *First 3 days: Decompression.* The pet may appear shut down, overly quiet, anxious, clingy, or, conversely, overstimulated. Eating, sleeping, and elimination patterns may be inconsistent.
- *First 3 weeks: Adaptation.* The pet begins to learn routines, test boundaries, and show more of their personality. Some behavioral challenges may emerge during this period.
- *First 3 months: Integration.* The pet starts to feel secure, relaxes into the environment, and develops a sense of belonging within the household.

While this framework is helpful, counselors must emphasize that every pet is an individual. Some animals move faster; others need significantly more time. Progress is rarely linear, and temporary setbacks are normal.

12.4.2 Individualized Transition Guidance

Some shelter pets benefit from a showing plan, which helps counselors highlight specific behavioral considerations during adoption counseling. Others may require a more detailed take-home plan, outlining concrete steps adopters can follow to ease the transition.

These plans may include guidance on:

- Establishing predictable daily routines.
- Allowing the pet to acclimate at their own pace.
- Avoiding overwhelming introductions or experiences.
- Providing appropriate training, enrichment, and mental stimulation.
- Using environmental management to prevent problem behaviors.
- Gradually introducing resident pets, children, or new environments.

Clear, practical guidance empowers adopters and reduces the likelihood of misunderstandings or unrealistic expectations.

12.4.3 Aligning Expectations with Reality

Research consistently shows that many pet returns to the shelter stem from mismatched expectations, not from adopter unwillingness (Dolan et al. 2015; Powell et al. 2021). Some adopters expect dogs to arrive housetrained, familiar with basic cues, or instantly compatible with resident pets. Others underestimate the caregiver burden involved in meeting a pet's physical, emotional, and behavioral needs.

Adopters should understand that:

- Household routines must be taught – not assumed.
- Pets do not automatically "fit" into a household like a puzzle piece.
- Both humans and animals must adapt and accommodate one another.
- Rules about furniture, boundaries, and schedules must be clear and consistent.
- Pets need guidance on where to eliminate, what to chew, when to play, and how to rest.

Normalizing this learning process helps adopters approach challenges with patience rather than frustration.

12.4.4 Providing Tools and Resources for Success

Counselors should send adopters home with curated resources tailored to their new pet. These may include:

- Recommended training and behavior resources.
- Contact information for post-adoption support.
- Referrals to qualified trainers or behavior professionals.
- Written handouts or digital guides on decompression and transition.
- Access to shelter behavior or medical team members for follow-up questions.

Whenever possible, shelters should also support adopters with practical tools. Sending home a small amount of the pet's current food allows for a gradual diet transition. On-site retail options – or clear recommendations – can help adopters choose appropriate leashes, harnesses, collars, litter boxes, litter types, toys, and enrichment items such as puzzle feeders. These tools reduce stress, prevent unwanted behaviors, and set the household up for success from day one.

12.4.5 Clear Return Policies and Ongoing Support

Adopters should be informed – clearly and compassionately – about the organization's return policy and encouraged to reach out early if challenges arise. Open lines of communication reinforce that the shelter remains a partner after adoption, not a gatekeeper left behind.

Post-adoption support may take many forms:

- Follow-up emails or phone calls.
- Access to educational materials.
- Community training classes or referrals.
- Behavior advice from trained team members or volunteers.

This ongoing relationship strengthens trust and improves retention.

12.4.6 Reframing Returns: Not a Failure, but a Learning Opportunity

Leadership must set the tone that returns are not failures. While finding the right match is always the goal, not every placement will succeed. That reality must be approached with compassion rather than judgment.

When a pet is returned:

- The pet has often benefited from time away from the shelter.
- The organization gains valuable insights into how the pet behaves in a home.
- Counselors can use this new information to refine future matches.

Returns should be viewed similarly to an extended foster stay, both a chance for the pet to decompress and for the organization to learn more. Adopters should be welcomed back without shame or criticism. Many adopters choose to waive their adoption fee or donate it to support the pet's next placement, further reinforcing the shared commitment to the animal's wellbeing.

This process creates a true win-win: the pet receives better-informed placement support, the organization improves matchmaking accuracy, and adopters leave feeling respected and valued – even when the match was not right.

12.4.7 Building Relationships Through Honest Preparation

Preparing adopters for the post-adoption transition is not simply about preventing returns – it is about building resilient, informed, and supported relationships. Expectation setting aligns optimism with reality, reduces stress for both people and animals, and strengthens the partnership between adopters and the organization.

When shelters embrace transparency, education, and compassion throughout the transition period, they not only improve individual outcomes but also reinforce their role as trusted community resources dedicated to lifelong success for pets and the people who love them.

12.5 Preparing Adopters for Shelter Pets with Known Behavioral Challenges

Adopting a shelter pet with known behavioral challenges can be deeply rewarding – and it often requires more time, patience, and support than adopting a pet without identified concerns. The authors' experience has consistently shown that when adopters are fully informed and appropriately prepared, they tend to be more tolerant, resilient, and committed when challenges arise. In fact, during post-adoption follow-up calls, it is frequently not the behavior identified and addressed in the shelter that becomes problematic. Instead, new and unrelated behaviors may emerge, while the originally discussed concern is often well managed. This is an indicator of good matching and realistic expectation setting.

By contrast, adopters who expect a "perfect" pet – one who arrives fully housetrained, emotionally intuitive, and seamlessly integrated – are more likely to feel disappointed when normal adjustment challenges occur. Minor, expected behaviors can escalate emotionally and, at times, result in a return. This highlights the importance of framing adoption not as acquiring a finished product, but as beginning a relationship that will grow at the animal's pace.

12.5.1 Transparency and Preparation Are Essential

Adoptions involving pets with behavioral challenges require additional care in counseling – not to discourage adopters but to ensure they are truly prepared. Adopters should understand both:

- The known challenges the pet currently exhibits.
- The potential challenges that may arise during transition and adjustment.

Clear, honest communication builds trust and empowers adopters to make informed decisions. When adopters feel respected and supported – rather than surprised or misled – they are more likely to persevere through difficulties.

12.5.2 Distinguishing Normal, Developmental Behavior from Behavioral Disorders

A critical part of counseling is helping adopters understand the difference between normal but problematic behaviors and true behavioral disorders.

Many undesirable behaviors are developmentally normal and commonly seen in adolescent or immature animals, including:

- Dogs jumping up on people.
- Puppies chewing inappropriate items.
- Cats swatting at ankles or hands during play.
- Overexuberant play or poor impulse control.

These behaviors are typical for the species and age. They are often responsive to management and training and frequently improve with maturity.

By contrast, behavioral disorders may involve more persistent patterns, heightened emotional reactivity, or safety concerns that require structured intervention and ongoing management. Helping adopters understand where a pet falls along this continuum prevents unnecessary alarm and reduces mislabeling of normal behavior as pathology.

12.5.3 Reframing "Aggression" Through Context

Many behaviors perceived as aggression are better understood through context. Adoption counselors should help adopters interpret behavior accurately and safely, for example:

- A dog herding and biting at running children may be expressing normal herding behavior rather than intent to harm.

- A dog barking and air-biting during rough play between adults and children may be overstimulated rather than aggressive.
- A cat biting a child's hand after being teased is responding defensively, not unpredictably.

Providing this context does not excuse unsafe behavior, but it allows adopters to manage situations proactively and realistically. When adopters understand *why* a behavior occurs and how to prevent it, they are far more likely to succeed.

12.5.4 The Power of Post-adoption Support

Adopters are significantly more likely to keep pets with behavioral challenges when they are informed about:

- The behavior challenge before adoption.
- Where to seek support or help afterward.

Post-adoption support may include:

- Group or virtual training classes.
- Written or digital behavior management resources.
- Consultations with trained shelter behavior staff.
- Referrals to qualified trainers or behavior professionals.

Equally important is the reassurance that returning the pet to the shelter remains an option if the match ultimately proves unsuitable. Knowing that the shelter will receive the pet back without judgment can significantly reduce adopter stress. For many adopters, return is a last resort, but the availability of that option often makes them more willing to try.

12.5.5 When Support Is Not Enough

Shelter teams must also recognize that even with robust support – such as low-cost veterinary care, free food, or training – some adoptions will not succeed. Returns are often influenced by factors outside the organization's control, including:

- Financial hardship.
- Loss of pet-friendly housing.
- Changes in physical or mental health of the adopter or family members.
- Unexpected caregiver burden.

Additionally, some adopters arrive with unrealistic expectations that a pet will intuitively understand and emotionally support them. Pets are sometimes adopted in hopes they will function as emotional support animals, without recognition that not all animals are suited for this role. When expectations exceed what the pet can reasonably provide, disappointment and frustration can follow.

12.5.6 Matching with Realism and Compassion

Successful placement of pets with behavioral challenges relies on:

- Robust post-adoption support.
- Honest, compassionate communication.
- Clear differentiation between normal and disordered behavior.
- Leadership that frames returns as learning opportunities rather than failures.

When adopters are encouraged to meet pets where they are – rather than where they wish them to be – the resulting relationships tend to be stronger and more resilient. Adopters who understand that progress happens at the animal's pace are often more patient, adaptable, and successful.

Preparing adopters for behavioral challenges is not about lowering standards or increasing risk. It is about aligning expectations with reality, supporting informed consent, and honoring the complexity of both pets and people. When done well, this approach protects animal welfare, strengthens adopter trust, and leads to more sustainable, humane outcomes for all involved.

In summary, adoption counseling is a strategic partnership that supports animal wellbeing, reduces LOS, and strengthens organizational sustainability. It should be a collaborative conversation – not a screening exercise – focused on transparency, realistic expectations, and informed decision-making. By removing unnecessary barriers, addressing bias, and providing consistent communication and post-adoption support, shelters improve match quality and community trust. The goal is not perfection or zero returns, but sustainable placements that protect pets, support adopters, and allow shelters to help more animals over time.

References

ASPCA Pro (2024). Pet adjustment periods: the 3 days - 3 weeks - 3 months guide, [online] available at: https://www.aspcapro.org/resource/pet-adjustment-periods-3-days-3-weeks-3-months-guide (accessed 1 February 2026).

Bir, C., Widmar, N.J.O., and Croney, C.C. (2017). Stated preferences for dog characteristics and sources of acquisition. *Animals* 7 (8): 1–19. https://doi.org/10.3390/ani7080059.

Dinwoodie, I.R., Zottola, V., Kubitz, K., and Dodman, N.H. (2022). Selection factors influencing eventual owner satisfaction about pet dog adoption. *Animals* 12 (17): 1–15. https://doi.org/10.3390/ani12172264.

Dolan, E.D., Scotto, J., Slater, M., and Weiss, E. (2015). Risk factors for dog relinquishment to a Los Angeles municipal animal shelter. *Animals* 5 (4): 1311–1328. https://doi.org/10.3390/ani5040413.

Holland, K.E. (2019). Acquiring a pet dog: a review of factors affecting the decision-making of prospective dog owners. *Animals* 9 (4): 124. https://doi.org/10.3390/ANI9040124.

Nakamura, M., Dhand, N., Wilson, B.J. et al. (2020). Picture perfect pups: how do attributes of photographs of dogs in online rescue profiles affect adoption speed? *Animals* 10 (1): 1–12. https://doi.org/10.3390/ani10010152.

Powell, L., Duffy, D.L., Kruger, K.A. et al. (2021). Relinquishing owners underestimate their dog's behavioral problems: deception or lack of knowledge? *Frontiers in Veterinary Science* 8 (September): 1–11. https://doi.org/10.3389/fvets.2021.734973.

13

Keeping Pets in Their Homes

13.1 Post-Adoption Support and Resources

Adoption does not end when the pet leaves the shelter. In many ways, it is the beginning of the most important phase of the organization's responsibility to both the animal and the adopter. Ongoing post-adoption support is one of the most effective tools shelters have to reduce returns, strengthen the human–animal bond, and ensure long-term success in the home.

Once a pet has been adopted, timely follow-up helps identify concerns early, before frustration, confusion, or fear escalate into crises. While some adopters are experienced and confident, others are new to pet ownership and may need reassurance, guidance, and normalization of common challenges. Both groups benefit from knowing that the organization remains available, invested, and supportive.

13.1.1 Why Post-Adoption Support Matters

Many returns occur not because adopters are unwilling, but because they feel overwhelmed, uncertain, or isolated. Early challenges – such as housetraining accidents, destructive behavior, vocalization, or difficulty integrating with resident pets – can feel alarming without context. Post-adoption support helps adopters:

- Feel confident that they made the right decision.
- Access help before challenges feel unmanageable.
- Understand what is normal during the adjustment period.
- Recognize when to intervene and when to give the pet time.

Reassurance alone can significantly increase retention.

13.1.2 Core Components of Post-Adoption Support

Every shelter, regardless of size or resources, can implement meaningful post-adoption support using scalable tools. At a minimum, organizations should offer support in the following forms:

Handouts (printed and/or digital).

Written materials allow adopters to revisit information at their own pace. Effective handouts may cover:

- Housetraining and litterbox basics.
- Enrichment, exercise, and routine building.

- Decompression and adjustment timelines.
- Introducing pets to children or resident animals.
- When, how, and where to seek professional help.
- Normal stress-related behaviors and how to manage them.

These materials may be created in-house and branded with the organization's identity. Alternatively, they can carefully be curated from reputable sources that emphasize humane, science-based practices.

13.1.2.1 Video Tutorials

Short, accessible videos can be particularly helpful for visual learners and busy families. Topics may include:

- Reading basic body language.
- Setting up a safe space at home.
- Managing common early challenges.
- Using enrichment tools and puzzle feeders.
- Teaching foundational skills with positive reinforcement.

Videos can reduce the need for repeated explanations and ensure consistent messaging.

13.1.3 Helplines (Phone, App, or Email Support)

A dedicated post-adoption helpline – whether staffed by trained team members or volunteers – can create a vital safety net. Knowing that help is only a call or email away can prevent impulsive decisions during stressful moments.

For organizations without in-house trainers or behavior specialists, a scripted response guide addressing the most common post-adoption questions can be invaluable. These scripts help ensure that adopters receive calm, consistent, and supportive guidance while allowing team members to recognize when a concern may be escalating.

13.1.4 Commitment to Humane, Evidence-Based Guidance

All post-adoption materials and conversations should promote positive reinforcement-based training methods. The use of punitive techniques or aversive equipment should be actively discouraged, as these approaches are associated with increased fear, anxiety, and aggression directed toward caregivers or family members (Herron et al. 2009), as well as overall deterioration of the human–animal bond between the pet and its owner (Kwan and Bain 2013).

Clear guidance on what *not* to do is just as important as instruction on what *to* do. Many adopters turn to online sources or well-meaning acquaintances for advice, which may include outdated or harmful practices. By proactively providing evidence-based alternatives, shelters protect both the pet and the adopter relationship.

13.1.5 Training the Team for Consistent Support

Post-adoption support is only as effective as the people delivering it. Team members and volunteers should be trained to:

- Avoid minimizing adopter concerns.
- Use empathetic, nonjudgmental language.

- Normalize common post-adoption challenges.
- Reinforce that help-seeking is encouraged, not discouraged.
- Recognize when referral to a trainer, veterinarian, or behavior professional is needed.

Consistency matters. Mixed messages erode trust, while calm, predictable support strengthens confidence and loyalty to the organization.

13.1.6 Building a Lifelong Relationship

Post-adoption support transforms the shelter from a one-time service provider into a long-term partner. It reinforces that the organization's commitment does not end at adoption but continues for the lifetime of the pet. This relationship benefits everyone involved, adopters feel supported, pets remain in stable homes, and shelters see improved retention, stronger community trust and better overall outcomes.

Despite best efforts, shelters can only control some of the factors that influence post-adoption success; changes in housing, finances, health, family dynamics, and life circumstances remain outside the organization's control and can affect outcomes even when strong support systems are in place. Keeping pets in their homes is not about preventing returns at all costs, it is about supporting people early, honestly, and compassionately, so fewer returns are needed.

13.2 What Adopters Can Do to Support a Successful Dog Adoptions

Adoption is a relationship, not a transaction. One of the most important things adopters can do – before ever selecting a pet – is to be honest with themselves about their readiness, expectations, and lifestyle. This self-reflection lays the groundwork for long-term success.

The authors often frame this question simply: **"Do you want a dog—or do you want *this* dog?"**

In practice, many adopters do not begin their search by thinking, *"I would like to adopt a dog – let's see which dog best fits my lifestyle."* Instead, they see a particular dog online or in the shelter and feel an immediate emotional connection. A photograph, a short video, or a brief interaction in a kennel can feel like love at first sight. This emotional response is powerful and entirely human, and it can lead to wonderful adoptions.

However, selecting a pet based solely on an instant connection can also carry risks. When adopters fall in love with a specific dog first, they may be less open to considering whether that dog's needs, energy level, behavioral challenges, or long-term management requirements truly align with their lifestyle. The desire to "*make it work*" can unintentionally override realistic self-assessment.

Adoption is most successful when emotional connection is paired with thoughtful reflection. Counselors should help adopters pause and consider whether they are able and willing to adapt to what *this* dog needs, rather than expecting the dog to adapt to an idealized vision of life in the home. In some cases, remaining open to different sizes, ages, appearances, or even species may lead to a more sustainable and fulfilling match.

Love at first sight can be the beginning of a strong bond, but long-term success depends on compatibility, flexibility, and informed commitment, not just the initial spark. Choosing *this* dog may come with specific needs, limitations, or management requirements that do not perfectly align with an adopter's original vision. The critical question then becomes: *Can you adapt to what this dog needs?* Or would you be better served by staying open to differences in appearance, size, age – or even species – when searching for the right match?

Being flexible in expectations often leads to stronger, more resilient relationships. Once a pet has been chosen, preparation is key. Bringing a new animal home is exciting, but it is also a disruption to normal routines for both people and pets. Thoughtful planning helps ease this transition and supports success for everyone involved.

13.2.1 Establishing a Consistent Routine for Success

13.2.1.1 Create a Predictable Home Base

Adopters should establish a consistent setup from the start. This may include:

- An exercise pen or crate.
- A designated sleeping area such as a dog bed.
- A quiet space where the dog can rest undisturbed.

Dogs should be calmly rewarded for choosing and resting in the dedicated area. Many shelter dogs are not crate trained, and crates should be introduced gradually and positively. At night, dogs should be confined in a crate, exercise pen, or the bedroom with the adopter to prevent wandering, inappropriate elimination, or chewing. Many dogs will naturally adjust their sleep schedule to match their owners'.

13.2.1.2 Housetraining and Elimination Routines

All dogs – especially newly adopted ones – benefit from a clear, consistent elimination schedule.

- Puppies: A general rule of thumb is that a puppy can hold their bladder for roughly their age in months ±1 hour.
  - For example, a two-month-old puppy will typically need to eliminate every two to three hours.
  - Adopters should plan frequent outdoor trips and, if a yard is not available, provide an appropriate indoor elimination option such as potty pads.
- Adult dogs: Most adult dogs should be taken out every three to four hours initially.

  Adopters should:

- Use a consistent elimination cue.
- Reward the dog immediately *after* elimination with food or praise.
- Take the dog out after meals and right before bedtime and upon waking up.
- Closely monitor for early signs of needing to eliminate (sniffing, pacing, whining, heading toward doors, and squatting).

Accidents are part of the learning process. Punishment for indoor accidents should be avoided, as it can increase fear and anxiety around elimination.

13.2.1.3 Exercise, Play, and Independence

Dogs need a balance of activity, enrichment, and rest. Adopters should:

- Schedule structured and appropriate play sessions.
- Set consistent times for exercise (walks, yard play, and hikes).
- Provide independent enrichment opportunities such as safe chew items and puzzle toys.

Toys should be rotated every two to three days, offering two to four different types made from varied materials to maintain novelty and engagement (see Chapter 8 for additional enrichment guidance).

Keep in mind that teaching a dog to settle independently is just as important as play and exercise.

13.2.1.4 Building Comfort with Being Alone

Gradual exposure to brief separations helps prevent distress:

- Start by leaving the dog alone for one to two minutes in another room.
- Repeat two to three short sessions daily, gradually increasing duration over weeks.
- Practice brief departures from the home once the dog is comfortable indoors.

Many adopters use home cameras to observe how their dog responds when alone. Signs such as vocalizing, pacing, panting, or scratching at doors and windows may indicate separation distress. Early intervention is encouraged, and adopters should seek professional guidance if these signs appear.

13.2.1.5 Training and Social Learning

Adopters should be encouraged to enroll in training classes. Even experienced dog owners benefit from structured classes, which:

- Build confidence in new environments.
- Provide safe exposure to people and other dogs.
- Strengthen communication between dog and owner.
- Help prevent small challenges from becoming larger problems.

Training classes support both learning and relationship-building and are an excellent investment in long-term success.

13.2.1.6 A Shared Responsibility for Success

Adopters play a central role in making adoption work. Honest self-assessment, flexibility in expectations, and proactive preparation help ensure that the relationship starts on solid footing. By meeting pets where they are – and committing to consistent routines, patience, and learning – adopters greatly increase the likelihood of a stable, rewarding bond that benefits both the animal and the family for years to come.

13.3 What Adopters Can Do to Support a Successful Cat Adoption

While breed and size are often less influential in cats than in dogs, successful feline adoptions still depend heavily on thoughtful self-assessment, realistic expectations, and preparation. Cats vary widely in age, energy level, sociability, medical needs, and tolerance for change. Taking time to reflect on these factors *before* adoption significantly improves the likelihood of a lasting match.

13.3.1 Choosing the Right Cat for Your Lifestyle

Adopters should begin by asking honest questions about their home, schedule, and preferences:

- Kitten or adult?
  Kittens are active, curious, and require significant time for supervision, play, and training. Adult and senior cats often have more predictable personalities and lower activity needs, which may better suit quieter households or busy adopters.

- Single cat or multiple cats?
  Some kittens benefit from being adopted in pairs, particularly if there are no other cats in the home. In contrast, some adult cats prefer to be the only cat. Understanding existing pets and household dynamics is essential.
- Energy level and interaction needs
  Highly energetic cats require daily interactive play and creative enrichment. Adopters should consider whether they enjoy playing, engaging, and inventing new enrichment activities or whether a more independent, lower-energy cat would be a better fit.
- Medical considerations
  Adopters should reflect on their capacity to manage medical needs. For example, a cat with Feline immunodeficiency virus (FIV) may be an excellent choice for a single-cat household, while other medical conditions may require ongoing care, medication, or monitoring.
- Behavioral considerations
  If adopting a cat with known behavioral challenges, adopters must be willing to follow recommended management strategies – such as using specific litter types or adding additional litter boxes – to support success.
- Affection preferences
  Some people want a highly cuddly cat; others are perfectly content with a "see-but-don't-touch" companion. Neither preference is wrong, but mismatches between expectation and personality often lead to frustration. Being honest about what kind of relationship is desired is critical.

The hardest and most important work happens *before* adoption: identifying what can realistically be provided rather than what is hoped for. Adoption counselors can help guide this reflection, but the most successful adoptions occur when adopters enter the shelter already knowing what they are looking for.

13.3.2 Establishing a Consistent Routine for Success

13.3.2.1 Preparing the Home for a New Cat

Preparation before the cat arrives home reduces stress and helps the transition go smoothly.

Litter Box Setup

Adopters should be counseled on proper litter box selection and placement:

- Clean litter boxes 1–2 times daily
- Use 2–4 inches of unscented clumping litter
- Provide one litter box per cat plus one additional box
- In multi-story homes, place at least one litter box per floor
- Place boxes in quiet, low-traffic areas, avoiding hallways or entryways
- Kittens may start with smaller boxes, but as they grow, boxes should be at least 1.5 times the length of the cat

Appropriate litter management is one of the most effective ways to prevent litter box issues, especially in multicat households or cats with known sensitivities.

13.3.2.2 Feeding, Enrichment, and Daily Routine

Cats thrive when their natural behaviors are supported.

- Feeding
  Cats benefit from multiple small meals (3–5 per day) to mimic natural hunting patterns. In the wild, cats may spend 17–46% of their time seeking food (Beaver 2003; Horwitz et al. 2009).

  - Dry food can be offered in puzzle feeders to encourage foraging.
  - Wet food can be divided into small portions and placed in multiple locations to promote "food hunting."
- Play and exercise
  Cats should receive 10–15 minutes of high-intensity interactive play daily – running, jumping, and stalking – using toys such as wand or fishing-pole toys. Toys should be rotated every two to three days, offering two to four different types each time to maintain novelty.
- Training and mental stimulation
  Some cats enjoy and benefit from clicker training, particularly food-motivated individuals. Training can improve confidence, strengthen the human–animal bond, and provide mental enrichment.

13.3.2.3 Environmental Enrichment and Resource Distribution

A well-designed environment reduces stress and supports emotional wellbeing:

- Provide multiple resting areas using beds of different materials.
- Offer cat trees, perches, and elevated spaces to promote safety and confidence.
- Include hides, covered beds, or simple cardboard boxes.
- Supply multiple scratching options, including vertical posts and cardboard scratchers.
- In multicat households, distribute resources throughout the home to reduce competition (Figure 13.1; Box 13.1).

In summary, selecting a new family member is a complex and deeply personal decision. Adoption choices are influenced by many factors, including the pet's appearance, sociability, behavioral history, and the adopter's lifestyle, experiences and biases. Trained team members play a crucial role in facilitating thoughtful matchmaking by helping adopters reflect honestly on their needs and capacities.

Open, effective communication – paired with transparency, realistic expectation setting, and supportive language – improves the adopter experience, reduces returns, and strengthens trust between shelters and their communities. When adopters are prepared, homes are ready and support continues beyond adoption day, both pets and people are far more likely to thrive together in their new life.

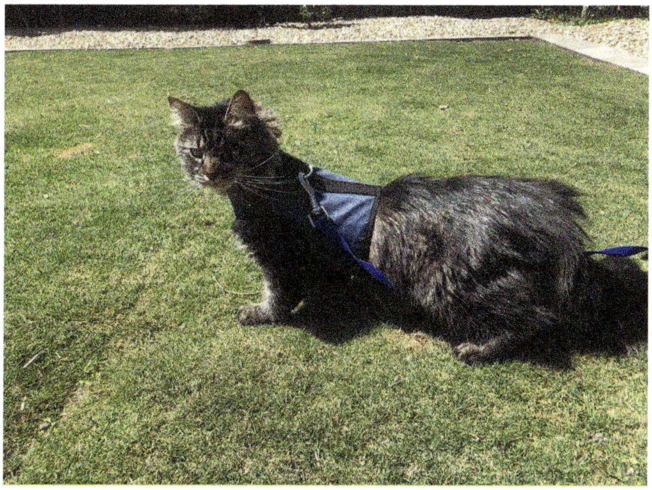

Figure 13.1 Cat in Harness

Box 13.1 Adventure Cats

Some adopters are interested in so-called **adventure cats** – cats that are trained and comfortable exploring the outdoors on leash, in backpacks, or during carefully curated outings. While these experiences can be enriching and fun for both cat and caregiver, they are only appropriate for cats with confident, outgoing temperaments that genuinely enjoy novelty and handling. Not every cat is suited for this role, making thoughtful matching essential for safety, welfare, and long-term success.

13.4 The Role of the General Practice Veterinarian

While shelters and adopters play central roles in making adoptions successful and keeping pets out of shelters, the general practice (GP) veterinarian is a critical and often underrecognized partner in this effort. GP veterinarians are uniquely positioned at the intersection of animal health, behavior, and caregiver capacity. Their relationship with adopters often begins within the first days or weeks after adoption, precisely when stress, uncertainty and adjustment challenges are most likely to surface.

Thoughtful, compassionate veterinary guidance during this vulnerable transition period can normalize common post-adoption challenges, prevent misinterpretation of stress-related behaviors, and redirect families away from frustration or blame. By providing early medical oversight, reinforcing realistic expectations, identifying emerging medical or behavioral concerns, and guiding families toward appropriate support, GP veterinarians can dramatically influence whether an adoption stabilizes or begins to unravel.

Private veterinary practices have an enormous and often underestimated impact on overall animal welfare. According to the 2023–2024 APPA National Pet Owners Survey, approximately 65.1 million U.S. households own at least one dog (American Pet Products Association 2023). In contrast, an estimated 6.5 million animals enter U.S. shelters annually. Even allowing for uncertainty in these figures, the disparity is striking: shelter animals represent only a small fraction of the total companion animal population receiving care in private veterinary practice.

This perspective underscores the critical role GP veterinarians play long before a pet ever enters a shelter. GP veterinarians are frequently the first and sometimes only professional resource available to pet owners when concerns arise. Through preventive care, early behavioral guidance, and timely intervention for emerging medical or emotional issues, veterinarians can help address problems before they escalate to the point of relinquishment.

Central to this impact is the veterinarian–client–patient relationship (VCPR). A strong VCPR fosters trust, open communication and collaborative problem-solving. When owners feel supported and heard, they are more likely to seek help early, adhere to recommendations, and remain committed during challenging periods. By identifying risks, offering reassurance and knowing when to refer for additional behavioral or medical support, GP veterinarians serve as a critical line of defense in keeping pets in their homes.

Because GP veterinarians are primarily focused on the daily care, evaluation, and treatment of owned animals, they understandably may not have the time or opportunity to consider the broader shelter population in their routine clinical work. This chapter aims to encourage veterinarians to think beyond the "shelter box" in order to recognize that their decisions can profoundly influence the welfare and outcomes of shelter animals. As a practitioner who bridges both private practice and shelter medicine, my goal is to raise awareness of how a veterinarian's actions or inactions can shape an animal's fate even before it enters the shelter system.

By educating clients about responsible pet ownership, including the importance of spaying and neutering, microchipping, and preventive health, veterinarians can directly influence community animal welfare. Furthermore, private practices play a critical role beyond routine veterinary care. They can provide medical and behavioral guidance that help reduce shelter intake, give post-adoption support, and improve adoption success.

It is important to recognize that an estimated 50–80% of shelter animals – a minimum of 3.2 million pets each year (exact figures vary by state and shelter system) – will eventually return to the owned pet population, either through reunification with their families or adoption into new homes (ASPCA 2024). In this way, shelter animals ultimately remain part of our collective patient population, reinforcing the idea that the connection between GP and shelter medicine is not separate but continuous.

Animals that are not adopted may be placed with rescue groups, transferred to other shelters, or sanctuaries or, in some cases, humanely euthanized. Regardless of the resolution, these animals continue to require veterinary oversight and care. GP veterinarians can play a vital role in this process by partnering with shelters, rescues, and sanctuaries caring for these animals and providing medical expertise, guidance, and support. Their involvement helps ensure that even animals outside of traditional adoption pathways receive compassionate and evidence-based care.

By applying the Pareto principle (1896) – often called the 80/20 rule, which suggests that roughly 80% of outcomes come from 20% of efforts – GP veterinarians can prioritize the small set of high-impact interventions that meaningfully reduce shelter admissions and improve animal wellbeing. High-impact strategies include supporting spay/neuter initiatives to decrease the number of unwanted litters, participating in trap–neuter–return (TNR) programs for community cats and offering (discounted) post-adoption examinations to ensure successful transitions into new homes. Additionally, focusing on pet retention efforts, such as addressing early behavioral and medical concerns, helps prevent animals from being surrendered in the first place.

By prioritizing these key areas, GP veterinarians can make a measurable difference by reducing admissions, improving welfare, and increasing positive outcomes for shelter pets and the communities they serve.

There are approximately 4100 brick-and-mortar animal shelters in the United States caring for an estimated 6 million homeless animals each year (Shelter Animals Count 2025). This means that, in theory, on average, each shelter will accommodate around 730 animals for adoption (assuming a 50% adoption rate) and another 730 animals on a temporary or long-term basis, awaiting reunification with an owner, transfer to another organization, or humane euthanasia due to medical, behavioral, or space limitations.

In contrast, as of 2025, there were an estimated 34,296 small animal veterinary practices in the United States (American Veterinary Medical Association 2025). If each of these practices could prevent just 100 adoptable pets per year from entering shelters – through early intervention, client education, and proactive care – the number of homeless animals would drop dramatically.

Reducing shelter admissions do not only relieve overcrowding but also allow shelters to direct resources sustainably toward treatment, enrichment, and rehabilitation for the pets in their care. This approach supports better health and behavioral outcomes, decreases stress, and increases adoption success. Ultimately, prevention and retention strategies strengthen the human–animal bond and improve the overall welfare and the quality of life for animals within the community. Additionally, these animals stay in the community and remain patients of the clinic, providing job security and representing good business sense for the GP veterinarian.

Through collaboration with shelters, ongoing education of adopters and proactive support during key transition periods, GP veterinarians become powerful allies in sustaining adoptions. Their role strengthens the human–animal bond, improves individual welfare outcomes, and contributes meaningfully to reducing shelter intake, benefiting animals, families, and the sheltering system as a whole.

13.4.1 Five Ways Veterinary Practitioners Play an Active Role in the Shelter Case Trajectory Strategy

13.4.1.1 Population Control

An obvious solution to pet overpopulation is surgical sterilization, which involves removing the gonads and thereby eliminating reproductive capacity. Most veterinarians are well-trained and comfortable performing spay and neuter surgeries on dogs and cats. A wide variety of accepted techniques exist for both male and female animals. Whether to perform ovariohysterectomy (OVH) or ovariectomy (OVE) for females or a pre-scrotal vs. a scrotal procedure for neutering depends on the size, age, and preference of the surgeon. It is important to understand that each of these procedures comes with risks, benefits as well as potential complications (Peeters and Kirpensteijn 2011; Lee et al. 2013; Pereira et al. 2018).

GP veterinarians should discuss the benefits and risks of sterilization with owners of intact pets as early as possible. In my experience, the initial puppy or kitten visit is the most effective time to introduce this topic. My goal is to understand the owner's perspective on sterilization and assess their knowledge about the procedure, all in a nonjudgmental and educational manner. Early discussions also allow for individualized recommendations regarding the optimal timing of gonadectomy, which may vary depending on the species, breed, and specific circumstances.

In some cases, the cost of surgical sterilization at a GP exceeds pet owners' budgets. Low-cost spay/neuter clinics may be available in your area. Ideally, a GP veterinarian should be familiar with such resources and direct clients to such resources if requested. Low-cost veterinary clinics that specialize in spay/neuter procedures, such as those offered by local municipal shelters, and animal non-profit organizations, are good places to start. While costs are typically lower than at a veterinary clinic, wait times may be significantly longer. Owners should be educated about the importance of scheduling such procedures way in advance.

A pet's shelter journey can be profoundly influenced by whether it has been sterilized prior to entering a shelter. Studies estimate that between 53% and 83% of dogs in shelters originally entered as strays (Wenstrup and Dowidchuk 1999; Lepper et al. 2002; Marston et al. 2004). Intact pets are at a significantly higher risk of roaming, becoming lost or being surrendered due to behavioral and management challenges (Hart and Hart 1985; Patronek et al. 1996a,b; Neilson et al. 1997; New et al. 2000; Weiss et al. 2012). Furthermore, neutered animals are more likely to be successfully reunited with their owners, highlighting the role of sterilization not only in population control, but also in improving individual animal welfare and shelter outcomes.

As stray dogs and cats enter the shelter without a history of their reproductive status, determining whether or not they have already been spayed or neutered can be challenging. This is particularly true for female pets. There are times when the scars left by a spay procedure are difficult to see or palpate in female animals. Moreover, an abdominal scar does not necessarily indicate that a pet has been altered. Abdominal surgery could have been performed for another medical reason. Although two palpable testicles indicate that a male pet is intact, the absence of these findings does not prove neuter status, since the male could be a cryptorchid (testicles in the abdominal or inguinal area). A greater amount of time and resources must be devoted to animals that are intact or presumed to be intact.

An effective and simple method for identifying sterilized animals is to use a standardized permanent visible identifier, which is easily recognizable during the shelter's admissions examination. This method can be used by any veterinarian to influence shelter pets' journey. As a result of such tattoos, animals with alter status can bypass the shelter's spay-neuter (SN) pathway and can be moved directly to the adoption pathway or returned to their owners without further process or fines. Most well-run shelters can reduce LOS for animals by two to seven days with this simple identification process. Even though it may not seem like much for an individual animal, when this number is multiplied by an average daily shelter population, it can easily add up to hundreds of care days per year.

In summary, altered animals that are clearly identified by a tattoo will save the shelter time and resources, allowing the organization to focus on addressing animals in need. Additionally, it will improve a pet's overall health and wellbeing by not undergoing another unnecessary surgical procedure. It is therefore imperative that veterinarians who perform surgical sterilization on owned and unowned pets tattoo a small, permanent marker that identifies them as altered. According to a survey of private veterinary practices, 5% of veterinarians tattooed owned dogs and cats and 11% tattooed unowned pets during sterilization (Mielo et al. 2022). This suggests significant changes could be made for the fate of shelter pets. This simple green line, which can be applied in seconds on the abdomen of male and female pets during surgery, has a significant impact on animal welfare.

Several techniques can be used for applying ink, and standardized locations are recommended regardless of where the incision is made (Griffin et al. 2016). Male dogs should have their tattoos placed parallel to the prepuce in the pre-scrotal region. Whether a flank approach to OVH is used for female cats, female dogs, or male cats, the recommended tattoo site is on the ventral abdomen just caudal to the umbilicus. In male cats, the ventral midline is selected because a common error during surgical preparation is to mistake a neutered male cat for a female. The tattoo will be visible upon shaving for a spay surgery or exploration for cryptorchidism (Box 13.2).

A sterilization tattoo is applied postoperatively adjacent to the incision in female cats and female dogs, on the ventral midline in male cats and in the pre-scrotal region in male dogs. In this technique, the surgical blade from the surgery is used to make a short, shallow incision through the dermis. By using a disposable sterile item such as a paper sterility identifier strip or a toothpick, a small amount of green tattoo paste is applied and the incision is sealed with glue.

Ear tipping is another visual identifier widely used for sterilized cats, particularly in community cat and TNR programs. It provides a clear indicator that a cat has been altered and can often be seen from a distance, helping caregivers and volunteers quickly identify sterilized individuals.

It is important that the ear tip is sufficiently large to be easily visible, especially in long-haired cats. In regions with cold temperatures, care should be taken to differentiate between an intentionally tipped ear and frostbite, as frost-damaged tissue can resemble an ear tip. Proper technique and postoperative monitoring help ensure the tip remains a reliable marker of sterilization.

Box 13.2 Tattoo Male Cats After Castration

Tattoo males too please – This procedure is just as significant for males as for females.

Cryptorchidism: during castration surgery, remove the retained testicle first, followed by the descended testicle. The tattoo should be applied after the surgery is completed and after BOTH gonads have been successfully removed.

13.4.1.2 Pet ID

Visual pet identification (tags and collars) and microchipping together with spay and neuter have been demonstrated to be important tools in reuniting lost pets with their owners (Lord et al. 2007; Weiss et al. 2011). Microchipping is a permanent identification method and can't be lost or easily removed. This increases the likelihood of reuniting lost pets with their owners, as shelters and veterinarians can quickly access the contact information associated with the chip. Additionally, microchipping can serve as proof of ownership. Pet owners in private practice need to be educated about the importance of identification. A microchip is an electronic transponder enclosed in a glass cylinder implanted under the skin of a pet, usually in the neck/interscapular region. Microchips transmit individual identification numbers when activated by waving a scanner over corresponding body areas. An identification number appears on the screen of the scanning wand. By educating owners on the importance of tags and permanent identification with implanted microchips, GP veterinarians influence the shelter pathway of a stray pet. Microchipped animals are far more likely to be returned to their owners, according to a study of more than 7,700 stray animals at animal shelters in 23 states. Microchipped stray dogs were returned to their owners at a rate more than twice that of all stray dogs. Even more dramatic was the difference in return rates for stray cats.

The American Veterinary Medical Association recommends veterinarians scan patients' microchips at least once a year. At that time owners can be reminded that it is important to register the chip and to maintain up-to-date identification tags on the pet's collar along with microchips for permanent identification. When microchipped animals weren't returned to their owners, errors or disconnected owners' telephone numbers were the most common reasons (Box 13.3).

13.4.1.3 Preventatives

These regular wellness exams are essential in establishing a relationship between the owner and veterinarian. When assessing an apparently healthy animal regularly, the veterinarian can inquire about any physical and behavioral health concerns that owners may not bring to a veterinarian's attention at a sick exam or until it is too late for intervention. It is only through this relationship that an owner can reach out for expert guidance if he is thinking about surrendering his pet. A veterinarian can also provide advice and ensure that pets are healthy and receive the best possible chance to remain in their homes.

Most of a GP veterinarian's time is spent discussing preventative care for pets in homes, knowing that regular preventative care can help to ensure the pet lives a long and healthy life. Vaccination against the most prevalent infectious diseases and prevention of parasitic conditions are probably the two most important topics veterinary professionals discuss on a daily basis. Veterinarians are crucial in ensuring vaccine efficacy by administering vaccinations correctly and at the appropriate time.

Vaccines are an important tool in the fight against many infectious diseases and are an essential tool for disease control and animal welfare. Vaccines are a necessity for all pets in homes to prevent illness, but the importance of adequate immunization for animals entering a shelter cannot be

Box 13.3 Tip Box

Offer microchipping as an automatic part of puppy visits or sterilization procedures, allowing owners to opt out rather than opt in. This approach increases uptake and helps ensure more pets can be reunited if lost. Be sure to educate owners about the importance of registering the microchip after it is implanted, as an unregistered chip cannot help return their pet home.

overstated. For this reason, some shelters have changed their intake requirements and will ask for an animal to be vaccinated at least two weeks before admission if at all possible. Consequently, the welfare of all shelter animals can be greatly improved.

It is imperative to vaccinate animals against highly contagious diseases, especially when they are in close contact with other animals. In some shelters, the constant turnover of animals and the need for group housing introduce various pathogens, making vaccination absolutely essential for maintaining shelter populations' health. Shelters are generally considered "high-risk environments" because they often house large numbers of animals in close proximity, increasing the likelihood of disease transmission. Additionally, animals in shelters are likely stressed, which can weaken their immune systems and make them more susceptible to infections. Vaccinations are the most effective way to keep animals healthy. The most cost-effective way of preventing infectious diseases in shelters is to prevent them through vaccinations.

Parasitic infectious diseases can also be easily avoided by regular preventative care. High-density housing such as in shelters can lead to infections and skin irritations. These are very common problems caused by fleas and other external parasites that infests dogs and cats. In the United States, flea allergy dermatitis (FAD) is the most common dermatological disease in dogs (Dryden 2024). The likelihood of developing FAD in dogs with atopic dermatitis is increased. Besides transmitting tapeworms, fleas can also cause anemia in young and sick animals and infest the environment. Geographical and seasonal differences affect tick exposure and tick-borne diseases. Heartworm disease can be fatal, and treating this condition is time-consuming, costly, and painful. Fortunately, heartworm infections are completely preventable.

Provided with proper preventative care, any pet can live longer in the home, but in a shelter, the chances of it surviving are multiplied. General practitioners can significantly influence the fate and welfare of animals that might enter shelters by ensuring their patient population stays up to date on core vaccinations and anti-parasitics. These preventative protocols not only support the overall health and stability of the community's pet population but may also reduce shelter intake due to preventable illnesses (Box 13.4).

13.4.1.4 Training and Behavior Support

Supporting humane training methods and providing behavior resources, incorporating positive reinforcement techniques, such as rewarding desired behaviors with treats or praise, is not only a very effective approach to training pets, it also improves the human–animal bond between the pet and its owner (Kwan and Bain 2013). Next to medical conditions, behavior concerns are a major reason for surrendering to a shelter (Patronek et al. 1996a; Scarlett et al. 1999; Salman et al. 2000; Wells and Hepper 2000; Christensen et al. 2007; Jensen et al. 2020; Kisley et al. 2024).

It is crucial that owners are educated early on about the importance of utilizing humane training tools and positive reinforcement, best discussed during their puppy's or kitten's first presentation at the clinic. The result is a significantly higher chance to stay in the home. It may not be feasible for a GP veterinarian without the time or expertise to coach pet owners, but clinics can provide accessible resources, support qualified positive reinforcement trainers, and refer owners early on to veterinary behaviorists to foster a community focused on humane animal training

Box 13.4 Quote

"Just because it's routine doesn't mean it's not essential," Animal Humane Society's Chief Veterinarian, Dr. Graham Brayshaw.

Box 13.5 Resources

Find a veterinary behaviorist here: https://www.dacvb.org/.

How to find a trainer here: https://www.ccpdt.org/dog-owners/certified-dog-trainer-directory/.

methods. In addition, practicing and demonstrating such techniques in the clinic will help build trust between veterinarians and owners. This will reduce the risk of owners relying on aversive techniques. Ultimately, this can result in improved animal welfare for pets (Box 13.5).

13.4.1.5 Veterinary Care Costs

Our clients' financial constraints are a daily reality for veterinarians. It is heartbreaking to witness owners unable to afford needed medical treatments or procedures because they are unaware of the costs involved in caring for pets. A rise in veterinary health care costs often puts pets at risk for premature euthanasia or surrender to shelters (Croney et al. 2025). The owners of animals that require extensive, financial-intensive, or long-term medical treatment may believe that they are not capable care takers and a shelter will be able to provide the care and find a new home for the pet. Although some shelters can handle extensive medical cases, most are not equipped to do so. As a result, animals surrendered to shelters for medical reasons often suffer poor welfare. Caretaker burden on owners with animals diagnosed with complex problems should be openly discussed and realistic options should be considered. In some cases, owners should be given the option or permission to euthanize an animal with a poor prognosis. It is also important to allow pet owners to make informed decisions about their pet's health that are financially feasible and within their budget.

In the event of an unexpected veterinary bill resulting from an animal's illness or injury, pet insurance can be an excellent way to keep them in their homes. It helps alleviate the financial burden on pet owners, allowing them to afford necessary treatments without stressing about high costs. Pet insurance also gives owners peace of mind, knowing they can provide the best possible care for their animals. Additionally, some care plans cover preventative care and therefore encourage proactive health management. As part of my standard history, I ask about pet insurance information upfront. It provides pet owners with a clear understanding of their financial responsibilities and options. This proactive approach can lead to quicker decision-making during a potential emergency, ensuring pets receive timely care. Owners are often surprised when I tell them I have pet insurance for my own pets. This frequently prompts a conversation about veterinary care costs, especially in an emergency situation. I then suggest that clients without pet insurance do some research into the various available options to learn if that is something they should consider. The importance of securing pet insurance while pets are still healthy cannot be overstated, as most policies do not cover preexisting conditions. Having this foresight may ultimately save pet owners from unexpected expenses and prevent surrender or premature euthanasia.

Many veterinary clinics offer financial support options such as third-party credit programs that can be used for routine care or unexpected needs, including surgery or advanced treatment, when clients qualify. Access to these options can provide pet owners with reassurance and flexibility during stressful situations. For individuals who do not qualify for credit-based assistance, grants, subsidies, or community-based support programs may be available. Establishing strong relationships with local organizations dedicated to helping pets and their families during financial hardship is an important component of comprehensive care.

Equally important is the thoughtful use of a spectrum of care approach. While it is appropriate to present the gold-standard diagnostic and treatment plan, veterinarians should also be prepared to discuss alternative, medically sound options when cost is a limiting factor. Offering tiered levels of care – clearly explaining what each option includes, its benefits, limitations, and potential outcomes – allows clients to make informed decisions without feeling judged or dismissed. When pet owners believe that inability to afford the most extensive or expensive option makes them "bad" caregivers, they may disengage entirely. A spectrum of care model preserves the VCPR, supports animal welfare and often prevents delayed care, relinquishment, or euthanasia driven by financial distress.

In summary, the role of the GP veterinarian in the shelter journey of a surrendered pet cannot be overestimated. Fortunately, only a small proportion of the pet population ever experiences shelter life, but even one avoidable shelter stay is one too many. Simple interventions – such as spay/neuter, proper preventative care, and identification – can significantly change an animal's fate, improve animal wellbeing, and reduce LOS in a shelter.

References

American Pet Products Association (2023). *2023–2024 APPA National Pet Owners Survey*. Stamford, CT: American Pet Products Association.

American Veterinary Medical Association (2025). *2025 AVMA Report on the Economic State of the Veterinary Profession*. Schaumburg, IL: American Veterinary Medical Association.

ASPCA (2024). Pet statistics: shelter intake and surrender [online]. Available at: https://www.aspca.org/animal-homelessness/shelter-intake-and-surrender/pet-statistics (accessed 31 January 2026).

Beaver, B.V. (2003). *Feline Behavior: A Guide for Veterinarians*, 2e. Philadelphia: Saunders.

Christensen, E., Scarlett, J., Campagna, M. et al. (2007). Aggressive behavior in adopted dogs that passed a temperament test. *Applied Animal Behaviour Science* 106: 85–95. https://doi.org/10.1016/j.applanim.2006.07.002.

Croney, C., Applebaum, J.W., Delgado, M., and Stella, J. (2025). How does access to veterinary care relate to animal welfare? *Advances in Small Animal Care* 6 (1): 209–221. https://doi.org/10.1016/j.yasa.2025.06.014.

Dryden, M.W. (2024). Flea allergy dermatitis in dogs and cats [online]. MSD Veterinary Manual. Available at: https://www.msdvetmanual.com/integumentary-system/fleas-and-flea-allergy-dermatitis/flea-allergy-dermatitis-in-dogs-and-cats (accessed 1 February 2026).

Griffin, B., Bushby, P.A., McCobb, E. et al. (2016). The Association of Shelter Veterinarians' 2016 Veterinary Medical Care Guidelines for Spay-Neuter Programs. *Journal of the American Veterinary Medical Association* 249 (2): 165–188.

Hart, B.L. and Hart, L.A. (1985). Selecting pet dogs on the basis of cluster analysis of breed behavior profiles and gender. *Journal of the American Veterinary Medical Association* 186 (11): 1181–1185.

Herron, M.E., Shofer, F.S., and Reisner, I.R. (2009). Survey of the use and outcome of confrontational and non-confrontational training methods in client-owned dogs showing undesired behaviors. *Applied Animal Behaviour Science* 117 (1–2): 47–54. https://doi.org/10.1016/j.applanim.2008.12.011.

Horwitz, D., Soulard, Y., and Junien-Castagna, A. (2009). The feeding behavior of the cat. In: *Encyclopedia of Feline Clinical Nutrition* (ed. P. Pibot, V. Biourge, and D.A. Elliott), 441–453. Royal Canin.

Jensen, J.B.H., Sandøe, P., and Nielsen, S.S. (2020). Owner-related reasons matter more than behavioural problems—a study of why owners relinquished dogs and cats to a Danish animal shelter from 1996 to 2017. *Animals* 10: 1064. https://doi.org/10.3390/ani10061064.

Kisley, M.A., Chung, E.J., and Levitt, H. (2024). Investigating the reasons behind companion animal relinquishment: a systematic content analysis of shelter records for cats and dogs, 2018–2023. *Animals* 14: 2606. https://doi.org/10.3390/ani14172606.

Kwan, J.Y. and Bain, M.J. (2013). Owner attachment and problem behaviors related to relinquishment and training techniques of dogs. *Journal of Applied Animal Welfare Science* 16 (2): 128–183. https://doi.org/10.1080/10888705.2013.768923.

Lee, S.-S., Lee, S.-Y., Park, S.-J. et al. (2013). Comparison of ovariectomy and ovariohysterectomy in terms of postoperative pain behavior and surgical stress in dogs. *Journal of Veterinary Clinics* 30 (3): 166–171.

Lepper, M., Kass, P.H., and Hart, L.A. (2002). Prediction of adoption versus euthanasia among dogs and cats in a California animal shelter. *Journal of Applied Animal Welfare Science* 5 (1): 29–42.

Lord, L.K., Wittum, T.E., Ferketich, A.K. et al. (2007). Search methods that people use to find owners of lost pets. *Journal of the American Veterinary Medical Association* 230 (12): 1835–1840. https://doi.org/10.2460/javma.230.12.1835.

Marston, L.C., Bennett, P.C., and Coleman, G.J. (2004). What happens to shelter dogs? An analysis of data for 1 year from three Australian shelters. *Journal of Applied Animal Welfare Science* 7 (1): 27–47. https://doi.org/10.1207/s15327604jaws0701_2.

Mielo, M.R., Amirian, E.S., and Levy, J.K. (2022). Identification of spayed and neutered cats and dogs: Veterinary training and compliance with practice guidelines. *The Veterinary Journal 285*: 105856. https://doi.org/10.1016/j.tvjl.2022.105856.

Neilson, J.C., Eckstein, R.A., and Hart, B.L. (1997). Effects of castration on problem behaviors in male dogs with reference to age and duration of behavior. *Journal of the American Veterinary Medical Association 211* (2): 180–182. https://doi.org/10.2460/javma.1997.211.180.

New, J.C., Salman, M.D., King, M. et al. (2000). Characteristics of shelter-relinquished animals and their owners compared with animals and their owners in U.S. pet-owning households. *Journal of Applied Animal Welfare Science* 3 (3): 179–201. https://doi.org/10.1207/S15327604JAWS0303_03.

Pareto, V. (1896). *Cours d'économie politique*. Lausanne: F. Rouge.

Patronek, G.J., Glickman, L.T., Beck, A.M. et al. (1996a). Risk factors for relinquishment of cats to an animal shelter. *Journal of the American Veterinary Medical Association* 209 (3): 582–588.

Patronek, G.J., Glickman, L.T., Beck, A.M. et al. (1996b). Risk factors for relinquishment of dogs to an animal shelter. *Journal of the American Veterinary Medical Association* 209 (3): 572–581.

Peeters, M.E. and Kirpensteijn, J. (2011). Comparison of surgical variables and short-term postoperative complications in healthy dogs undergoing ovariohysterectomy or ovariectomy. *Journal of the American Veterinary Medical Association* 238 (2): 189–194. https://doi.org/10.2460/javma.238.2.189.

Pereira, M.A.A., Gonçalves, L.A., Evangelista, M.C. et al. (2018). Postoperative pain and short-term complications after two elective sterilization techniques: ovariohysterectomy or ovariectomy in cats. *BMC Veterinary Research* 14: 335. https://doi.org/10.1186/s12917-018-1657-z.

Salman, M.D., Hutchison, J., Ruch-Gallie, R. et al. (2000). Behavioral reasons for relinquishment of dogs and cats to 12 shelters. *Journal of Applied Animal Welfare Science* 3 (2): 93–106. https://doi.org/10.1207/s15327604jaws0302_2.

Scarlett, J.M., Salman, M.D., New, J.G. Jr., and Kass, P.H. (1999). Reasons for relinquishment of companion animals in U.S. animal shelters: selected health and personal issues. *Journal of Applied Animal Welfare Science* 2 (1): 41–57.

Shelter Animals Count (2024). *The State of Pet Sheltering in 2023: National Data Report*. [online] Available at: https://www.shelteranimalscount.org/data-reports (accessed 31 January 2026).

Thompson, K.F., McBride, E.A., and Redhead, E. (2010). Training engagement and the development of behaviour problems in the dog: a longitudinal study. *Journal of Veterinary Behaviour: Clinical Applications and Research* 5 (1): 57. https://doi.org/10.1016/j.jveb.2009.013.

Weiss, E., Slater, M.R., and Lord, L.K. (2011). Retention of provided identification for dogs and cats seen in veterinary clinics and adopted from shelters in Oklahoma City, OK, USA. *Preventive Veterinary Medicine* 101 (3–4): 265–269. https://doi.org/10.1016/j.prevetmed.2011.05.008.

Weiss, E., Slater, M., and Lord, L. (2012). Frequency of lost dogs and cats in the United States and the methods used to locate them. *Animals* 2 (2): 301–315. https://doi.org/10.3390/ani2020301.

Wells, D.L. and Hepper, P.G. (2000). Prevalence of behaviour problems reported by owners of dogs purchased from an animal rescue shelter. *Applied Animal Behaviour Science* 69: 55–65.

Wenstrup, T.R. and Dowidchuk, L. (1999). Pet overpopulation: data and measurement issues in shelters. *Journal of Applied Animal Welfare Science* 2 (4): 303–319. https://doi.org/10.1207/s15327604jaws0204_4.

14

Ethical and Legal Considerations of Modern Animal Sheltering

14.1 Ethical Dilemmas when Adopting Pets with Behavioral Disorders

Modern animal sheltering increasingly recognizes behavioral health as an integral component of animal welfare. However, placing pets with known or suspected behavioral dysregulations into adoptive homes presents complex ethical dilemmas that require careful, transparent, and humane decision-making.

Shelters increasingly encounter pets whose behavioral challenges extend beyond overt aggression and include severe fear and phobia, separation-related distress, compulsive behaviors, chronic anxiety, and generalized reactivity. Behavioral disorders may result in persistent psychological distress, impaired functioning, or an inability to cope not only with typical shelter but also a traditional home environment. These conditions can significantly compromise a pet's wellbeing while also creating care burdens for adopters.

Adopting out pets with significant behavioral disorders – especially aggression – raises serious ethical dilemmas for shelters, veterinary teams, and adopters. The decision is not simply about "*finding a home*" or finding the "*right*" home. These dilemmas often sit at the intersection of animal welfare, human safety, adopter rights and responsibilities, as well as organizational liability and societal trust.

Ethical evaluation must therefore consider not only the adoptability of the animal but also the likelihood that intervention will meaningfully improve quality of life within a reasonable timeframe. Ethical decision-making in such cases requires shelters to balance their lifesaving mission with their duty to provide humane care, prevent foreseeable harm, and allocate limited organizational resources responsibly.

Prolonged confinement, repeated placement attempts, or ineffective treatment plans may unintentionally exacerbate suffering rather than resolve it. Resource allocation is an unavoidable ethical factor. Shelters operate within constraints related to staffing expertise, physical space, time, funding, and the emotional labor placed on care teams. Animals with intensive behavioral needs often require specialized handling, individualized treatment plans, extended lengths of stay (LOS), and ongoing professional behavioral oversight. When resources are insufficient to meet these needs, continuing treatment or placement efforts may compromise care for other animals or contribute to professional burnout and moral distress. Ethical stewardship requires recognizing when resource limitations materially affect welfare outcomes and decision feasibility.

Equally important is the responsibility to avoid transferring disproportionate risk or burden to adopters. Ethical placement decisions must account for the average adopter's experience level, living environment, access to qualified professional support, and financial capacity. Transparency and informed consent are essential components of ethical practice; however, they do not absolve shelters of responsibility when foreseeable risks remain high or when an animal's needs exceed what most private homes can reasonably provide.

At the same time, one of the greatest challenges in behavioral decision-making lies in the inherent unpredictability of outcomes. Shelters and behavior professionals have all witnessed animals who exceed expectations and thrive in adoptive homes despite significant concerns during assessment. Behavioral change following placement is influenced by variables that cannot be fully replicated or measured in the shelter environment, including environmental stability, human–animal bonding, and individualized management.

Previous chapters emphasize the importance of using the best available information and data to guide these decisions. Nevertheless, it is neither possible nor realistic to anticipate every outcome. Errors in judgment – both in placing pets who ultimately struggle and in declining placement for pets who might have succeeded – are inevitable. Acknowledging this uncertainty should not discourage thoughtful placement efforts, nor should retrospective doubt paralyze organizational decision-making.

Instead, shelters have an ethical obligation to continually improve the quality and consistency of the information used to inform decisions. This includes applying a Problem-Oriented Veterinary Behavior Record (POVBR) approach and engaging in strategic behavioral care trajectory planning. It also requires regularly evaluating behavior and wellbeing over time and maintaining thorough, accurate documentation. While this framework cannot eliminate uncertainty, it increases the likelihood of sound, defensible decisions and reduces preventable harm.

Ultimately, the goal is not perfection, but progress – getting decisions right more often by grounding them in evidence, reflection, and ethical accountability. In recognition of the increasing number of shelter animals presenting with complex behavioral and medical comorbidities, this chapter is intentionally included to foster open discussion, shared responsibility, and institutional support for shelter teams navigating these difficult and emotionally demanding decisions.

Below is a structured overview of the key ethical issues that shelters must consider when determining a care trajectory for pets with serious behavioral challenges, not only aggression. These issues arise when behaviors – such as severe fear, separation-related distress, compulsive disorders, or excitability and arousal – impact both the animal's wellbeing and the safety of the community. Ethical decision-making requires balancing the shelter's mission to save lives with its responsibility to ensure humane treatment, minimize suffering, and prevent foreseeable risks to adopters, teams, and other animals. It also requires protecting and allocating organizational resources reasonably, recognizing that time, staffing skills, emotional burden on care teams, space, and financial limitations can affect the quality of care and the feasibility of long-term treatment for pets with serious behavioral needs.

14.1.1 Duty to Protect Public Safety

Shelters have an ethical and legal obligation to ensure that animals placed into the community do not pose a foreseeable risk to adopters, neighbors, children, or other animals.

- Adopting out any pet, particularly a dog, with a known history of aggression can directly or indirectly expose people and other animals to harmful situations.
- Failing to disclose, minimizing, or otherwise downplaying behavioral risks undermines public trust and can jeopardize the shelter's credibility and mission and with this its future.

14.1.1.1 Ethical Conflict

Shelters must continually balance the desire to save a pet's life with their obligation to protect people and the community from injury.

14.1.2 Animal Wellbeing vs. Life Preservation

While saving pets is a core shelter mission, placing an animal into an environment where it is likely to fail – or where it may pose a risk – can lead to significant negative outcomes, including:

- Return to the shelter, often in a worse behavioral or emotional condition.
- Increased stress and deterioration of behavior, making rehabilitation more difficult.
- Further aggressive or problematic incidents, putting people and other animals at risk.
- Potential legal and liability consequences for the adopter and the shelter.
- Euthanasia following a bite or severe incident, which results in more suffering for the pet and emotional trauma for professional teams, volunteers, and adopters (who may never want to adopt an animal again).

14.1.2.1 Ethical Conflict

Is preservation of life always the highest good, even when it may cause more suffering for the pet?

14.1.3 Informed Consent and Transparency

Even with extensive information, adopters often underestimate what it means to care for an animal with serious behavioral concerns. Without full and transparent disclosure, meaningful informed consent is not possible. If adopters cannot realistically understand or manage the risks involved, proceeding with placement may be ethically inappropriate.

Ethically, adopters must be given full, honest, and understandable disclosure of:

- All known behavioral history, including observed behaviors in the shelter and any information from previous homes.
- Bite incidents, regardless of severity, context, or frequency – POVBR can to be summarized and shared. Discharge plans need to be available.
- Known triggers or situations likely to elicit aggression, fear, or other problem behaviors.
- Management requirements, including environmental setup, safety tools, handling limitations, and supervision needs.
- Prognosis and realistic expectations, outlining the likelihood of improvement, potential setbacks, and the level of ongoing support required.

14.1.3.1 Ethical Conflict

How much information to provide and how to present it without discouraging adoption?

14.1.4 Potential for Unfair Burden on Adopters

These may be unrealistic or unfair expectations for most adopters.

Pets with serious aggression often require:

- Skilled handling.
- Strict environmental management.

- Ongoing behavior modification.
- Long-term medication.
- Financial resources.
- A highly controlled home environment.
- Appropriate veterinary and medical handling plans, which can result in suboptimal veterinary care if not provided.

14.1.4.1 Ethical Conflict

Is it ethical to expect a private individual to manage the lifelong risks and demands associated with such a pet?

14.1.5 Strict Liability for Dog Bites

Many jurisdictions have adopted strict liability statutes for dog owners, changing the traditional "*one bite*" rule.

- Owners are liable for dog bites regardless of knowledge of the dog's dangerous propensities.
- Defenses such as contributory negligence and assumption of risk may apply depending on the jurisdiction.
- Some jurisdictions require owners of dangerous animals to confine them to reduce risk.

14.1.5.1 Ethical Conflict

Is it ethically defensible to transfer this level of long-term responsibility, liability, and risk to a private adopter?

14.1.6 Liability and Organizational Responsibility

Failure to fully disclose known dangerous behavior may create legal exposure for shelters and result in lasting reputational damage.

14.1.6.1 Ethical Conflict

Should preserving one pet's life come at the expense of community safety and public trust?

14.1.7 Resources and Opportunity Cost

A pet requiring months of intensive behavior therapy, single-person handling, and specialized training may consume resources that could otherwise support animals who are safer, more readily treatable, more adoptable, and equally in need.

14.1.7.1 Ethical Question

Is it fair to allocate limited shelter resources to a single high-need case at the expense of the broader animal population?

14.1.8 Quality of Life for the Pet

Certain behavioral disorders – particularly those marked by chronic fear, unpredictability, or severe aggression – may stem from neurological conditions, genetic predispositions, early trauma, inadequate socialization, or lifelong triggers. When an animal cannot safely function in a typical home environment, even with appropriate treatment, its quality of life may remain significantly compromised.

14.1.8.1 Ethical Question
Is prolonging life in a highly restricted or managed environment truly humane?

14.1.9 The Risk of Moral Distortion ("Save at All Costs" Culture)

External and internal pressures can distort decision-making and increase the risk of unsafe or unethical placements. Shelter teams may feel compelled to

- Avoid euthanasia.
- Meet live-release targets.
- Satisfy donor expectations.
- Uphold a "*save every pet*" culture.

14.1.9.1 Ethical Question
Does prioritizing live-release metrics undermine sound ethical judgment?

Given these realities, can adopting an animal with considerable behavioral challenges or known aggression be ethically justified?

Adopting Out a Dog May Be Ethically Defensible When
- Triggers can be reliably controlled.
- Robust safety measures are in place.
- A humane endpoint is clearly defined.
- The animal has a reasonable prognosis.
- The behavior is predictable and manageable.
- Veterinary behavior professionals support the plan.
- The adopter is highly experienced, fully informed, and adequately resourced.

Adoption Is Generally Not Ethical When
- The prognosis for improvement is poor.
- The adopter lacks advanced behavioral expertise.
- The animal experiences persistent fear or distress.
- Aggression is severe, generalized, or unpredictable.
- Resources and professional support are insufficient.
- Placement poses a significant risk to people or other animals.
- There is a history of serious injury, particularly to children or the face and hands.

14.1.9.2 Ethical Bottom Line
Shelters must balance compassion with responsibility. Preserving life should never come at the expense of public safety or prolonged animal suffering. Ethical sheltering prioritizes transparency, safety, animal welfare, realistic outcomes, professional behavioral assessment, and humane alternatives when adoption is not appropriate.

Furthermore, there is currently very little legal material addressing behavioral considerations in dogs and cats and virtually no statutory or regulatory guidance concerning the role of veterinary behavior professionals in shelters and rescue organizations. Likewise, the legal implications surrounding animals that display significant behavioral challenges while in shelter care – or following adoption – remain poorly defined and inconsistently addressed across jurisdictions.

As a result, many shelters are left to navigate complex ethical and liability considerations without clear legal frameworks to guide decision-making. This gap places organizations, teams, and adopters in a vulnerable position when managing animals whose behavioral needs may affect well-being, safety, or long-term outcomes.

The next part of this chapter is authored by Bob McNair, an attorney with specialized insight into animal welfare and liability issues. The following sections are intended to provide shelters and adopters with a clearer understanding of the legal landscape as it currently exists, identify areas of risk and responsibility, and support informed, ethical decision-making in the absence of comprehensive legal standards.

14.2 Legal Implications for Organizations and Adopters

Responsibilities, duties, and potential liabilities attach to most of life's relationships and activities. For example, if you are licensed to operate a motor vehicle, that license is conditioned on your willingness to abide by the laws and obligations associated with the privilege of driving on public streets and highways. Generally, drivers are expected to know and obey the rules of the road, operate their vehicle in a safe manner, and maintain their vehicle so as not to cause harm or injury to others or damage to private or public property. Failure to do so may result in fines, penalties, or even civil or criminal actions for damage to property or injury to others caused by the negligent or reckless operation of a vehicle. The same is true of owning a pet. Pet owners are expected to care for the animals under their charge, providing food, water, shelter, and necessary medical care; to neither be negligent nor cruel in the treatment of such pets; and to ensure that the animals are kept safely under the owner's control in a manner that does not pose a threat of damage to property or injury to others. Just like with driving a car, the neglect or intentional breach of a pet owner's duties and responsibilities can result in fines and other penalties, or can leave the pet owner liable for damages to the property of another, or for injuries to others caused by their pet. The following outlines some of the basic legal factors central to responsible pet ownership, all of which should be considered before adopting or purchasing a domestic animal.

14.2.1 Cruelty to Animals

Cruelty to animals is morally and ethically repugnant and legally forbidden. Legal actions against an offending party are normally prosecuted as criminal offenses, initiated by a local or state animal services agency, or other police authority (Soehnel 1992). Occasionally, a cruelty offense can present both a criminal and civil action when the circumstances involve, or include, someone's pet or domestic animal being subject to an act of cruelty by a third party. However, most modern animal cruelty statutes expressly provide for criminal prosecution by government authorities. Such prosecutions focus on the wrongdoer's intent.

This means that the act of cruelty must have been malicious, voluntary, intentional, and/or reckless and done with knowledge of the cruel nature of the act. In addition to overt acts of cruelty (such as beating, shooting, or other forms of abusive mistreatment of animals), animal cruelty may also be based on a *failure* to act, such as not providing sufficient food, water, or shelter, or failing to provide proper medical care.

Criminal cruelty charges can also be brought related to dog or other animal fighting contests, but such circumstances are beyond the scope of this outline. Actions can also be brought against animal hospitals, animal shelters, breeders, etc., in proper circumstances under animal cruelty statutes, but, again, these are beyond the scope of this discussion.

14.2.2 Strict Liability Statutes

The old saying that a dog is allowed "*one bite*" no longer applies under modern strict liability statutes. These statutes generally provide that, if a dog bites someone, the owner is liable to the injured person, with only limited defenses available. In places where there is no strict liability statute, the general theory of liability (imposing a measure of "strict liability") is that an owner of a domestic animal who knows, or has reason to know, that the animal has "*unusually dangerous propensities*," is liable for harm done by the animal, even if the owner has taken "*extraordinary precautions*" to prevent such harm. The difference here is that the latter requires an owner's knowledge of the dog's dangerous nature, while the former does not. Additionally, in jurisdictions *without* strict liability statutes, some courts have removed the requirement of scienter (the knowledge of the owner) of a dog's dangerous or vicious nature, thereby imposing liability for dog bite injuries more in line with the strict liability standard. Needless to say, all of this has significantly blurred the lines between strict liability and common law jurisdictions.

There are also variations within different strict liability jurisdictions themselves. In one state, the strict liability statute *presumes* the fault of the dog owner in dog bite cases, subject only to proof that the bite was not actually caused by another. In other strict liability states, the statutes contain provisions requiring owners of dangerous or vicious animals to confine or restrict such animals in a manner that severely reduces or eliminates the exposure of these animals to potential dog bite victims. Given all of the above, it should be clear that the nature, extent, and elements of strict liability statutes, or the different interpretations of older common law principals that impose some measure of strict liability on dog owners, are in no way uniform (Miller 1987).

In addition to the various forms of dog bite liability throughout the United States, the defenses to these actions also differ from state to state. These defenses provide dog owners with a potential path that can either reduce their exposure for damages or eliminate liability for dog bite injuries altogether. Traditionally, defenses such as contributory negligence and assumption of the risk have been available to dog owners if the circumstances of the specific incident warrant it. Contributory negligence, simply stated, provides that the actions of the dog bite victim in a specific case can be, of themselves, negligent in a way that contributed to the injury suffered by that victim. Assumption of the risk holds that if a person is aware of the potential danger of a certain situation or condition and elects to expose themselves to such possible danger, then they voluntarily assume the risk of potential injury by doing so. Depending on the state, the existence (or absence) of a strict liability statute and/or the form of common law actions that may be permitted, these defenses may or may not be available to dog owners who are sued by an alleged dog bite victim. Additionally, defense theories have developed and been implemented to relieve dog owners from statutorily imposed strict liability for dog bite injuries. One prevalent defense in strict liability cases is where the bite victim has provoked the dog in a manner that caused the dog to attack. Proof of such provocation will, in many instances, exonerate the dog owner from liability for the victim's injuries (this defense is discussed in more detail below). Ultimately, it will be the court that decides if a victim's behavior toward the dog constitutes a provocation sufficient to permit the dog owner to invoke this defense. In some states, another defense in strict liability cases is the victim's status as a trespasser on the dog owner's property. Some courts will allow a dog owner to escape judgment under a strict liability statute by the owner's posting of warning signs on the dog owner's property. Given all of the above, as with other legal issues involving dog ownership, it is important to be familiar with the statutes and ordinances in your own state and city to insure that you, as the pet owner, take reasonable steps to eliminate, or at least minimize any injuries or damage inflicted or done by your dog and the liability that may result.

14.2.3 Provocation of Dog as a Defense

When someone is bitten by a dog, it seems reasonable that the dog owner should be held liable. However, it would be unjust to make the dog's owner pay for injuries in cases where the bite was actually the fault of the victim. Because of this possibility, the wording of many dog bite statutes (holding the dog owner strictly liable for dog bites) provides that a victim's *provocation* of the dog is a defense to claims based on a resulting dog bite or other injury. However, it is often unclear if, under such statutory provisions, a victim's contributory negligence and/or assumption of the risk are also available as defenses. Some courts have ruled that where dog bite statutes are "*unambiguous*," and do not provide for defenses other than provocation, the other defenses cannot be "*read into*" these statutes by the courts. Other decisions have even permitted the defense of provocation where the victim is a small child, reasoning that dog bite statutes are to be "*strictly construed*," and where there is no exception within the statute to the defense for children victims, then the courts should not insert one. On the other hand, under common law actions based on negligence, other courts have stated that young children *cannot* be contributorily negligent, nor can they "*assume the risk*" in dog bite cases (since children are deemed incapable of making mature, informed, or rational decisions, or of appreciating the real hazards of most dangerous situations). In addition, various courts have ruled (regarding the provocation defense) that where strict liability statutes do not differentiate between intentional and unintentional acts (of provocation), either may constitute provocation. This means that even an *unintentional* act by a victim may provide a defense under a dog bite statute, unless the dog's reaction is deemed excessive (such as in cases of a vicious attack). There are a variety of cases dealing with differing circumstances from touching or petting a dog, to kicking a dog, attempting to ride a dog, or pushing a dog out of the way with a knee, hand, or foot. Each of these incidents resulted in a dog bite, and each raised questions as to whether there was a defense of provocation, or contributory negligence, on the part of the victim. The point is to be aware that, even under statutes that hold a dog owner strictly liable for dog bites or other harm and injuries to persons, there is usually at least one recognized defense (i.e. provocation of the dog by the victim) within such statutes that may prevent recovery, depending on the circumstances of the case (Zitter 1993).

But this creates new and different problems under these strict liability statutes. For example, when a bite victim yells, screams, or stamps their feet at an advancing, aggressive dog, do such actions constitute provocation, or are they reasonable under the circumstances to defend oneself (or others)? What about someone yelling at a dog's owner who is then bitten by the dog? Could that constitute provocation of a dog sufficient to provide a defense under a dog bite statute? Could such actions constitute contributory negligence on the part of the victim, if the victim brings an action on a negligence theory? Facts of each case will always matter and can dictate the outcome. Kicking a dog maliciously without justifiable cause will likely constitute provocation. Kicking at a dog in self-defense when the dog appears aggressive and potentially dangerous may be deemed reasonable and justified.

Different circumstances are presented with guard or watchdogs, which are often trained to attack strangers who come onto the owner's property. If these dogs bite a trespassing intruder, it could be argued that any resulting bite or injury was the fault of the intruder. Some cases support this position. Others reach different conclusions, especially where the victim is a child.

But what about circumstances where there is no direct interaction with a dog that results in a dog bite? For example, when someone is walking next to a fenced property and a dog approaches, unnoticed by the pedestrian, and bites them when the pedestrian did not say anything and did not come onto the property at the time of the bite, is the dog owner liable? How might that differ from the pedestrian placing his or her hand or head over the fence, resulting in a bite? These two instances are not the same. The former does not appear to provide a claim of provocation or contributory negligence, while the latter certainly may. Still other dog bite cases involve victims who approach dogs that are either tethered or roaming inside of yards or porches at or near residences or businesses. Several cases that have considered defenses of provocation, contributory negligence, or assumption of the risk have permitted such defenses where the victim ignored properly posted warning signs, the barking of the dog, or other aggressive canine behavior when the victim entered the property. Other courts have ruled differently when the warning signs were deemed to be inconspicuous or that otherwise failed to adequately warn the victim of the danger. Still other cases involve victims who enter buildings and approach dogs kept inside. Again, defenses of provocation, contributory negligence, or assumption of the risk will depend on the facts of each case.

But what about when a dog bite victim merely walks or rides a bicycle by a dog on a city street? Here, defenses of provocation, contributory negligence, or assumption of the risk are generally not permitted. The principle is that the dog owner is responsible for keeping his or her dog under control in such environments, and will usually be held liable for any unprovoked bite or attack. Other dog bites or attacks may occur when a victim opens a door to a house or other building where a dog or dogs are located. Issues of liability and available defenses to the dog owner will many times depend on whether the victim had permission to enter and whether the victim ignored warning signs or other indications that dogs were present behind the closed door. Instances involving veterinarians, dog trainers, groomers, and other animal workers acting in their professional capacity create additional issues. For example, some courts have reasoned that any dog may bite, especially when in a strange place, being handled by strange people. These courts have held that veterinary workers assume the risk of injury from dog bites in the course of treating the dog. Dog groomers may also be deemed to have assumed the risk of dog bites during grooming for the same reasons. An exception may arise where the dog owner knows of their dog's propensity to bite, but fails to inform the veterinarian, groomer, or trainer of such propensity. On the other hand, unnecessary rough handling of an animal by an animal professional may present a possible defense of provocation or contributory negligence on the part of that professional. Although general legal principles in different jurisdictions will govern how liability for dog bites and dog-related injuries is determined, the facts and circumstances of each case will also play a large role in deciding to what extent the owner may be liable, or whether the victim assumed the risk of injury, was contributorily negligent, or had provoked the dog in a manner that presented a legitimate defense.

14.2.4 Liability of Those Who Keep and Harbor Dogs

The distinction between one who keeps a dog and one who harbors a dog is critical within the context of dog bite liability. A keeper is someone who has temporary control over a dog, such as a friend or employee who takes care of the dog. A harborer, on the other hand, is someone who provides shelter or refuge for the dog, such as a landlord or friend who allows the dog to stay at their home. Keeping a dog has a proprietary aspect with the keeper exercising some measure of care, custody and control over the dog. Harboring, on the other hand, does not have the same kind of proprietary interest associated with keeping. As noted, harboring is usually defined as sheltering or giving refuge to a dog. Both keeping and harboring carry different levels of liability (Ludington 1988).

When a host allows a house guest to bring his or her dog into the house, the host is probably not the keeper of the guest's dog. This is because the guest retains primary control and custody of the dog. But what about when a dog owner leaves town without his or her dog and enlists someone to care for the animal in the owner's absence? Is the caretaker the dog's keeper? If the caretaker cares for the dog on the caretaker's own property, then the caretaker is the dog's keeper; if the dog is left on the owner's property, and the caretaker goes there to take care of it, the caretaker is *not* the dog's keeper.

Family dog cases are the most common and sometimes, the most complicated. A dog may be owned by the parents, or by a son or daughter, or even by some other relative. One or all of these family members may (or may not) care for the dog in various ways; some family members may leave and return, or be at home only on weekends or during the summer. The dog itself may come and go, eating and sleeping at home or away, outside, inside, on the porch or even at one of the parent's work places. The question arises, "Who among all these people is keeping or harboring the dog, or are all of them doing so?" This is a factual question left for courts and jurors to decide. If only one spouse owns the dog, but both spouses jointly care for it, the non-owning spouse is a joint keeper of the dog. If only one spouse owns the dog, and the other spouse does not help care for it, but controls the premises where they live with the dog, the "premises-controlling" spouse is a keeper of the dog. However, if one spouse owns the dog and the other spouse neither cares for the dog and does not control the premises, then the non-owner spouse is *not* the dog's keeper. If a son or daughter owns a dog which is kept at the parents' home, the parents may also be the dog's keepers.

Another common case is that of employer-employee. When an employee brings his or her dog onto the employer's premises, the question becomes whether the dog is there for the employee's convenience or for the employer's benefit. If it is for the employer's benefit, then the employer is probably the keeper of the dog. If it is there only for the employee's convenience, then the employer is probably not the dog's keeper. If the employer owns the dog, the question becomes whether the employee's duties require them to care for the dog. If so, then the employee is the dog's keeper; if not, then the employee is not a keeper or harborer of the employer's dog.

A final group of cases involve landlord-tenant situations. Absentee landlords have been held not to be the keepers or harborers of their tenants' dogs, even though the landlord may have the authority to forbid tenants to keep dogs, or to make rules governing the keeping of dogs on the premises. Additionally, a landlord's manager is not the keeper or harborer of the tenant's dogs, despite having similar authority to that of the landlord. However, on-premises landlords who live with or share business premises with their tenants have been held to be keepers or harborers of their tenants' dogs.

Why is any of this important? Because if an injured party wants to hold someone other than the actual owner of a dog liable for injuries or damage caused by a dog, it will be necessary to determine not only who the owner is, but whether another person, by virtue of having possession, custody and/or control over the dog (or by providing shelter or refuge for the dog), qualifies as a keeper or harborer of that dog during or at the time that the injury or damage occurred.

14.2.5 Liability for Injuries to Social Guests

What about guests, invited to and attending social gatherings or events at a dog owner's home or property who, in the course of that social event, are bitten by the host's dog? In order to appreciate various degrees of liability for injuries to persons entering another's property, legal distinctions need to be made between those classified as invitees, licensees, and trespassers. Invitees fall into two categories: business invitees and public invitees. Business invitees are invited onto the owner's premises for business dealings with the property owner or possessor (such as restaurant patrons and retail store customers). Public invitees are members of the public who have the right to be on the premises. This would include people who, for example, visit a public park or library. Property owners and possessors owe invitees the highest duty of care. This means they must keep their premises reasonably free of dangerous conditions and fix any hazards in a reasonable amount of time, or clearly post visible warnings of any such hazards. Like invitees, licensees are invited onto the owner's premises, but not for the benefit of the property owner. Most social guests, for example, are considered licensees. Even if a licensee is formally invited onto a property, they are not owed the same duty of care as are invitees. While property owners must still notify licensees about known hazards, they don't have a duty to inspect the premises before allowing a licensee to enter. Trespassers, unlike invitees and licensees, do not have a lawful right to be on the premises. Although it may seem unfair, property owners still owe a duty of care to trespassers. They cannot, for example, set traps to injure trespassers to deter them from coming onto the property. Additionally, if there's an attractive nuisance on the premises (i.e. a swimming pool), the property owner must take reasonable steps to protect children who might trespass because of the attraction; otherwise, the owner may be held liable for any injuries or deaths that may result (Zitter 1985).

It should be clear that social guests at the home or property of another are legally considered to be licensees. So, what happens when someone invites a friend to go with him to visit someone at a home, where the owner of the home also owns a dog? In one such case, two people approach the home from a pathway commonly used to access the house from the back. As they approached, a dog rushed out of the back door and bit the visitor's friend. Is the home/dog owner liable to the bite victim? In this case, there was a strict liability statute in effect, holding the owner of the dog liable for the dog bite that, in fact, occurred. Second, under common law, the dog owner had a duty to warn a licensee of a known hazard (such as a potentially dangerous dog that might attack). Finally, if it is shown that the dog bite victim exercised reasonable care in approaching the house (i.e. did not provoke the dog and did not ignore warnings that a dog was on the property or that it could be dangerous), then the home/dog owner would probably be held liable, either under the strict liability statute, or under the common law (if the owner knew of the dog's dangerous tendencies).

In another instance, a social guest was bitten by the host's dog when the guest offered the dog some food. The court held the guest was entitled to recover damages from the host because the host failed to restrain the dog. Here, the guest was a first-time visitor at the host's home, and the host had even warned the guest that their dog would snap if petted. Still, the host allowed the dog full run of the house, even though he was aware of the dog's "snapping" behaviors and knew that the dog had one previous biting incident. The court in this case ruled that the dog should have been secured in the presence of a stranger. These examples, which are not exhaustive, should at least suggest that, if a dog owner knows of their dog's tendency to snap at or bite strangers, or knows that their dog has any dangerous or vicious behaviors, the smart course of action would be to restrain or confine the dog when others visit, whether as an invitee or as a social guest.

14.2.6 Liability for Injury to Trespasser from Attacks by a Vicious Dog

What happens when the victim of a vicious dog attack is trespassing on the dog owner's property at the time of the attack? Some courts focus on the wrongful conduct of the dog owner (in keeping a vicious dog), concluding that the dog's owner may be liable for injuries to a trespasser, regardless of the care exercised in controlling and/or confining the animal. Other courts focus on the wrongfulness of the trespasser, concluding that the dog owner is merely under a duty to exercise some degree of care to avoid injuring trespassers. Under the strict liability theory, many cases involving injuries to trespassers have been decided on the grounds that a vicious dog is a nuisance, the keeping of which (with knowledge of its vicious tendencies) is so wrongful, that the owner is responsible for any harm caused by the animal, including harm to trespassers (Trenkner 1975a). Other decisions have held that the mere keeping of a vicious dog, of itself, constitutes negligence of such a degree that the owner is liable to a trespasser injured by the dog, regardless of the way the animal is kept or confined. Although in many states, courts have held that owners of vicious dogs are subject to strict liability statute, including for injuries suffered by trespassers, there are other cases where courts have ruled that the "*cautious*" use of a vicious dog at night, as a necessary protective measure against criminal wrongdoers, is justifiable under the common law principal that a person may use such force as is necessary to protect his property. In one case, the court determined that the strict liability dog bite statute did not apply when the person injured was trespassing on the dog owner's property after dark or who was engaged in some unlawful activity on the dog owner's property during the daytime. Further, several cases (which support the strict liability theory) have held that the ordinary contributory negligence of a trespasser bars recovery of damages from the dog owner. A few contrary rulings, however, have reasoned that it is logically inconsistent to hold that ordinary contributory negligence is a proper defense against claims based on strict liability. Some jurisdictions that have not embraced the strict liability theory have even rejected the position that the keeping of a vicious dog is akin to using spring guns and traps against trespassers. One case stated that there is no useful purpose served by prohibiting a person from taking reasonable steps to protect his property from intrusions. Some decisions, under the negligence theory, have even required a showing of a higher degree of fault on the part of the dog owner for a trespasser to be entitled to recovery for his dog bite injuries.

All of the above only emphasize the need to determine the laws in effect in the jurisdiction where you live and keep a dog. In states with strict liability dog bite statutes, liability usually exists for dog bite injuries regardless of the vicious or dangerous nature of the dog or the owner's knowledge of such vicious or dangerous tendencies. Still, liability factors involving attacks by vicious dogs of trespassers that enter onto the dog owner's property can vary greatly from one locale to another.

14.2.7 Dog Owner's Liability to Victims of "DOG FRIGHT"

In cases involving actions brought by "*dog fright*" victims, courts have traditionally applied the same principles used in dog bite cases to assess a dog owner's liability (Lewter 1984). For example, it has generally been the law that, unless otherwise provided by statute, the essential element in any action to recover damages for injuries caused by a dog, whether by biting, or otherwise, is the knowledge that the dog is vicious or dangerous, or has mischievous tendencies. Regardless of the nature of the injury caused by a dog and suffered by a third party, the general rule is that the dog's owner may be liable if the third party is exposed to unreasonable risk of harm by the foreseeable actions of that person's dog. The concept of "*foreseeability*" implies that the owner of the dog would need to know that dog's propensities and general behavior (in order to determine if such propensities and behaviors might give rise to a potential risk of harm to another). Courts seem to generally apply such rules in cases where the injury that resulted was not from any physical contact between the dog and the victim, but from fright engendered by the victim's encounter with a menacing dog. The outcome of each case, of course, will depend on the specific facts, the locale of the incident, and the role and legal status of the injured person. For example, different results have been reached in cases where an injured party was a customer or business invitee within the premises of the dog owner. The same is true for cases where a social guest or visitor to a dog owner's home was injured when startled by the owner's dog lunging at the visitor. The more frequent instances occur where a pedestrian or traveler on a public road or walkway has been injured when scared by a threatening or leaping dog. Here, some courts have concluded that the dog owner's liability was established where the owner was negligent in allowing his or her dog to be in a position to frighten a passerby. Since these types of claims against dog owners are not based on a physical injury, but are an emotional injury (causing fright, shock, and distress) that may exacerbate a pre-existing anxiety disorder, the measure of damages could range anywhere from a nominal award, to one much more significant, depending on the severity of the dog's behavior and the nature and degree of the trauma suffered by the victim. Of course, the jurisdiction in which such a claim is brought will also determine the availability of such actions, and can affect the likelihood of success, as well as the measure of damages, if any, that might be awarded.

14.2.8 Intentional Infliction of Emotional Distress

It is generally recognized that pets are many times treated as "*members of the family*" that owns, keeps, and cares for the pet. Still, what is seen as a beloved pet by one can be perceived as a menace to another. Disputes can arise between pet owners and others that can escalate into confrontations, where strong force ends up being used to restrain the animal involved in such confrontations. There are many cases dealing with both negligent and even the intentional injury or killing of pets. In extreme cases, where the pet is treated with disproportionately harsh and vicious measures, or in an outrageous manner, the pet's owner may claim to have suffered severe emotional distress as a result. Disputes exist over whether one can legally recover for negligent or intentional infliction of emotional distress in such cases. Some courts say no, as pets are only "*property*" under the law, and one cannot recover for an "*emotional connection*" with property. Other courts reason that the affectionate bond between a pet owner and their pet is real, and a malicious injury or destruction of that pet provides an element of damages that the owner should be allowed to recover. The latter of these opposing judicial positions has even permitted claims against veterinarians, shelters, animal hospitals, breeders, and animal boarders, as well as against others involved in the care of animals. The basis of these emotional distress actions is that the owner entrusted their pet to these persons or entities and they somehow cruelly violated that trust. Where such claims are permitted, the circumstances and specific facts will determine if the pet owner can, in fact, recover damages on the legal theory of emotional distress. A central element in these cases is that the actions (or failure to act) on the part of the defendant must rise to the level of outrageous or egregious conduct in order to warrant recovery of damages (Zitter 2001). In one case, a court found for the pet owner where a transporter left the animal in a hot place for too long, and the animal died. This court rejected the defendant's claim that the pet owner could not recover because she did not witness the incident. However, another court denied a pet owner's claim on similar facts, holding that the transporter's actions, however negligent, were not intentionally directed at the animal's owner. If one who is entrusted with the care of another's pet mistakenly has the animal put down, the court may not permit recovery for emotional distress, since the conduct was negligent, not intentional, and the conduct was neither extreme nor outrageous. Confrontations between animals and persons other than veterinarians, shelter personnel, or caretakers (i.e. neighbors) can sometimes result in the animal being injured or killed. Further, someone who becomes fearful of a wandering dog may call the police. The officers responding to such a call may have to make a split-second decision regarding what must be done to protect the public from what might be a vicious, dangerous, or even diseased animal. Such actions, again, made in the spur of the moment by the police, probably do not rise to the level of extreme, egregious, or outrageous conduct that would permit recovery by the animal's owner. In disputes over the repeated misbehavior or trespass by a neighbor's dog, the result may be that the dog is hit, beaten, or even shot by the offended party. The pet owner may very well have a strong emotional response to such actions, but the courts in such cases have reached different conclusions depending on the severity or outrageousness of the offended party's behavior, and the circumstances that brought such behavior about in the first place.

14.2.9 Animal Noise (as a Private or Public Nuisance)

The law of nuisance restricts a landowner's use of property so that it will not unreasonably interfere with another's use and enjoyment of their land and/or residence. Nuisance law attempts to balance the right of landowners to use land as they see fit against the duty not to do so in a way that will cause injury to others. Nuisance law covers intentional harm, as well as harm created by negligence, recklessness, or hazardous conduct. Nuisances can be public or private, or both. A private nuisance is a civil wrong, based on a non-trespassory invasion or disturbance of rights in land and affecting an individual or limited number of people. A public nuisance depends on an interference, not with land, but with the rights of the community at large. These differences are not based on the nature of the nuisance, but the scope of its injury and its effect. The principal difference is that public nuisances are usually brought to court by government entities, while individuals can bring an action to abate a private nuisance, seek damages caused by the nuisance, or both. The private nuisance is normally brought by a landowner, or landowners, affected by the nuisance. A public nuisance is an unreasonable interference with a right common to the general public.

Animals, as a rule, are not regarded as nuisances *per se*, but they, or the places they are kept, can become a nuisance (White 2001). For example, noises made by animals, or odors created by keeping certain kinds of animals, may be enjoined as a nuisance when they become detrimental to the comfort of those living in the neighborhood. Although courts recognize that the keeping of dogs is pervasive and generally accepted, many cases also acknowledge that "*man's best friend is not necessarily the best friend of man's neighbors.*" To that end, many courts have ruled that the keeping of dogs may become a private nuisance subject to equitable relief, such as an injunction, when it interferes with nearby residents' comfortable enjoyment of their homes or yards, or where the value of their property has been reduced. Although a large number of these cases have involved commercial operations that house dogs in kennels, the courts have also recognized that even one or two dogs may create sufficient interference with the sleep of neighbors, or with the enjoyment of their property, to constitute a private nuisance. To constitute a nuisance, the noise, odors, or other undesirable aspects of keeping domestic animals must be shown to materially offend persons of ordinary sensibilities and habits. In some private nuisance cases, the courts have considered the relative financial investment of the parties, the economic importance of the defendant's operation, the general nature of the area (urban, rural, or mixed use), and local zoning ordinances as factors to be considered in private nuisance cases. Several cases demonstrate that courts seem willing to grant some form of relief where a neighbor shows that the noises, sights, or odors caused by the neighboring animals are, in fact, offensive, unjustly, and/or unnecessarily intrusive and are continuously disruptive of the neighbor's quiet enjoyment of their adjoining or nearby properties.

14.2.10 Animals as Attractive Nuisance

Most jurisdictions under the *Attractive Nuisance Doctrine* ("AND") hold that one who maintains premises with certain conditions, instrumentalities, or agencies that are dangerous to children of tender years (i.e. that are unable to apprehend the peril of such conditions) that may attract children to the premises, has a duty to protect such children against the dangers of the attraction. A majority of jurisdictions have held that AND is not applicable, as a matter of law, to injuries caused by animals (Trenkner 1975b). They reason that dogs, for example, cannot constitute an attractive nuisance since they are too "common" to be inherently dangerous to a child. Some courts, however, have ruled that the issue is not whether the condition is "common," but whether that condition poses an unreasonable risk of harm to a child. For example, a German Shepherd, although a common animal, could be an attractive nuisance if its past behavior would lead a reasonable person to believe that the dog was sufficiently dangerous to potentially cause injury at some later date. Further, such danger must be foreseeable, and a single incident usually does not put the dog owner on notice that the dog is dangerous or vicious (unless the nature of that single incident would lead a reasonable person to conclude that the dog was sufficiently dangerous to likely cause harm or injury to a person in the future). Again, when keeping animals, including pets, on your property, it is best to know the law in your city and state regarding liability for animals that may be considered an attractive nuisance. Armed with such knowledge, it is also best to err on the side of caution in how and where you keep such animals, where it is possible that children may come onto your property.

14.2.11 Considerations Regarding Animal Shelters and Rescues

The following is not an outline of the legal structure, or specific statutes and ordinances governing the operation of municipal animal shelters, or of for-profit and non-profit animal rescue organizations. Rather, this discussion concerns factors to be considered when dealing with (including adopting dogs and cats from) any of these organizations. Animal shelters are government entities that normally operate at a local (city/county) level. They are authorized by law (state statutes and/or local ordinances) to enforce animal safety and welfare laws and regulations within their jurisdiction. Such activities may include policing the community for stray, potentially diseased, and "at large" animals, and then sheltering, feeding, and caring for such animals or, when legally appropriate, disposing of certain animals under their control. Many times the shelters have programs for members of the community to adopt available and unclaimed animals and may even provide vaccination and spay and neuter services for adopted animals. Other duties of shelters may include enforcing regulations for rabies or other animal vaccinations as well as licensing requirements, investigating animal-related incidents, making determinations about dangerous or vicious animal cases, impounding animals from (1) hoarding situations, (2) animal fighting contest environments, and (3) other animal abuse, neglect, or cruelty situations. The shelters may also accept surrendered animals from local residents. Services provided by shelters will vary greatly, depending on the size of the shelter's staff, its budget, facilities, policy dictates and constraints, as well as the availability of volunteer workers to assist with shelter functions and duties. A major concern regarding shelters is the space constraints (for housing animals) that almost always exist. When a shelter takes in more animals than it can house, the only options are: (1) adoption or fostering of animals by the public; (2) animal rescue organizations taking excess animals from the shelter; (3) transferring animals to other shelters (if permitted); or (4) euthanasia of the excess number of animals (including animals that have been at the shelter for an extensive period of time and/or animals that have developed behavioral problems from shelter stress). Most shelters cannot select the number, types, breeds, health, age, or condition of the animals it takes in.

As noted above, shelters also cannot keep more animals than it can safely house and care for without compromising the health and welfare of the shelter's overall animal population. Given all of these circumstances, adopting a dog or cat from a local shelter should at least be considered, if you are thinking of acquiring a pet. Many, if not most, of the shelter animals available for adoption would make wonderful pets and usually did nothing wrong to warrant their current circumstances. Further, as noted above, many shelters will assist with vaccines, spay and neuter services, and discounts for initial veterinary exams for adopted pets. Even if such services are not available, the adoption fees at shelters are usually considerably lower than the cost of purchasing an animal from a breeder or store. Another excellent source to consider for animal adoptions is animal rescue organizations. These organizations, from national entities, such as the SPCA, to local dog and cat rescues, are usually non-profit organizations that exist for the sole purpose of taking in dogs or cats at risk for euthanasia from over-crowded shelters, and even taking owner surrenders, providing interim housing, fostering, and care for such animals until a suitable person or family can be found to adopt them into a "forever home." Adoption fees with rescues will vary, as will potential services for vaccinations, spay and neuter and initial veterinary visits for the newly adopted pet. Again, even though the fees may be somewhat higher than fees at a local shelter, they will normally be lower than acquiring a dog or cat from a breeder. Two remaining issues should also be addressed. First, animals (especially dogs) in shelters and even rescues may have developed a variety of behavioral issues through no fault of their own. These issues can vary from anxiety, depression, behaviors caused by past trauma inflicted on the animal, self-protective behaviors based on fear or existing pain, and even aggressiveness or other issues resulting from a lack of training or socialization and stress. Because of overcrowding issues, policy mandates, staff and supervisory decisions, liability concerns, and the absence of professional veterinary behavior professionals, many otherwise good shelter dogs are removed from consideration for adoption by members of the public or for transfer to a rescue organization because of perceived behavioral problems observed in dogs brought into the shelter. Should you find a potential canine companion at a shelter (or rescue) that isn't behaviorally "perfect," it could be beneficial to include an analysis by a veterinary behavioral expert (possibly with your initial veterinary exam) to determine the true nature and extent of the behavioral issues that have been observed and the potential treatment avenues that might be available. So many perfectly marvelous, personable, and loving dogs are passed over because they need a little help. For such dogs, a veterinary behaviorist would be a terrific place to start. Finally, one other factor for those who are considering adopting a dog or cat is the importance of spaying and neutering your new "four-legged" (or "tri-pod") companion. The overpopulation of dogs and cats in the United States is at a crisis level, so much so that we cannot cure the problem through rescuing animals from shelters and rescue organizations. An intentional, nation-wide program aimed at spaying and neutering our pet animals is needed. Certainly, advocating for such programs with your local and state representatives is important. Even more important is ensuring that each of us is doing our part, as responsible pet owners, by having our pets spayed or neutered before they have an opportunity to add to the overpopulation crisis among dogs and cats in this country. It is the only practical way we can eliminate overcrowded shelters, rescues that are full to capacity, and the high euthanasia rates for dogs and cats at shelters that result from such overwhelming conditions.

In summary, when considering the variety of issues surrounding responsible pet ownership, together with all the various potential liability issues that could affect even the most diligent of pet owners, it is important to remember the gift that dogs and cats are and the joy and companionship they bring into our lives. These companions do not care what we look like, where we live, or how much money we have in the bank. They provide unconditional love and loyalty to us in exchange for some attention, a little affection, and the food and care that we have to give. That's a pretty good deal, even within the mandates of responsible pet ownership, as discussed above.

References

Lewter, V.G. (1984). Liability of dog owner for injuries sustained by person frightened by dog. *American Law Reports 4th* 30: 986–999. (Supp. 2019).

Ludington, J.P. (1988). Who "harbors" or "keeps" dog under dog liability statute. *American Law Reports 4th* 64: 963–1000. (Supp. 2019).

Miller, W. (1987). Modern status of rule of absolute or strict liability for dog bite. *American Law Reports 4th* 51: 446–471. (Supp. 2019).

Soehnel, S.A. (1992). What constitutes offense of cruelty to animals – modern statutes. *American Law Reports 5th* 6: 733–882. (Supp. 2019).

Trenkner, T.R. (1975a). Liability of owner of dog known by him to be vicious for injuries to trespasser. *American Law Reports 3rd* 64: 1039–1064. (Supp. 2019).

Trenkner, T.R. (1975b). Animals as attractive nuisance. *American Law Reports 3rd* 64: 1069–1074. (Supp. 2019).

White, P. Jr. (2001). Keeping of domestic animals as constituting public or private nuisance. *American Law Reports 5th* 90: 619–686. (Supp. 2019).

Zitter, J.M. (1985). Liability to adult social guest injured otherwise than by condition of the premises. *American Law Reports 4th* 38: 214–224. (Supp. 2019).

Zitter, J.M. (1993). Intentional provocation, contributory or comparative negligence or assumption of the risk as defense to action for injury by dog. *American Law Reports 5th* 11: 127–217. (Supp. 2019).

Zitter, J.M. (2001). Recovery of damages for emotional distress due to treatment of pets and animals. *American Law Reports 5th* 91: 545–584. (Supp. 2019).

15

Future Trends and Innovations

15.1 The Evolving Role of Behavioral Medicine in Animal Shelters

Behavioral medicine is one of the most critical pillars of modern animal sheltering. While housing, medical care, and adoption placement remain essential, it is increasingly clear that behavioral health determines welfare, safety, length of stay (LOS), team wellbeing, and long-term outcomes more than any other single factor.

Behavior cases are consistently the most controversial, emotionally taxing, and ethically complex situations that shelters face. Animals with behavioral challenges often remain in care the longest, receive the most attention, and generate the strongest emotional attachments among team members, volunteers, and foster caregivers. These cases carry a disproportionate burden of moral distress, particularly when outcomes are uncertain or difficult decisions must be made. For this reason alone, behavior cannot be treated as an afterthought or secondary concern.

Historically, shelters have focused on safely housing animals, addressing immediate medical needs, assessing public safety risk, and moving animals toward adoption as efficiently as possible. While this approach has saved countless lives, it has also revealed a critical limitation: animals with unmet behavioral needs in animal shelters deteriorate over time, become less adoptable, more stressed, and more challenging to manage. In many cases, delayed behavioral intervention unintentionally worsens prognosis – leading to prolonged confinement, increased risk to staff, and emotionally devastating end-of-life decisions.

15.1.1 Why Early Behavioral Focus Is Essential

Behavioral health must be addressed early, proactively, and systematically – not reactively when a case reaches crisis. The immediate admission period represents the most vulnerable phase of an animal's shelter journey. Stress is highest, coping capacity is lowest, and behavior can rapidly shift in response to confinement, noise, unpredictability, and loss of control. Early identification of risk factors, paired with timely intervention, can prevent mild stress responses from becoming entrenched behavioral pathology.

Focusing on behavior early:

- Reduces LOS.
- Improves wellbeing and emotional stability.
- Supports ethical, defensible decision-making.

- Increases adoptability and placement success.
- Lowers team member injury risk and professional burnout.

Behavioral medicine allows shelters to move beyond a binary view of animals as either "*adoptable*" or "*not adoptable*." Instead, it facilitates dynamic, wellbeing-centered trajectories that evolve with the pet's needs and response to care.

15.1.2 Ethical Consistency Across Organizations

One of the most pressing needs in sheltering is the application of consistent ethical standards across organizations.

Euthanasia due to behavior conditions, prolonged confinement, sanctuary placement, and long-term medication use are often judged differently depending on an organization's philosophy, public pressure, and available resources. These inconsistencies create public confusion, internal conflict, and emotional strain for the professionals responsible for making difficult welfare decisions. In many regions, strong opposition to behavior-related euthanasia – except in the most extreme cases, such as severe or egregious bites – makes it challenging to provide appropriate welfare for animals whose needs cannot be met within the shelter environment.

Municipal shelters, in particular, are often held to standards that are unrealistic given their staffing, physical space, intake volume, and financial limitations, especially when compared to well-resourced nonprofit or private shelters. When euthanasia for behavior conditions is not considered an acceptable option – unlike medical conditions where an animal's suffering is more readily acknowledged – shelters may be forced into prolonged confinement, inadequate housing, or unsafe management strategies. None of these align with modern welfare expectations or team members' wellbeing. This is particularly problematic given that animals with severe behavioral conditions may experience levels of suffering comparable to those with serious medical illness, yet this suffering is often less visible and less readily accepted.

Addressing these disparities requires acknowledging the ethical complexity and operational realities of behavior cases, ensuring that welfare-based decisions are supported rather than stigmatized. It is crucial in promoting consistent, transparent standards that protect both pets and the people who care for them.

Behavioral medicine provides a framework for:

- Objective welfare assessment.
- Risk evaluation grounded in evidence.
- Transparent documentation and decision-making.
- Ethical alignment across shelters, rescues, and municipal agencies.

Applying behavioral standards with the same rigor used in medical decision-making ensures that behavioral suffering is taken as seriously as physical illness.

15.1.3 Prevention, Early Intervention, and Multimodal Care

The future of shelter behavioral medicine lies in prevention and early intervention, supported by multimodal treatment plans. Research is increasingly focused on:

- Targeted enrichment and decompression strategies.
- Thoughtful use of nutraceuticals and psychopharmacology.

- Standardized intake assessments paired with welfare tracking.
- Integration of training, environmental modification, and handling protocols.

Critically, more research is needed that focuses specifically on shelter populations, rather than extrapolating from privately owned pets. Shelter animals face unique stressors, time constraints, and care realities that demand tailored behavioral strategies.

15.1.4 Interdisciplinary Collaboration and the Role of Social Work

Behavior does not exist in isolation, neither for animals nor for people. The expansion of interdisciplinary collaboration, particularly with social workers and human services professionals, is reshaping shelter practice. Integrating behavioral medicine with social work aligns directly with the One Welfare model, strengthening outcomes for both animals and people and reinforcing, instead of separating, the human–animal bond. This is especially relevant for pets belonging to unhoused individuals. These animals often experience significant distress and reduced wellbeing when removed from their caregivers and placed in shelters, and many enter the system due to the interface between homelessness and law enforcement rather than true neglect.

Forward-thinking, One Welfare-aligned approaches prioritize keeping pets with their people whenever safely possible through community-based support, behavioral and medical outreach and partnerships with social services. More research is needed, but emerging evidence suggests that these strategies improve welfare, reduce shelter intake, and support both members of the human–animal dyad.

Social workers can:

- Support community-based interventions that keep pets with families.
- Assist in crisis situations involving domestic violence or mental health.
- Address human factors driving relinquishment (housing insecurity, trauma, and financial strain).
- Provide support for team members experiencing compassion fatigue, moral injury, and professional burnout.

Integrating behavioral medicine with social work strengthens outcomes for both pets and people, reinforcing the human–animal bond rather than treating animal welfare in isolation.

15.1.5 Design, Education, and Access to Expertise

Shelter design is increasingly informed by behavioral science. Lighting, acoustics, and spatial layout have profound effects on stress and coping. Even older facilities can implement low-cost, evidence-based changes that significantly improve welfare.

At the same time, technology is expanding access to expertise via:

- Virtual staff training and mentorship
- Shared data platforms and benchmarking
- Artificial Intelligence (AI)-supported behavioral documentation
- Teleconsultations with veterinary behaviorists, trainers, or other consultants

These innovations allow shelters of all sizes to engage in continuous improvement, regardless of geographic or financial limitations.

15.1.6 Innovation: AI, Data, and Predictive Behavioral Care

A major emerging trend is the integration of AI and advanced data analytics into shelter behavioral medicine. These tools have the potential to revolutionize how shelters identify, monitor, and respond to behavioral needs.

AI-driven systems can:

- Detect early indicators of stress, shutdown, or escalation.
- Analyze behavioral, medical, and environmental data at scale.
- Monitor posture, movement, vocalization, sleep patterns, and activity.
- Flag animals at risk of deterioration before behavior becomes severe.

Computer vision and sound-analysis technologies can support continuous, objective welfare monitoring, particularly in group housing environments where subtle changes may be missed. These tools are not intended to replace human judgment, but rather to augment professional expertise, improve consistency, and reduce reliance on subjective interpretation alone.

15.1.7 Looking Forward

Behavioral medicine is no longer optional, it is foundational to humane animal sheltering. By prioritizing behavior alongside medical care and housing, shelters can reduce suffering, improve outcomes, support their teams, and make ethically grounded decisions with confidence.

The future of sheltering lies in early behavioral focus, interdisciplinary collaboration, and thoughtful innovation. While no shelter can eliminate all stress or resolve every behavioral challenge, embracing behavioral medicine as a core discipline offers a sustainable and compassionate path forward – for pets, professionals, and the communities they serve.

Central to this evolution is ethical consistency: the principle that animal welfare should be held as the primary concern across all settings, even though the *means* to support that welfare will differ by shelter size, staffing, expertise, and resources. Ethical consistency does not imply identical outcomes or capabilities. Rather, it acknowledges that some medical and behavioral conditions can be humanely managed in certain settings but not in others. In those cases, continuing treatment at the expense of an animal's quality of life – or the safety and wellbeing of teams – does not represent ethical care.

A welfare-centered framework allows shelters to make defensible, compassionate decisions grounded in the animal's lived experience, not in external pressure or unrealistic expectations. By aligning behavioral and medical ethics, shelters can move toward transparent, humane, and sustainable practices that respect both animal suffering and human capacity. Ultimately strengthening trust within the community and within the profession itself.

15.2 Future Research Directions: Behavioral Medicine, Community Needs, and Innovation

Animal sheltering is undergoing a profound transformation, driven by advances in behavioral medicine, welfare science, data analytics, and interdisciplinary collaboration. Future research must balance compassion with evidence-based practice, ensuring that animal welfare, public safety, team member wellbeing and organizational sustainability evolve together. The following priority areas represent the most critical directions for innovation and inquiry in modern sheltering.

15.2.1 Understanding Generational and Cultural Differences in Pet Ownership

Pet ownership expectations are not universal. They vary significantly across generations, cultures, and social identities – shaping how people relate to animals, interpret behavior, and engage with animal shelters.

- Generational differences can influence priorities and decision-making. The "*fur baby*" mindset shapes expectations around ethical treatment, sustainability, transparency, individualized care, and the emotional integration of pets into daily life. Younger generations, particularly Millennials and Gen Z's, often emphasize sustainability, ethical treatment, transparency, and integration of pets into family and identity, while older generations may prioritize reliability, routine, and traditional care models (Philpotts et al. 2024; Xie 2025).
- Cultural, geographical, and racial identities influence beliefs about animals, acceptable behaviors, housing norms, and help-seeking behaviors. Research initiatives examining multicultural pet ownership are revealing meaningful differences in trust, expectations, and engagement with animal welfare organizations.
- Cross-cultural welfare studies demonstrate that attitudes toward animals – and tolerance for certain behaviors – are shaped by social norms and lived experience, underscoring the need for context-specific approaches rather than one-size-fits-all messaging.

Future research in this area will allow shelters to design adoption counseling, outreach, education, and diversion programs that reflect what communities actually value and need – rather than relying on assumptions rooted in dominant cultural norms.

15.2.2 Diversity, Equity, and Inclusion (DEI) in Animal Welfare Systems

Diversity, equity, and inclusion (DEI) is increasingly recognized as essential to both ethical practice and effective service delivery in animal welfare.

- Structural inequities – such as housing restrictions, income disparities, language barriers, and systemic bias – directly affect access to veterinary care, training resources, and the ability to retain pets.
- Research suggests that workforces reflecting the communities they serve improve communication, trust, and engagement, ultimately benefiting both animals and people (AVMA 2025; Maxwell 2025).
- Emerging studies are beginning to document racial and ethnic disparities in shelter procedures and outcomes, including relinquishment pathways, adoption screening, and enforcement practices.

Future research must move beyond values statements to empirically examine how DEI initiatives affect:

- Animal welfare outcomes.
- Access to care and adoption equity.
- Community trust and engagement.
- Team member retention and morale.

Understanding how intersectional identities shape both pet ownership and professional experiences is essential for building inclusive, humane shelter systems.

15.2.3 Expanding "Pets with Purpose": Second Careers and Support Roles

A growing area of innovation reframes successful outcomes beyond traditional adoption. Some shelter animals may thrive in structured, purpose-driven roles that better match their temperament and needs.

Potential pathways include:

- Service work, such as psychiatric, mobility or assistance.
- Detection and conservation.
- Search-and-rescue and disaster response.
- Working cats in barns, bodegas, warehouses, and other community areas.
- Therapy and facility animals in schools, hospitals, senior centers, domestic violence shelters, and community spaces.
- Educational, vocational, or rehabilitation programs, including prison-based initiatives.

Research priorities include:

- Establishing ethical selection criteria and care trajectory strategies (CTS).
- Comparing welfare outcomes of second-career placements vs. prolonged shelter stays.
- Developing reliable behavioral and emotional assessment tools to identify appropriate candidates.

This strength-based approach recognizes that some animals flourish with structure, engagement, and predictable routines – even when they struggle in conventional pet homes.

15.2.4 AI, Facial Recognition, and Welfare Monitoring

When applied thoughtfully, ethically, and transparently, AI offers significant promise. Computer vision and facial-recognition technologies may allow animal shelters to:

- Identify individual animals in group housing.
- Detect early indicators of stress, illness, or social conflict.
- Ensure equitable access to resources in shared environments.
- Track feeding access, enrichment use, social interactions, and movement.

These novel systems could help flag pets who are:

- Avoiding food or enrichment.
- Becoming socially withdrawn.
- Experiencing rising stress before overt behavior change occurs.

Predictive analytics may further support:

- CTS and LOS forecasting.
- Data-informed resource allocation.
- Optimized foster placement timing.
- Early identification of behavioral decline.

Critical research needs include validating accuracy across breeds and species, preventing algorithmic bias and ensuring AI augments – rather than replaces – professional judgment.

15.2.5 What Adopters Really Want: Decision Psychology and Behavior-Centered Matching

Adopter expectations are often misaligned with animal shelter messaging. Research increasingly shows that adopters prioritize:

- Post-adoption support.
- Lifestyle compatibility.
- Predictable behavior in the home.
- Honest, clear behavioral information.

Key research questions include:

- How adopters interpret behavioral labels and risk.
- How transparency affects satisfaction, retention, and return rates.
- The impact of structured post-adoption support on long-term outcomes.
- Whether videos, real-life observations, and enrichment histories improve match success.

Understanding adopter psychology allows shelters to shift from "selling pets" to facilitating informed, resilient matches that reduce returns and improve wellbeing. There are studies that have examined adopter psychology. This is important research that needs to be conducted on a regular basis after economic and political changes or major world events that affect people's lifestyle and economy. For example, the COVID-19 pandemic changed the world and how people interacted and kept companion animals. The changes the pandemic produced may have long-lasting generational effects on people's relationship with their pets.

15.2.6 Integrating Human Services: Social Work and Public Health

Behavioral medicine increasingly recognizes that animal welfare and human welfare are inseparable. Embedding social workers within animal shelter systems can:

- Support adopters and pet owners in crisis.
- Reduce trauma associated with surrender decisions.
- Mitigate compassion fatigue, moral distress, and professional burnout among team members.
- Address root causes of relinquishment (housing insecurity, domestic violence, and financial hardship).

Future research should evaluate:

- Reductions in repeat relinquishments.
- Team member wellbeing and retention.
- Cost-effectiveness and community-level impact.
- Outcomes of integrated human–animal support programs.

This model reframes animal shelters as community support hubs, rather than solely intake and placement facilities. Many municipal shelters are currently located on the outskirts of communities – often near prisons or waste treatment plants. This can reinforce negative public perceptions. Shifting this narrative should begin at the local government level, with intentional investment in shelter placement, visibility, and integration into the community.

15.2.7 Measuring What Matters: Next-Generation Welfare Metrics

The next phase of shelter innovation requires moving beyond intake and outcome statistics.

Priority research areas include:

- Continuous welfare scoring systems for various aspects for sheltering and fostering, including group play, enrichment, training, etc.
- Ethical frameworks for humane endpoints in shelter pets.
- Behavioral recovery and resilience metrics for the entire shelter pet population.
- Quality-of-life benchmarks during shelter stays.

These tools support proactive, humane decision-making rather than reactive crisis management.

15.2.8 The Effect of Legislation on Pet Ownership and the Ethical Human–Animal Bond

Legislation increasingly plays a significant role in shaping pet ownership, sourcing, and public attitudes toward the human–animal bond. Several cities and states have enacted laws that restrict or ban the sale of certain animals in pet stores. In California, recent legislation has placed additional limitations on pet brokers, including prohibitions on selling animals under one year of age, requirements to disclose the origin of animals, and bans on nonrefundable deposits (California State Assembly 2025a,b). These measures are intended to curb large-scale commercial breeding practices, increase transparency, and protect consumers and animal welfare.

Future research should examine the downstream effects of this legislation on animal sheltering, including:

- Whether adoption rates from shelters increase as access to commercially sold pets becomes more limited.
- Whether relinquishment rates to municipal shelters are affected by changes in pet sourcing and expectations.

Greater transparency may empower prospective pet owners to make more informed decisions and could reduce impulse purchases that later result in relinquishment. At the same time, restricting the number of animals bred and sold commercially may shift public focus toward adoption from local shelters, potentially strengthening community engagement and reinforcing the ethical human–animal bond through more intentional, informed pet ownership.

15.2.9 Nutrition and Metabolic Health

Nutrition and metabolic health represent one of the most under-researched yet increasingly critical areas of shelter animal welfare. While advances in behavioral medicine, enrichment, and population management have improved outcomes, comparatively little is known about how stressed, confined, or behaviorally compromised animals should be fed to support both physical and emotional wellbeing. As shelter populations change, these gaps are becoming impossible to ignore.

15.2.9.1 Caloric Needs in Stressed and Confined Animals

Current feeding recommendations for dogs and cats are largely extrapolated from healthy, owned pets living in stable environments. These guidelines do not account for the profound metabolic effects of chronic stress, confinement, disrupted sleep, or limited agency – all common features of the shelter experience. Stress alters energy expenditure, appetite regulation, insulin sensitivity, and hormone signaling, yet there is limited evidence to guide caloric intake for animals experiencing acute or prolonged stress.

Key research questions include:

- How does chronic stress affect metabolic efficiency and weight gain or loss?
- Do stressed shelter animals require fewer or more calories than standard maintenance estimates?
- Are current feeding guidelines contributing to unintended obesity or muscle loss during shelter stays?

Without evidence-based answers, shelters risk both overfeeding and underfeeding animals, each leading to serious welfare consequences.

15.2.9.2 The Rise of Obesity in Shelter Populations

Twenty years ago, obesity was relatively uncommon in shelter pets. Today, shelters increasingly admit overweight and obese dogs and cats, reflecting broader societal trends in pet ownership. Obesity complicates shelter care by increasing the risk of orthopedic disease, cardiovascular strain, heat intolerance, dermatologic conditions, and decreased mobility, factors that directly affect wellbeing and adoptability.

Obese animals also present unique behavioral and management challenges:

- Increased frustration or discomfort during handling.
- Slower response to behavior modification due to pain or fatigue.
- Reduced willingness or ability to engage in enrichment and exercise.

Research is urgently needed to determine:

- How to balance metabolic health with emotional wellbeing and adoptability.
- Safe and humane weight-management strategies in short-term, high-stress environments.
- Whether caloric restriction during shelter stays improves or worsens stress and behavior.

15.2.9.3 Nutrition, Anorexia, and Medical Risk

At the opposite extreme, many shelter animals – particularly cats – experience stress-related anorexia. In obese cats, even brief periods of reduced food intake can precipitate hepatic lipidosis, which is a life-threatening condition that increases the risk of morbidity and mortality in shelter settings.

The tension between encouraging food intake, managing dietary preferences, and avoiding excessive food switching, while minimizing food waste and reducing the risk of attracting rodents, remains a daily clinical challenge.

Future research should focus on:

- Early predictors of appetite suppression in stressed animals.
- The role of palatability, texture, temperature, and feeding context in restoring appetite.
- Optimal feeding strategies to prevent hepatic lipidosis without increasing gastrointestinal (GI) upset.

15.2.9.4 Allergies, Food Sensitivities, and Behavioral Overlap

Food allergies and intolerances add another layer of complexity. Animals with dermatologic or GI disease often exhibit behavior changes such as irritability, withdrawal, or increased reactivity. This can be misinterpreted as purely behavioral problems. In shelters, limited diet options and frequent food changes can exacerbate both physical symptoms and stress.

Research priorities include:

- How food sensitivities influence behavior and stress expression.
- Best practices for managing elimination or novel-protein diets in shelters.
- The impact of dietary inconsistency on welfare, behavior, and adoptability.

15.2.9.5 The Gut–Brain Axis and Behavioral Health

One of the most promising frontiers in welfare research is the gut–brain axis. Emerging evidence shows that the gut microbiome influences stress reactivity, anxiety, cognition, immune function, and emotional regulation through neural, endocrine, and immune pathways. Shelter animals experience frequent disruptions to gut health due to stress, diet changes, medications, and illness, yet the behavioral consequences of these disruptions remain poorly understood.

Critical research questions include:

- How does shelter stress alter the microbiome? How quickly can those changes occur?
- How does gut health influence response to enrichment, training, or psychopharmacology?
- Can targeted nutrition, prebiotics, probiotics, or diets mitigate stress-related behavioral deterioration?

Understanding the gut–brain connection may fundamentally reshape how shelters approach both nutrition and behavioral care.

15.2.9.6 Nutrition as Behavioral and Welfare Medicine

Nutrition should no longer be viewed as a logistical necessity alone, but as an integral component of behavioral medicine and welfare science. Food choice, feeding method, timing, and composition all influence stress, predictability, agency, and emotional state. For many animals, feeding is one of the few daily events over which they can exercise control.

Future innovation must explore:

- Feeding as enrichment and agency.
- Individualized nutrition plans based on stress level, medical status, and behavior.
- Integration of nutritional data into welfare scoring and behavioral tracking systems.

15.2.9.7 Looking Ahead

As shelter populations become more medically complex, behaviorally diverse, and metabolically vulnerable, nutrition science must evolve alongside behavioral medicine. Evidence-based feeding strategies that account for stress physiology, obesity, allergies, and the gut–brain axis are essential for improving welfare, reducing disease, and supporting recovery.

Importantly, the relationship between stress and disease in shelters is no longer theoretical. High arousal, chronic fear, and lack of enrichment directly compromise immune function, increasing susceptibility to conditions such as canine infectious respiratory disease complex (CIRDC) and feline upper respiratory infection (URI). We frequently discuss population density, ventilation, and housing design as disease determinants, but behavioral health and environmental enrichment are equally influential. Programs that reduce barking, lower arousal, increase choice, and provide predictable routines have been associated with measurably lower rates of respiratory disease, faster recovery, and reduced need for medical intervention.

These connections provide a strong justification for investment in behavioral enrichment, stress-reducing housing strategies, and nutrition plans tailored to the physiological effects of chronic stress.

Investment in shelter-specific nutrition and behavioral health research is no longer optional. It is a necessary step toward truly humane, integrated, and forward-thinking animal care.

In summary, the future of animal sheltering lies in the integration of behavioral medicine, technology, DEI-informed practice, adopter psychology, and human services. No single innovation will solve the complex challenges shelters face. Progress depends on a shared commitment to evidence-based compassion, ethical consistency, transparency, and continuous learning. By advancing research in these areas, shelters can evolve into systems that better serve animals, support professionals, and meet the real needs of the communities they exist to help.

References

American Veterinary Medical Association (AVMA) (2025). Why diversity is good for business, [online] available at: https://www.avma.org/resources-tools/diversity-and-inclusion-veterinary-medicine/why-diversity-good-business (accessed 1 February 2026).

California State Assembly (2025a). AB-519 Pet broker sales: chaptered, California Legislative Information. Available at: https://leginfo.legislature.ca.gov/faces/billNavClient.xhtml?bill_id=202520260AB519 (accessed 1 February 2026).

California State Assembly (2025b). AB-506 Pets: sales of dogs, cats, and rabbits: chaptered, California Legislative Information. Available at: https://leginfo.legislature.ca.gov/faces/billNavClient.xhtml?bill_id=202520260AB506 (accessed 1 February 2026).

Maxwell, S. (2025). Embracing the power of diversity, equity, and inclusion in the veterinary industry, *dvm360*, [online] available at: https://otto.vet/dei-veterinary-industry/ (accessed 1 February 2026).

Philpotts, I., Blackwell, E.J., Dillon, J. et al. (2024). What do we know about dog owners? Exploring associations between pre-purchase behaviours, knowledge and understanding, ownership practices, and dog welfare. *Animals* 14: 396. https://doi.org/10.3390/ani14030396.

Xie, J. (2025). Comparative study of consumer behavior patterns among different pet owner groups. *SHS Web of Conferences* 225: 01020. https://doi.org/10.1051/shsconf/202522501020.

Appendix A

Leadership Books, Frameworks, and Professional Resources

This appendix brings together resources that have accompanied the authors through the real, often unglamorous work of leadership. Many of these books were not discovered in quiet moments of reflection, but during long commutes across the Bay Area – listened to hour after hour in traffic, offering perspective, reassurance, and clarity when the work felt heavy or uncertain. Later, many of those same titles arrived in the mail and took their place on well-worn bookshelves, continuing to serve as trusted references long after the commute ended.

These resources helped shape how the authors approached leadership during moments of doubt, fatigue, and difficult decision-making. They provided language when words were hard to find, frameworks when problems felt overwhelming, and reminders that growth, both personal and organizational, is rarely linear.

The materials shared here reflect our recommendations, not a comprehensive list, for current and aspiring leaders in animal welfare and other mission-driven fields. They are offered not as abstract theory but as tools that have been lived with, listened to during long commutes, revisited during difficult seasons, highlighted, annotated, and returned to when leadership was challenging or uncomfortable.

Over time, these resources supported the development of emotional intelligence, collaboration and ethical, sustainable leadership rooted in responsibility rather than authority. Many of these lessons were reinforced – and sometimes challenged – through the guidance of mentors and professional coaches in our careers, whose perspective helped turn insights into practice.

Ultimately, leadership is a personal journey. Where you begin matters far less than your willingness to start where growth feels most uncomfortable.

A.1 Foundational Leadership and Management

Behar, H. (2007). *It's Not About the Coffee: Lessons on Putting People First from a Life at Starbucks.* New York: Portfolio.

Brown, B. (2018). *Dare to Lead: Brave Work. Tough Conversations. Whole Hearts.* New York: Random House.

Collins, J. (2001). *Good to Great: Why Some Companies Make the Leap. . . and Others Don't.* New York: HarperBusiness.

Covey, S.R. (1989). *The 7 Habits of Highly Effective People: Powerful Lessons in Personal Change.* New York: Free Press.

Covey, S.R. (1991). *Principle-Centered Leadership.* New York: Simon & Schuster.

De Pree, M. (2004). *Leadership Is an Art*. New York: Doubleday.
Grove, A.S. (1995). *High Output Management*. New York: Vintage Books.
Kouzes, J.M. and Posner, B.Z. (2017). *The Leadership Challenge: How to Make Extraordinary Things Happen in Organizations*, 6e. Hoboken, NJ: Wiley.
Sinek, S. (2009). *Start with Why: How Great Leaders Inspire Everyone to Take Action*. New York: Portfolio.
Sinek, S. (2014). *Leaders Eat Last: Why Some Teams Pull Together and Others Don't*. New York: Portfolio/Penguin.
Willink, J. and Babin, L. (2015). *Extreme Ownership: How U.S. Navy SEALs Lead and Win*. New York: St. Martin's Press.

A.2 Leadership Development and Team Effectiveness

Chapman, G. and White, P. (2011). *The Five Languages of Appreciation in the Workplace: Empowering Organizations by Encouraging People*. Chicago, IL: Northfield Publishing.
Covey, S.R. (1991). *Principle-Centered Leadership*. New York: Simon & Schuster.
Lencioni, P. (2002). *The Five Dysfunctions of a Team: A Leadership Fable*. San Francisco, CA: Jossey-Bass.
Lencioni, P. (2012). *The Advantage: Why Organizational Health Trumps Everything Else in Business*. San Francisco, CA: Jossey-Bass.
Maxwell, J.C. (2001). *The 17 Indisputable Laws of Teamwork: Embrace Them and Empower Your Team*. Nashville, TN: Thomas Nelson.
Maxwell, J.C. (2005). *The 360° Leader: Developing Your Influence from Anywhere in the Organization*. Nashville, TN: Thomas Nelson.
Maxwell, J.C. (2007). *The 21 Irrefutable Laws of Leadership: Follow Them and People Will Follow You*, 10e. Nashville, TN: Thomas Nelson.
Maxwell, J.C. (2011). *The Five Levels of Leadership: Proven Steps to Maximize Your Potential*. New York: Center Street.
Maxwell, J.C. (2014). *Good Leaders Ask Great Questions: Your Foundation for Successful Leadership*. New York: Center Street.
Townsend, P.L. (1995). *Leadership Beyond Reason*. New York: McGraw-Hill.
Tracy, B. (2010). *How the Best Leaders Lead: Proven Secrets to Getting the Most Out of Yourself and Others*. New York: AMACOM.
Wiseman, L. (2010). *Multipliers: How the Best Leaders Make Everyone Smarter*. New York: HarperBusiness.

A.3 Negotiation, Influence, and Difficult Conversations

Fisher, R. and Ury, W. (2011). *Getting to Yes: Negotiating Agreement Without Giving In*, 3e. New York: Penguin Books.
Patterson, K., Grenny, J., Maxfield, D. et al. (2013). *Crucial Accountability: Tools for Resolving Violated Expectations, Broken Commitments, and Bad Behavior*, 2e. New York: McGraw-Hill.
Patterson, K., Grenny, J., McMillan, R., and Switzler, A. (2012). *Crucial Conversations: Tools for Talking When Stakes Are High*, 2e. New York: McGraw-Hill.

Stone, D. and Heen, S. (2014). *Thanks for the Feedback: The Science and Art of Receiving Feedback Well.* New York: Viking.

Stone, D., Patton, B., and Heen, S. (2010). *Difficult Conversations: How to Discuss What Matters Most*, 2e. New York: Penguin Books.

Ury, W. (2007). *Getting Past No: Negotiating with Difficult People*, rev. ed. New York: Bantam Books.

Voss, C. (2016). *Never Split the Difference: Negotiating as If Your Life Depended on It.* New York: HarperBusiness.

A.4 Change Leadership, Strategy, and Organizational Culture

Bridges, W. (2009). *Managing Transitions: Making the Most of Change*, 3e. Philadelphia, PA: Da Capo Press.

Conner, D.R. (1993). *Managing at the Speed of Change: How Resilient Managers Succeed and Prosper Where Others Fail.* New York: Villard Books.

Connors, R. and Smith, T. (2011). *Change the Culture, Change the Game*. New York: Portfolio/Penguin.

Doran, G.T. (1981). There's a S.M.A.R.T. way to write management's goals and objectives. *Management Review* 70 (11): 35–36.

Grenny, J., Patterson, K., Maxfield, D. et al. (2013). *Influencer: The New Science of Leading Change*. New York: McGraw-Hill.

Heath, C. and Heath, D. (2010). *Switch: How to Change Things When Change Is Hard*. New York: Broadway Books.

Johnson, S. (1998). *Who Moved My Cheese? An Amazing Way to Deal with Change in Your Work and in Your Life*. New York: G.P. Putnam's Sons.

Kotter, J.P. (1996). *Leading Change*. Boston, MA: Harvard Business School Press.

Kotter, J.P. and Rathgeber, H. (2006). *Our Iceberg Is Melting: Changing and Succeeding Under Any Conditions*. New York: St. Martin's Press.

Laloux, F. (2014). *Reinventing Organizations: A Guide to Creating Organizations Inspired by the Next Stage of Human Consciousness*. Brussels: Nelson Parker.

Patterson, K., Grenny, J., Maxfield, D. et al. (2011). *Change Anything: The New Science of Personal Success*. New York: McGraw-Hill.

Peters, T.J. and Waterman, R.H. (1982). *In Search of Excellence: Lessons from America's Best-Run Companies*. New York: Harper & Row.

Pink, D.H. (2009). *Drive: The Surprising Truth About What Motivates Us*. New York: Riverhead Books.

A.5 Emotional Intelligence, Communication, and Human Behavior

Cain, S. (2012). *Quiet: The Power of Introverts in a World That Can't Stop Talking*. New York: Crown Publishers.

Clear, J. (2018). *Atomic Habits: An Easy & Proven Way to Build Good Habits & Break Bad Ones.* New York: Avery.

Coyle, D. (2018). *The Culture Code: The Secrets of Highly Successful Groups*. New York: Bantam Books.

Dweck, C.S. (2006). *Mindset: The New Psychology of Success*. New York: Random House.

Goleman, D. (1995). *Emotional Intelligence: Why It Can Matter More Than IQ*. New York: Bantam Books.

Goleman, D., Boyatzis, R., and McKee, A. (2002). *Primal Leadership: Realizing the Power of Emotional Intelligence*. Boston, MA: Harvard Business School Press.

Rosenberg, M.B. (2003). *Nonviolent Communication: A Language of Life*, 2e. Encinitas, CA: PuddleDancer Press.

Stone, D. and Heen, S. (2014). *Thanks for the Feedback: The Science and Art of Receiving Feedback Well (even when it is off base, unfair, poorly delivered, and, frankly, you're not in the mood)*. New York: Viking.

A.6 Animal Welfare Frameworks and Evidence-Based Practice

These frameworks anchor leadership decisions in science, ethics, and welfare outcomes.

American Veterinary Medical Association (AVMA) (2023). Animal welfare: guidelines and position statements. Available at: https://www.avma.org/resources-tools/animal-health-and-welfare/animal-welfare (accessed 28 December 2025).

ASPCA (2023). Shelter standards and animal welfare resources. Available at: https://www.aspcapro.org/essentials (accessed 28 December 2025).

Farm Animal Welfare Council (FAWC) (1979). Five freedoms. Available at: https://www.gov.uk/government/groups/farm-animal-welfare-committee-fawc (accessed 28 December 2025).

Humane Society of the United States (HSUS) (2023). Animal sheltering and welfare standards. Available at: https://www.humaneworld.org/en/sheltering-adoption-and-fostering-resources (accessed 28 December 2025).

Maddie's Fund (2023). Shelter medicine and welfare resources. Available at: https://www.maddiesfund.org (accessed 28 December 2025).

Mellor, D.J. and Reid, C.S.W. (1994). Concepts of animal well-being and predicting the impact of procedures on experimental animals. Available via Five Domains overview at: https://www.fivedomainsmodel.com (accessed 28 December 2025).

Mellor, D.J. (2020). Updated Five Domains model: welfare assessment frameworks. Available at: https://www.fivedomainsmodel.com/the-five-domains-model (accessed 28 December 2025).

Royal Society for the Prevention of Cruelty to Animals (RSPCA) (2023). Shelter and rescue welfare standards. Available at: https://www.rspca.org.uk/whatwedo/strategy/our-strategy-2030/priorities/rescue-and-care?p_l_back_url=%2Fsearch%3Fq%3Dcare%2Bstandards&p_l_back_url_title=Search (accessed 28 December 2025).

University of Florida Shelter Medicine Program (2023). Shelter medicine resources. Available at: https://sheltermedicine.vetmed.ufl.edu (accessed 28 December 2025).

University of California, Davis – Koret Shelter Medicine Program(2023). Shelter medicine and welfare science. Available at: https://www.sheltermedicine.com/ (accessed 28 December 2025).

A.7 Leadership Tools, Assessments, and Practical Frameworks

Used for self-awareness, team development, and organizational alignment:

After-Action Reviews (AARs)
https://www.army.mil/article/159800/after_action_reviews
(Structured reflection and learning process originally developed by the U.S. Army)

CliftonStrengths (StrengthsFinder)
https://www.gallup.com/cliftonstrengths
(Strengths-based leadership and team development model by Gallup)

DiSC Assessment
https://www.discprofile.com
(Overview of DiSC personality styles, workplace applications, and certified assessments)

Enneagram
https://www.enneagraminstitute.com
(Personality framework focused on motivation, stress responses, and growth)

Kotter's 8-Step Change Model
https://www.kotterinc.com/methodology/8-steps
(Evidence-based framework for leading organizational change)

Lencioni's Team Health Model
https://www.tablegroup.com
(Team effectiveness framework, including the Five Dysfunctions of a Team)

Myers–Briggs Type Indicator (MBTI)
https://www.myersbriggs.org
(Official MBTI framework, type descriptions, and organizational use)

Psychological Safety Framework (Amy Edmondson)
https://www.hbs.edu/faculty/Pages/profile.aspx?facId=6451
(Research and resources on psychological safety in teams and organizations)

Situational Leadership Model (Hersey–Blanchard)
https://situational.com
(Leadership model focused on adapting style to follower readiness and task needs)

SMART Goals, OKRs, and the Eisenhower Matrix

- SMART Goals: https://www.mindtools.com/a4wo118/smart-goals
- OKRs (Objectives and Key Results): https://www.whatmatters.com
- Eisenhower Matrix: https://www.eisenhower.me/eisenhower-matrix

Appendix B

Species Differences and Their Role in Welfare and Behavioral Assessment – Why It Matters

Species differences play a critical role in welfare and behavioral assessment, as dogs and cats express stress, communication, and coping strategies in fundamentally different ways. Recognizing these differences is essential for accurate interpretation of behavior, appropriate care planning, and ethical decision-making throughout the shelter journey. A behavior observed in one species may signal something very different in the other; grounding assessments in species biology – rather than human assumptions – prevents misinterpretation and supports humane outcomes.

These distinctions align directly with the **Five Domains Model** of animal welfare (see Chapter 1). Species-specific behavior and communication influence each domain differently:

- Nutrition: Stress may reduce appetite in cats (often quietly), while dogs may continue to eat despite significant distress – making food intake an unreliable cross-species welfare indicator.
- Environment: Dogs often benefit from routine, social access, and activity, whereas cats prioritize environmental control, hiding options, vertical space, and predictability.
- Health: Behavioral signs of pain or illness can be overt in dogs but subtle or masked in cats, requiring species-tailored observation.
- Behavior: Social interaction, play, and training are enriching for many dogs; for cats, forced interaction can increase fear, while choice and control improve welfare.
- Mental state: The same outward behavior (e.g. freezing, avoidance, and vocalization) can reflect curiosity, fear, frustration, or distress depending on species context.

Applying the Five Domains through a species-specific lens ensures that welfare assessments reflect how dogs and cats actually experience their environment. This approach reduces unnecessary stress, improves safety, and leads to a more accurate, ethical case trajectory strategy (CTS) from admission through placement.

B.1 Examples of Misinterpretation Risks

B.1.1 Approaching the Front of the Kennel

Same Behavior, Different Meaning: Front-of-Kennel Positioning

Dog	Cat
Often represents a social invitation	May reflect stress rather than sociability
Many dogs move forward because humans are sources of comfort, information, or reinforcement	A cat at the front of the enclosure may be attempting to escape confinement or guard the threshold
Behavior may indicate interest in interaction, desire to go outside, curiosity, or excitement	May indicate environmental overstimulation, frustration, or heightened arousal
Typically paired with loose posture and affiliative signals	Often accompanied by outstretched paws, intense staring, or tail flicking
Generally interpreted as approach behavior	These accompanying signals often indicate irritation or defensive readiness

Why this matters: Team members may interpret a front-of-kennel cat as "friendly" and attempt contact, only to provoke swatting, biting, or escape attempts.

B.1.2 Eye Contact

Eye Contact: Same Signal, Different Meaning

Dogs	Cats
Brief eye contact is often affiliative or a request for interaction	Direct eye contact is frequently perceived as a social threat, especially in confined spaces
Many dogs naturally "check in" visually with humans for guidance or reassurance	Friendly intent is more commonly signaled through soft eyes or slow blinking
Sustained eye contact may still be tolerated in relaxed contexts	Hard, unblinking stares often indicate discomfort, arousal or defensive readiness
Eye contact often facilitates engagement and training	Eye contact can escalate stress or provoke defensive behavior

Why this matters: Approaching a cat with direct staring may escalate fear or aggression, while avoiding eye contact with a dog seeking engagement may be misread as disinterest or neglect.

B.1.3 Vocalizations

Vocalization: Similar Behavior, Different Meaning

Dogs	Cats
Barking often reflects excitement, attention-seeking, or barrier frustration rather than aggression	Vocalization may indicate distress, fear, demand, or social solicitation depending on context

Dogs	Cats
Frequency and tone can change with arousal or environmental stimulation	Type of vocalization (meow, yowl, growl, or hiss) carries distinct meaning
Barking alone is not a reliable indicator of threat	Yowling or growling typically signals a warning and increased risk
Often increases in social or high-arousal settings	Often escalates when a cat feels trapped, overstimulated, or threatened

Why this matters: Misinterpreting vocalizations can lead to unsafe handling or inaccurate behavioral labeling. Assuming a barking dog is aggressive may unnecessarily restrict opportunities for enrichment or placement, while failing to recognize warning vocalizations in cats can increase the risk of defensive aggression.

B.1.4 Body Orientation

Body Orientation: Same Posture, Different Meaning

Dogs	Cats
Turning sideways is commonly an appeasement or politeness signal	A sideways stance often reflects defensive readiness or escalation
A head-on approach is typical and not automatically aggressive	A direct approach may be territorial or investigative rather than affiliative
Often used to reduce social pressure during interactions	Frequently used to appear larger or prepare for confrontation
Usually paired with loose posture and curved body	Often accompanied by stiff posture, piloerection, or tail lashing

Why this matters: Misreading body orientation can result in unsafe handling and inaccurate behavioral assessments. Interpreting a cat's sideways stance as friendliness may increase the risk of defensive aggression, while mislabeling normal canine approaches as threatening can lead to unnecessary restrictions or stress.

B.1.5 Handling Tolerance

Handling Tolerance: Same Interaction, Different Thresholds

Dogs	Cats
Many dogs tolerate handling by unfamiliar people, even when mildly uncomfortable	Handling tolerance varies widely; overstimulation can occur quickly and sometimes abruptly
Discomfort is often communicated through more visible signals	Cats often communicate discomfort through subtle, easily missed signals
May continue to engage despite stress	May escalate rapidly once thresholds are exceeded
Tolerance can mask underlying stress	Stress may be hidden until a defensive response occurs

Why it matters: Assuming equal handling tolerance across species increases the risk of bites, scratches, and mislabeling behavior. Dogs may appear compliant while experiencing stress and cats may escalate defensively when early signals are overlooked. Species-appropriate handling and careful observation reduce injury risk, minimize fear, and support more accurate welfare assessments.

B.2 Understanding Species Differences Improves Wellbeing

Recognizing species- and breed-related behavioral differences is essential for accurate welfare and behavioral assessment in shelter settings. When behavior is interpreted through a species-appropriate lens, teams can reduce unnecessary stress, prevent defensive aggression and improve safety for animals and people alike. Accurate interpretation supports more effective CTS, guides appropriate enrichment, and improves adoption matching while reducing bites, scratches, and escape incidents.

Understanding baseline behavior allows teams to distinguish fear from frustration, prey drive from aggression, working drive from hyperactivity and stress-related pacing from normal breed-typical energy. Anticipating species- and breed-specific stressors also helps prevent behavioral deterioration, particularly for high-drive dogs or socially dependent cats who may struggle in traditional shelter environments.

Applying this knowledge enables the design of targeted health and wellbeing plans, such as structured outlets for herding breeds, scent-based enrichment for terriers, foster placement for social cats and low-touch environments for shy or fearful cats. Finally, recognizing typical response patterns improves safety by reducing misinterpretation – for example, understanding when freezing, darting movement, or swatting reflects stress or frustration rather than aggression.

Ultimately, species-informed assessment supports humane, effective, and ethical sheltering by aligning care, placement, and intervention decisions with how animals actually experience their environment.

Appendix C

Behavioral Health Assessment Staging (BHAS)

C.1 Behavioral Triage Guide for Shelter Use

BHAS 1 – Stable and Social
Severity: Minimal **Clinical Status**: Stable **Key Indicators** – Socially appropriate, behaviorally stable – Minimal fear, anxiety, or stress – Mild trigger responses with rapid recovery – Easily distractible and redirectable **Care and Management** – Routine care and standard enrichment – Managed by all trained staff and volunteers – Problem behaviors rare or near extinction (~2 weeks) – Psychoactive medications or supplements are rarely needed. **Adoption Status:** ✅ Available for adoption

BHAS 2 – Mild Behavioral Concern
Severity: Low **Clinical Status:** Stable with monitoring **Key Indicators** – Mild, situational fear, anxiety, or stress – Consistent improvement observed – Responsive to enrichment and early intervention **Care and Management** – Basic management and training plan – Teach foundation behaviors (sit, look, touch, and find it) – Simple behavior modification (DRA, counterconditioning) – Problem behaviors significantly reduced or near extinction (~2 weeks) – Psychoactive medications or supplements may be temporarily indicated to alleviate stress response **Adoption Status:** ✅ Available for adoption

BHAS 3 – Moderate Behavioral Disorder
Severity: Moderate **Clinical Status:** Guarded but treatable **Key Indicators** – Consistent fear, avoidance, anxiety, or low-level aggression – Moderate response intensity and recovery time – Distractible with effort and high-value reinforcement – Interferes with routine handling or care **Care and Management** – Structured management and training plan – Daily behavior/training sessions – Targeted behavior modification (alternative behaviors, DS/CC) – Progress primarily seen in the absence of triggers – Typically psychoactive medication(s) and supplements are useful to alleviate anxiety. **Adoption Status:** ⚠ Conditional – available for adoption

BHAS 4 – Severe Behavioral Disorder
Severity: High **Clinical Status**: Unstable – intensive care required **Key Indicators** – Significant fear, reactivity, aggression, or distress – Safety concerns during handling or husbandry – Requires experienced handlers and strict protocols **Care and Management** – Intensive intervention and close monitoring – Twice-daily behavior modification sessions – Veterinary behavioral oversight required – Safety equipment may be necessary (muzzle, head collar, and double leash) – Psychoactive medications are often prescribed and helpful to alleviate anxiety. **Reassessment Thresholds** – No progress at one week → modify plan – No progress at two weeks → explore alternative trajectories **Adoption Status**: ✕ Not available for adoption

BHAS 5 – Critical/Unstable Behavior
Severity: Critical **Clinical Status**: Behavioral emergency **Key Indicators** – Serious safety risk to people or animals – Escalating, unpredictable, or deteriorating behavior – Multiple bite incidents and/or severe aggression – Unable to cope with shelter environment – Often co-morbid with medical conditions **Care and Management** – Immediate veterinary and behavioral evaluation – Quality-of-life assessment and trajectory planning – Humane euthanasia considered when no viable alternatives exist – some cases are too severe for or refractory to psychoactive medications or supplements **Adoption Status**: ✕ Not available for adoption

C.2 Key Reminders

- BHAS stages describe **current clinical status**, not permanent traits
- Animals may move **up or down** the scale over time
- Consistent documentation supports safety and humane care
- When in doubt, consult behavior or veterinary leadership

Designed for rapid reference, cross-team communication, and welfare-based decision-making.

Appendix D

Risk Assessment Checklist with Scoring Weights for Shelter Pets with Behavioral Disorders

Purpose: To quantify **safety and welfare risk**, guide care trajectory decisions, and support ethical consistency.

1) **Trigger Predictability (0–3 points)**
   - ☐ Predictable, consistent trigger → **0**
   - ☐ Somewhat predictable → **1**
   - ☐ Inconsistent → **2**
   - ☐ Unpredictable/multiple triggers → **3**

Score: ___ /3

2) **Motivation for Behavior (0–3 points)**
   - ☐ Fear/anxiety without aggression → **0**
   - ☐ Defensive aggression → **1**
   - ☐ Frustration/barrier-related → **2**
   - ☐ Offensive/approach-oriented aggression → **3**

Score: ___ /3

3) **Frequency (0–3 points)**
   - ☐ Rare/isolated → **0**
   - ☐ Occasional → **1**
   - ☐ Frequent → **2**
   - ☐ Daily or escalating → **3**

Score: ___ /3

4) **Intensity/Interruptibility (0–2 points)**
   - ☐ Low intensity/can be easily interrupted/redirected → **0**
   - ☐ Moderate intensity/can sometimes be interrupted/redirected → **1**
   - ☐ Extreme intensity/cannot be interrupted/redirected → **2**

Score: ___ /2

5) **Bite Severity (0–5 points)**

   No Bite Behaviors (BSC Level 1)
   - ☐ **Dog:** Warning only (growl, freeze, and hard stare) → **0**
   - ☐ **Cat:** Hissing, growling, swatting (no contact), spitting, stomping → **0**

Escalation Without Injury (BSC Level 2)

- ☐ Bite without contact (dog) → **1**
- ☐ Contact with clothing or leash (dog)/contact without skin puncture (cat) → **2**

Bite Behavior (BSC Level 3–7)

- ☐ Single bite → **3**
- ☐ Multiple bites or escalating bites → **4**
- ☐ Severe bite (medical treatment required, face/head/neck or deep punctures) → **5**

Score: ___ /5

6) **Bite History and Pattern (0–3 points)**
   - ☐ No prior history → **0**
   - ☐ Single prior incident → **1**
   - ☐ Repeated incidents → **2**
   - ☐ Pattern across contexts → **3**

Score: ___ /3

7) **Warning Signals and Recovery (0–3 points)**
   - ☐ Clear warnings + fast recovery → **0**
   - ☐ Subtle warnings or slow recovery → **1**
   - ☐ Minimal warnings → **2**
   - ☐ No warning + prolonged arousal → **3**

Score: ___ /3

8) **Size and Physical Risk (Dogs) (0–3 points)**
   - ☐ Small → **0**
   - ☐ Medium → **1**
   - ☐ Large → **2**
   - ☐ Giant → **3**

   *(Cats: default **1 point** for handling risk)*

Score: ___ /3

9) **Medical and Contributing Factors (0–2 points)**
   - ☐ No contributing medical concerns → **0**
   - ☐ Possible pain/medical factor → **1**
   - ☐ Confirmed medical/neurologic/endocrine issue → **2**

Score: ___ /2

10) **Management Feasibility and Welfare (0–4 points)**
    - ☐ Safe handling feasible + good welfare → **0**
    - ☐ Management possible but resource-intensive → **1**
    - ☐ Chronic stress/declining welfare → **2**
    - ☐ Poor quality of life despite intervention → **3**
    - ☐ Ongoing risk + welfare deterioration → **4**

Score: ___ /4

TOTAL SCORE: ___ /31

Risk Category and Recommended Pathway

Low Risk (0–8 Points)

- **Recommended:**
  In-shelter behavior plan, enrichment, and adoption support
- **Focus:** Early intervention and monitoring

Moderate Risk (9–16 Points)

- **Recommended:**
  Structured behavior plan and foster/transfer consideration
- **Focus:** Risk mitigation, resource matching, and frequent reassessment

High Risk (17–23 Points)

- **Recommended:**
  Specialized foster and transfer to a behavior-capable organization
- **Focus:** Staff safety, welfare protection, and ethical review

Critical/Unacceptable Risk (24+ Points)

- **Recommended:**
  Compassionate behavioral euthanasia discussion
- **Focus:** Preventing suffering, injury, and moral harm

Note: Any **severe bite**, **unpredictable aggression**, or **rapid welfare decline** may warrant escalation regardless of total score.

Final Decision and Documentation

- Case trajectory selected: ☐ Manage/Behavior modification plan ☐ Foster ☐ Transfer ☐ Euthanasia
- Reviewed by: ☐ Medical ☐ Leadership ☐ Behavior (if available)
- Date: ____________________
- Next review (if applicable): ___________

Core Principle

High risk ≠ bad animal.
High risk = poor fit between needs, environment, and resources.
This tool supports **ethical clarity**, **organization protection**, and **animal and team wellbeing** – not punishment or blame.

Appendix E

Framework for a Decision Tree for Psychoactive Medication Selection Pathway in Shelters

A step-by-step clinical algorithm for the use of short-acting oral behavior medications in dogs.

1) **Start with fundamentals (always)**
   1) **Confirm medical status**
      - Rule out/address pain, nausea, pruritus, neurologic disease, gastrointestinal conditions and other medical drivers.
   2) **Implement safety + management first**
      - Do **not** use medication as a substitute for safe handling, avoidance, or environmental management.
   3) **Define the target**
      - Identify the *primary state*: Anxious/agitated, panic, and/or painful.
   4) **Baseline measure**
      - Document baseline: Arousal level, ability to eat treats, response to cues, pacing/vocalizing, and body language.
2) **First-dose monitoring protocol (applies to every branch)**
   5) Give **ONE** medication first (unless the algorithm specifies an add-on for panic).
   6) Observe 60–120 minutes after the first dose.
   7) For short-acting meds, observe during the efficacy window and record: better/same/worse (plus side effects).
   8) Never trigger on purpose to "test" the medication.
   9) Use medication to set the patient up for success (lower baseline distress and enable learning).

A) Dog is anxious and/or agitated AND non-painful

   Step A1 – Start trazodone
   - **<40 lbs**: 50–100 mg BID
   - **40–70 lbs**: 100–200 mg BID
   - **>70 lbs**: 200–300 mg BID

   Reassess (same day and daily until stable):
   - If too sedating → cut dose in half
   - If helps but not enough → increase 50–100 mg per dose daily
     - Max 10 mg/kg per dose, up to TID
   - If enough but wearing off → move from BID → TID
   - If does nothing or worsens → stop trazodone → go to A2

   Step A2 – Switch to/add clonidine
   - **Start 0.01–0.03 mg/kg BID**

Reassess:
- If helps but not enough → increase up to 0.05 mg/kg
- If wearing off → increase frequency: BID → TID → QID → switch to guanfacine
- If does nothing or worsens → stop clonidine → add gabapentin

(Continue monitoring individual response, welfare impact, and safety.)

B) Dog shows panic AND has NO history/signs of aggression to people or dogs *(e.g., hypersalivation, inconsolable, constant vocalization, and unable to settle)*

Step B1 – Start trazodone (same as A1)
- Begin trazodone dosing as above
- Reassess within a few hours

Step B2 – If not enough within a few hours, add clonazepam
- Add clonazepam 0.05–0.1 mg/kg BID

Reassess:
- If helps but not enough → increase in small increments (max dose 0.5 mg/kg BID)
- If paradoxical agitation, aggression, or worsens → stop clonazepam → go to B3

Step B3 – Use gabapentin instead (if clonazepam not tolerated or not available)
- **<20 lb**: 100–200 mg BID
- **20–40 lb**: 200–400 mg BID
- **>40 lb**: 400–600 mg BID

Reassess:
- If **helps but not enough** → increase by **100 mg increments** up to **50 mg/kg**

C) Dog is anxious and/or agitated AND painful

Step C1 – Start gabapentin
- **<20 lb**: 100–200 mg BID
- **20–40 lb**: 200–400 mg BID
- **>40 lb**: 400–600 mg BID

Reassess:
- If **helps but not enough** → increase by **100 mg increments** up to **50 mg/kg**
- If **enough but wearing off** → move to **TID**
- If **does nothing or worsens** → **stop gabapentin** → move to **trazodone pathway (A1)**

D) Dog has panic + pain AND no aggression

Step D1 – Start gabapentin (same as C1)
- Reassess within a few hours

Step D2 – If not enough, add clonazepam
- **Clonazepam 0.05–0.1 mg/kg BID**
- If needed, incrementally increase up to max dose **0.5 mg/kg BID**
- If paradoxical/agitated/aggressive → stop clonazepam → move to **trazodone pathway (A1)**

Ongoing Reassessment (All Branches)

1) Track side effects and function daily:
   - Eating, resting, social engagement, ability to train, and startle recovery
2) Once stable, adjust plan based on length of stay (LOS):
   - Short LOS → maintain short-acting protocol
   - Longer LOS expected (>4 weeks) → consider adding a long-term agent (per your broader chapter guidance)

These medications and dose recommendations are informed by the literature and adapted by the authors specifically for use in shelter pets. Always complete Steps 1 and 2 before initiating any medication. Each pet is an individual and may respond differently, requiring thoughtful monitoring and adjustment.

Index